The
Living Heart
DIET

Michael E. DeBakey

Antonio M. Gotto, Jr.

Lynne W. Scott

John P. Foreyt

RAVEN PRESS / A FIRESIDE BOOK
PUBLISHED BY SIMON & SCHUSTER, INC.
NEW YORK

Copyright © 1984 by Raven Press Books, Inc.
All rights reserved
including the right of reproduction
in whole or in part in any form
First Fireside Edition, 1986
Published by Simon & Schuster, Inc.
Simon & Schuster Building
Rockefeller Center
1230 Avenue of the Americas
New York, New York 10020
FIRESIDE and colophon are registered trademarks
of Simon & Schuster, Inc.
Designed by Carol Edelson
Manufactured in the United States of America
10 9 8 7 6 5 4 3 2 1
10 9 8 7 6 5 4 3 2 1 Pbk.

Library of Congress Cataloging in Publication Data

Main entry under title:

The Living heart diet.
    Includes indexes.
    1. Heart—Diseases—Diet therapy. 2. Heart—Diseases—
Diet therapy—Recipes. 3. Heart—Diseases—Nutritional
aspects. I. DeBakey, Michael E. (Michael Ellis), 1908–
[DNLM: 1. Diet. 2. Cookery. 3. Cardiovascular diseases—
Prevention and control. WG 100 L785]
RC684.D5L58   1984b   616.1'20654   84-10693

ISBN: 0-671-54127-7
ISBN: 0-671-61998-5 Pbk.

Preface

In 1977, we published a book for the general public on cardiovascular disease called *The Living Heart*. That book grew out of our personal experiences with patients and the many questions they and their families asked us about heart disease. The book was very well received, and we were pleased with the level of technical sophistication concerning heart disease that many of our readers exhibited. A few reviewers initially suggested that the book was too technical and that none other than scientists and physicians would bother to read it. Obviously, those reviewers were incorrect and underestimated our readers, because our book reached a wide audience. We believe that the book served a useful educational function for all who read it. The concluding chapter of that book dealt with preventive maintenance—providing useful, practical information for the individual interested in decreasing his or her risk of developing premature heart disease.

In the years since the publication of *The Living Heart*, it has become increasingly apparent that preventive maintenance plays a crucial role in maintaining the health of the heart. A study completed by the United States Federal Government in 1984 proved for the first time that the risk of coronary heart disease can be reduced by lowering blood cholesterol. This study, called the "Coronary Primary Prevention Trial," showed that reduction of blood cholesterol levels in middle-aged men was associated with reduced incidence of angina pectoris (heart pain), non-fatal heart disease, the need for coronary artery bypass surgery, and coronary heart disease death. A lower number of positive results from exercise stress tests was also shown with the reduced cholesterol levels. The investigators who participated in the trial believe that these findings can be extended to other age groups, both male and female. They estimate that if all Americans reduced their blood cholesterol levels by 25%, the incidence of coronary heart disease in the United States would drop by 50%.

Thus, *The Living Heart Diet* focuses on one of the most crucial aspects of preventive maintenance, namely, diet. In this book, we discuss in detail the functions of the heart and how diet can affect those functions. Following this explanatory section is a collection of recipes, menus, and diet guidelines organized in a cookbook format. Used together, these sections will enable one to evaluate his or her particular dietary needs and design a suitable diet. By "diet," here, we do not mean (necessarily) a weight-loss program, but rather a style of daily eating designed to promote a living heart.

The Living Heart Diet tells you how to cook the food that doctors tell you to eat. The comprehensive nature and the individualized approach of *The Living Heart Diet* set it apart from the many other books concerning diet that are now on the market:

- We provide, in the opening section, "Your Body and Its Relation to Diet," a thorough explanation of the role of diet in the healthy functioning of your heart. This is followed by a collection of over 500 recipes in the "Recipe" section. We conclude with the section entitled "Managing Your Diet," which contains menus and food guides. Used together, these three sections encourage you to learn what type of diet is best for your needs, how to prepare the foods that will comprise that diet, and how to put your new eating plan into effect.

- As there is no single diet that is appropriate for all people, we describe the different types of diets most often recommended by physicians for prevention and treatment of heart disease. In particular, we give guidelines for the basic LIVING HEART DIET, the LOW-CALORIE LIVING HEART DIET, the LOW-SODIUM LIVING HEART DIET, the DIABETIC DIET, the TYPES I TO V HYPERLIPIDEMIA DIETS, and the VERY LOW FAT DIET.

- A comprehensive collection of low-sodium recipes is located in a separate, readily accessible section for the many people who have been advised to restrict their sodium intake. To provide an even greater variety of recipes, we explain how recipes in other sections of the cookbook can be modified for sodium-restricted diets.

- Vital nutritional information is provided with each recipe in a format that allows you to use this information readily in planning your diet correctly. Serving size, nutrient analysis, food exchange value, and information about which type of specialized diet the recipe is particularly well suited for are included with each recipe.

- We explain a sensible and effective approach to weight loss for those of you who want to lose weight. And, of course, we include a set of menus to allow you to plan your weight-loss program most effectively.

- Only ingredients that are acceptable on the diet are included in the recipes of *The Living Heart Diet*. That is, there is no inclusion in the recipes of "a little sour cream" or "just one egg." All ingredients are low in cholesterol and saturated fat. This is especially important in light of the recent study, mentioned earlier, which shows that reducing high levels of cholesterol reduces the incidence of heart disease. Other cookbooks have allowed small portions of a food that is not acceptable on a diet designed for the health of your heart.

One of two deaths in our country each year is related to heart disease; this disease therefore affects virtually everyone in some way. Our book is intended first for patients and families of patients with cardiovascular disease and for those at high risk of developing heart disease. Next, our book will be of interest to individuals in good health who recognize the importance of diet in maintaining their health. We believe strongly that an unhealthy diet can contribute to the development of heart disease and, thus, that it is best to begin a healthy diet early in life—especially in families where there is a strong history of cardiovascular disease.

The subject of heart disease is of immense importance in our society, and the significance of being informed about the relationship between diet and a healthy heart grows each day. We expect that our readers will find this book extremely valuable in following their physician's recommendations and in answering the many questions of both a practical and a theoretical nature that occur when an individual attempts to adopt a more healthful diet.

THE AUTHORS

Acknowledgments

During the past seven years, many devoted individuals have contributed to the production of this book. Their efforts have made the actual writing of the text a pleasurable and satisfying experience for the authors.

We especially wish to thank Barbara Allen and Enid Edwards for their extraordinary and tireless efforts in coordinating the production of the book, their perseverance in editing, typing and proofing the manuscript, and the standard of excellence that they maintained throughout the project. Also, we are extremely pleased with our cover photograph. We thank our photographer Mel Reingold for his contributions to the cover.

Although the development, testing, and analyses of over 500 recipes are a labor of love, they are at times tedious tasks. Jacqueline Mitchell brought to this task a sincere interest in developing a large volume of excellent recipes and provided many invaluable suggestions. We thank her for her dedication and for the hundreds of hours spent working on these recipes.

We also wish to thank Susi LeBaron for her assistance in testing and typing the recipes. For their excellent assistance in preparing the recipes, we thank Lynn Baughman, Denise Tobias Garner, Rebecca Reeves, Patricia Pace, Karen Kennedy, Wanema Frye, Elizabeth Manis, and Janice Henske. We are especially grateful to L. A. "Al" Greene, Jr. for his interest and cooperation in helping us test many of the recipes.

Ruth Harvey initially developed and tested recipes under the direction of Clara McPherson. Valerie Knotts made possible the testing of recipes in the laboratory of the Nutrition and Food Sciences Department of Texas Woman's University in Houston, and her nutrition and dietetic students assisted in food preparation. We are grateful for their contribution.

We believed that an analysis of the nutrients for each recipe would be helpful to all readers in planning menus and would be particularly valuable to those persons with special dietary restrictions. We wish to thank Robert Mitchell for developing a program for the computerized nutrient analysis of each recipe and to express our appreciation for the many hours he devoted to this program.

A special thanks is expressed to Sharon Bonnot for typing the Food Guides, the Appendix, and many of the tables in the text.

About the Authors

Michael E. DeBakey, M.D., is one of the most eminent heart surgeons in the world. He was among the first to complete a successful heart transplant in the United States and has pioneered new methods for the diagnosis and treatment of heart disease. Among Dr. DeBakey's noted surgical accomplishments are the first successful resection and graft replacement of an aneurysm of the thoracic aorta and first successful coronary artery bypass. Currently, he is Chancellor of Baylor College of Medicine and also serves there as the Chairman of the Department of Surgery.

Antonio M. Gotto, Jr., M.D., D.Phil., is one of the world's most important specialists in research on fats in the blood and their role in the development of coronary heart disease. He serves as the Scientific Director of the Baylor College of Medicine, National Heart and Blood Vessel Research and Demonstration Center of the National Institutes of Health. Currently, he serves as the Chairman of the Department of Medicine at Baylor College of Medicine and The Methodist Hospital, both of Houston, Texas.

Lynne W. Scott, M.A., R.D., is a clinical researcher and is Chief Dietitian of the Diet Modification Clinic at Baylor College of Medicine and The Methodist Hospital, both of Houston, Texas. She is also Assistant Professor in the Department of Medicine at Baylor College of Medicine. She has worked with the American Heart Association on the development of their diet materials for the treatment of hyperlipidemia.

John P. Foreyt, Ph.D., is a clinical psychologist and the Director of the Diet Modification Clinic at Baylor College of Medicine and The Methodist Hospital, both of Houston, Texas. Currently, he is Associate Professor in the Departments of Medicine and Psychiatry at Baylor College of Medicine.

Contents

Your Body and Its Relation to Diet

The Heart and Its Vessels/Atherosclerosis or Arteriosclerosis?/How Does Atherosclerosis Begin?/Formation of Plaque and Its Consequences/Symptoms of Atherosclerosis/Progression of Atherosclerosis/Coronary Atherosclerosis, Angina Pectoris, and Heart Attack/Risk Factors/Blood Fats (Lipids): Cholesterol and Triglycerides/Lipoproteins: The Carriers of Cholesterol and Triglycerides in the Blood/The Families of Lipoproteins/Disposing of Cholesterol/ Hyperlipidemia and Hyperlipoproteinemia/Causes of Hyperlipidemia and a Description of the Various Types/How Do Hyperlipidemia and Hyperlipoproteinemia Relate to Diet?/Hypertension/Smoking/Secondary Risk Factors

The Low-Calorie Living Heart Diet/Fat in The Living Heart Diet/Fats in the Low-Calorie Diet/Cholesterol in The Living Heart Diet/Meat, Fish, and Poultry in The Living Heart Diet/Meat, Fish, and Poultry in the Low-Calorie Diet/Meatless Meals in The Living Heart Diet/Fiber/Eggs in The Living Heart Diet/Eggs in the Low-Calorie Diet/Dairy Products in The Living Heart Diet/ Dairy Products in the Low-Calorie Diet/Bread and Cereal Products in The Living Heart Diet/Bread and Cereal Products in the Low-Calorie Diet/Alcoholic Beverages/Nonstarchy Vegetables in The Living Heart Diet/Fruits in The Living Heart Diet/Fruits in the Low-Calorie Diet/Miscellaneous Foods/ Meals Away from Home/Eating on the Run/Low-Calorie Breakfast Ideas/ Lunch Box Ideas

Recipes

SECTION II. THE LIVING HEART DIET: LOW-SODIUM RECIPES

Low-Sodium Recipes/Low-Sodium, Low-Calorie Recipes/Low-Sodium Recipes for Diabetics/Low-Sodium Recipes for Types I–V Hyperlipoproteinemia Diets/Low-Sodium, Very Low Fat Recipes/Products Used in Low-Sodium Recipes

Managing Your Diet

THE LIVING HEART DIET: FOOD GUIDES 317

Meat, Fish, and Poultry Guide/Egg Guide/Dairy Products Guide/Bread and Cereal Guide/Fat Guide/Fruit Guide/Vegetable Guide/Miscellaneous Food Guide

Introduction

Due partly to an increasing interest in health and partly to the high premium placed on thinness, diet has become almost an obsession of our society. Although many books about diet continue to make the best-seller lists, most of the dietary regimens proposed can be classified only as fad diets. They offer hopes of achieving thinness and beauty—but only by radically changing one's diet and, all too frequently, only by risking one's health.

The LIVING HEART DIET is *not* a fad diet. It is a medically sound, clinically tested diet based on the highly successful Baylor College of Medicine and The Methodist Hospital nutritional management program for individuals at risk for or with heart disease. In *The Living Heart Diet* we begin by explaining, in nontechnical terms, the rationale behind our diet. To this end, we review the current medical evidence linking diet with arterial disease, high blood pressure (hypertension), and other cardiovascular problems; we analyze new data on the additional risk factors—smoking, obesity, diabetes, stress, and personality types—associated with heart disease; and we supply essential background information on food and nutrition. We believe that enough experimental evidence and data from major population studies are available to strongly recommend that *all* individuals follow a diet aimed at controlling their weight and one that is less rich in saturated fats and cholesterol. We therefore recommend the basic LIVING HEART DIET to the general population.

For people already afflicted with cardiovascular disease, little controversy exists concerning appropriate measures. A limited salt intake is mandatory, and most physicians recommend that saturated fat and cholesterol also be controlled. Obesity places an extra strain on the heart and worsens certain metabolic conditions, such as a tendency to high blood fats or diabetes, and so must be controlled. High blood pressure, a known risk factor in the development of cardiovascular disease, is exacerbated by both excess body weight and high salt consumption. A recent study by the United States Federal Government demonstrated that lowering blood cholesterol in people with high levels will reduce the risk of coronary heart disease. Thus, in addition to the basic diet, *The Living Heart Diet* presents therapeutic diets specially designed to treat high blood pressure, congestive heart failure, fluid retention (edema), high blood cholesterol and/or high triglycerides, and to achieve weight reduction in obese individuals. These dietary measures are clearly distinguished from those recommended to the general population.

We do not believe in crash weight-loss diets for those who wish to lose weight; all the diets we recommend are safe and designed to help you keep weight off once you have lost it. All diets, including weight-loss diets, should provide sufficient calories, nutrients, and vitamins to sustain good health, and should be varied enough to allow you to maintain the diet for as long as you wish. Our weight-loss approach, therefore, is a gradual one, aimed at achieving a weight reduction of one to two pounds per week. As our weight-loss program is an integral part of our overall diet, the diet followed during the period of weight loss can be easily adapted after weight reduction by simply increasing the intake of calories—either by modifying the weight-loss recipes or by enjoying more of the recipes found in *The Living Heart Diet*.

Even more than just focusing on the foods we eat, we must be concerned with our attitudes toward eating and the habits we have built up around food. Understanding these factors is just as important in adopting a healthy, permanent style of eating as knowing what and how much to eat. *The Living Heart Diet* features a special chapter—complete with helpful questionnaires—devoted to discussing your attitudes and behavior surrounding food and diet.

Our LIVING HEART DIET approach has been successful for many of our patients already. We encourage you to adopt it. There may be no single path to good health, but we believe that following the LIVING HEART DIET is an auspicious beginning.

THE AUTHORS

How to Use This Book

The Living Heart Diet is specially written to make it easy for you to have the necessary facts about your heart and nutrition, and to translate those facts into a diet that is healthy as well as enjoyable to prepare and eat. To help you maintain this healthy diet, we present over 500 recipes, display menus for complete meals, and include food guides for long-term planning and general reference. *The Living Heart Diet* is divided into three major parts:

> Your Body and Its Relation to Diet (Chapters 1 to 5)
> Recipes
> Managing Your Diet

All these parts work together to help you achieve the basic goals of the LIVING HEART DIET.

YOUR BODY AND ITS RELATION TO DIET (CHAPTERS 1 TO 5)

To learn about the LIVING HEART DIET that is right for you, turn to the first part of the book, Your Body and Its Relation to Diet. Chapter 1, "Atherosclerosis, Risk Factors, and Diet," explains how the heart and other components of the circulatory system function when they are working properly—and when they are not. It also describes the risk factors that may lead to the development of heart disease and how they can be controlled.

In Chapter 2, "The Living Heart Diet," we describe the basic LIVING HEART DIET in full detail. Also discussed is the LOW-CALORIE LIVING HEART DIET, recommended for two groups of people: those who want to lose weight, and diabetics. This chapter outlines specifically, for each of these two diets, what types of food you may eat, how they should be prepared, and in what quantities you may eat them. We describe how the LOW-CALORIE LIVING HEART DIET employs an "exchange list system," which enables you to plan your daily caloric and nutritional intake precisely, without having to count calories or make any elaborate lists. Each recipe found in the Recipes section of this book is accompanied by a table which will provide you with the nutritional information you need to use this simple system. Other commonly eaten foods are assigned values from this exchange list system in The Living Heart Diet Food Guides so that you may completely plan your daily caloric and nutritional intake on the diets that recommend such planning.

Chapter 3, "The Low-Sodium Diet," explains fully how to manage sodium intake on the LOW-SODIUM LIVING HEART DIET for those of you whose physician has recommended it. Instructions are provided for keeping track of your sodium intake by employing a simple point system. Directions are also provided for a selection of appropriate recipes from the section of Recipes devoted to the LOW-SODIUM LIVING HEART DIET.

If your physician has recommended that you adopt a diet to reduce high blood levels of fats (hyperlipidemia), turn to Chapter 4, "Dietary Treatment of Hyperlipidemia." *The Living Heart Diet* employs a stepwise, progressive approach to the treatment of hyperlipidemia, based on which type of hyperlipidemia you have. Instructions on how to select the appropriate recipes from the Recipes section are included in this chapter. Also included are instructions on how to manage a low-sodium diet and hyperlipidemia at the same time.

Chapter 5, "Losing Weight and Keeping It Off," outlines in eleven steps an effective and medically safe behavioral approach to weight loss. This approach can be combined with the LOW-CALORIE LIVING HEART DIET to achieve a gradual and permanent weight loss.

RECIPES

The second part of this book, Recipes, comprises the cookbook portion of *The Living Heart Diet*. A complete collection of recipes, from appetizers to desserts, is provided. This cookbook is divided into two sections:

> The Living Heart Diet: Recipes
> The Living Heart Diet: Low-Sodium Recipes

Such a division allows those of you on a sodium-restricted diet to find the appropriate recipes quickly and easily—without having to flip through hundreds of recipes you should not use and without having to modify each recipe in order to reduce the sodium content. Also, these dishes were intended from the start to be low in sodium; they will not taste as if they are *missing* salt.

Each recipe in this book is directly followed by important nutritional information. For example, turn to the recipe for Stir-Fried Vegetable Medley on page 155. Directly beneath the recipe directions, you will see a table of nutritional information.

First, each table lists the quantity of food to which the nutritional information applies. In most cases, this is one serving of the recipe. In other cases, nutritional information is supplied for a specific quantity of food—for example, 1 tablespoon.

Second, each table lists the number of *calories*, and the quantities of *protein, fat, carbohydrate, saturated fat, monounsaturated fat, polyunsaturated fat, cholesterol*, and *sodium* found in the specified amount of that recipe. In the bottom, right-hand corner of every odd-numbered page, you will find a footnote that explains the abbreviations used in these tables for the units of measurement:

> *Abbreviations:* **Cal,** calories; **Prot,** protein; **Carb,** carbohydrate; **Sat,** saturated fat; **Mono,** monounsaturated fat; **Poly,** polyunsaturated fat; **Chol,** cholesterol; **Na,** sodium. Protein, fat, carbohydrate, saturated fat, monounsaturated fat, and polyunsaturated fat are expressed in *grams*. Cholesterol and sodium are expressed in *milligrams*.

If your particular LIVING HEART DIET suggests that you count your daily intake of any of these nutritional items, these numbers will enable you to do so.

Third, you will find a row entitled "Exchanges," where an exchange value of each recipe is provided. This "exchange value" is used in the "exchange list system" (described in Chapter 2) by those on the LOW-CALORIE LIVING HEART DIET. In the case of Stir-Fried Vegetable Medley (page 155), the exchange value is 1 vegetable plus ½ fat.

Fourth, you will see a row entitled "Recommended for," which lists all the diets that this recipe is particularly well suited for. As you can see, Stir-Fried Vegetable Medley is recommended for the LIVING HEART DIET; LOW-CALORIE LIVING HEART DIET; and TYPES IIA, IIB, III, AND IV HYPERLIPIDEMIA DIETS. One important point to remember is that it is assumed that all the low-sodium recipes can be used by those of you on the LOW-SODIUM LIVING HEART DIET.

MANAGING YOUR DIET

The third part of the book, Managing Your Diet, opens with the Living Heart Diet Menus. Here you will find 7 days of each of the following menus:

> Living Heart Diet Menus
> Low-Calorie Menus
> Low-Sodium Menus

Each day's menu has been designed to give you the proper caloric and nutritional values specified for the appropriate diet. In fact, these values are listed alongside each day's menus. Every recipe included in these menus is from the *Recipes* section; each is marked with an asterisk (*) to identify recipes given in the book. The recipes can be located by looking up the title of the recipe in the Recipe Index. These menus constitute only a few of the menu possibilities to be found in *The Living Heart Diet*. Refer to the guidelines specific to your diet outlined in Your Body and Its Relation to Diet (Chapters 1 to 5) in order to design your own menus.

The *Living Heart Diet Food Guides* follow next; they cover the major food categories: Meat, Fish, Poultry Guide; Egg Guide; Dairy Products Guide; Bread and Cereal Guide; Fat Guide; Fruit Guide; Vegetable Guide; and Miscellaneous Food Guide. You will find that each guide lists acceptable ("Yes") and unacceptable ("No") foods; that is, those foods (and how much) that are allowed on the LIVING HEART DIETS, and those that are not recommended.

An *Appendix* is provided following the Food Guides. Included are tables of information, which are referred to frequently in the five chapters comprising Your Body and Its Relation to Diet. The *Glossary* defines all terms used in this book that may be unfamiliar to you.

The book concludes with two indexes: *Subject Index* and *Recipe Index*. The Subject Index lists terms and topics covered in Chapters 1 to 5 (Your Body and Its Relation to Diet), and in the Menus, Food Guides, and Appendix (Managing Your Diet). The Recipe Index, as its name indicates, references all recipes in the cookbook portion (Recipes). Each recipe is indexed by title, by main ingredient(s), and, when possible, by the category of food appropriate to the recipe. For example, Stir-Fried Vegetable Medley will be found under "Stir-Fried Vegetable Medley," and under "Squash" because squash is the main ingredient. In the Recipe Index, all low-sodium recipes are set in italics to differentiate them clearly.

We hope that you will use *The Living Heart Diet* frequently—as a general reference of information concerning your heart and diet, and as a specific guide to planning a healthy diet daily.

The Living Heart Diet

Your Body and Its Relation to Diet

Keeping the complex processes of our bodies in perfect working order is not a simple matter. We do, however, have direct influence over some of these processes. Educators will tell you that the first step to proper care of our bodies is understanding the mechanisms involved. That is what this section is about.

We are interested primarily in the heart (which pumps the blood) and its tributaries (which carry the blood to the far reaches of our bodies). If anything disturbs this exquisite mechanism at *any* point, then the rest of the body will suffer from a lack of the nutrients and oxygen the blood normally delivers to it.

Diet plays a large part in maintaining the good condition of the body's life-sustaining pump (the heart) and its network of circulatory vessels (arteries, veins, and capillaries). Although this fact has been widely advertised by the merchants of low-cholesterol, low-calorie foods, and has very probably been thoroughly discussed by your own physician, there still seems to be a lack of understanding among the general population of exactly how this all works. Therefore, before presenting our recipes and menus, we will briefly discuss the ways in which your heart and circulation function—and how diet actually affects this mechanism, from the very day you are born.

Incidentally, if words are used whose meanings are unclear, please consult the *Glossary* at the end of the book. Anything you do to provide yourself with a better chance of living a longer and healthier life can only be enhanced by your fully understanding the whys and wherefores of your body and how what you eat affects it.

1

1

Atherosclerosis, Risk Factors, and Diet

THE HEART AND ITS VESSELS

The "circulatory system" consists of the heart plus all of the body's blood vessels (arteries, veins, and capillaries). This system serves to pump and circulate blood throughout the body. The heart plays a central role in this system: It pumps the blood, which the blood vessels then carry to the vital organs as well as the rest of the body. Because the terms "heart disease" and "heart attacks" are in general usage, they are used interchangeably in this book to refer to virtually all forms of cardiovascular disorders.

About 30 million people in the United States suffer from cardiovascular disease, and almost one million die from it each year. Of these deaths, about two-thirds are due to disorders of the blood vessels that supply blood directly to the heart. Known as coronary (meaning crown) arteries, these vessels are arranged in a ring around the heart, and blockage of one of them may lead to a heart attack.

Another 200,000 deaths each year are caused by a disturbance of one of the arteries supplying the brain—either blockage of that artery or hemorrhage (uncontrolled bleeding) from it. This type of attack is called a stroke, shock, or a cerebrovascular accident. The rest of the deaths related to the circulation are largely due to high blood pressure, a malformation of the heart itself, infection of the heart valves, weakness of the heart

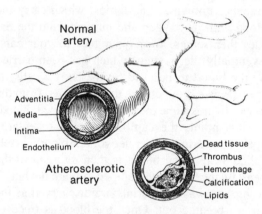

FIG. 1. The three layers of the arterial wall are: the intima (closest to the blood), the media (smooth muscle cells which contract to squeeze blood through the vessel), and the adventitia (the nerve and blood supply). The endothelium is a layer of cells which protects the intima. The inner surface of the normal artery is smooth and shiny whereas the wall of the atherosclerotic artery protrudes into the interior of the vessel and partially blocks the flow of blood. This protrusion in the atherosclerotic artery is called plaque and contains dead tissue, blood clots, calcified tissue and fats (lipids).

muscle, trauma to the heart, and blood clots which break loose and are carried to the lungs.

Although the allusion to a "broken heart" is familiar to all of us, in truth most circulatory or heart problems are caused not by the heart itself but, rather, by the arteries that feed it. The artery itself consists of three "layers" (Fig. 1). The innermost layer (intima), which is closest to the blood, is lined with a layer of cells (the endothelium) that serve as a protective covering. The middle layer of the artery wall (media) contains certain cells—smooth-muscle cells (so called because of their uncluttered microscopic appearance)—which can contract if the artery needs to squeeze more blood through it. The outermost layer (the adventitia) contains the nerve and blood supply to the vessel wall itself. These arteries form networks of vessels which carry blood pumped from the heart to the brain, lungs, and other vital organs and tissues of the body (Fig. 2). Arteries ultimately narrow into smaller branches known as capillaries, which carry the blood with its oxygen and nutrients into the tissues themselves, from your toes to your ears. Eventually the oxygen, which has been carried by the blood to be used by the body's cells, is spent; waste products are then collected from the tissues by this same (now oxygen-depleted) blood. At this point, the capillaries begin to enlarge again and form another network of blood vessels called veins. The blood is then returned to the heart by the veins and pumped through the lungs, where the waste materials are discharged as the air we breathe out. Once the blood is freed of wastes, it can and does replenish itself with oxygen from the air we breathe in—and the cycle begins all over again. (The newly oxygen-supplied vessels, now once again called arteries, carry the oxygen to the body, etc.)

ATHEROSCLEROSIS OR ARTERIOSCLEROSIS?

Most circulatory disease is caused by a blockage in an artery. The underlying disease responsible for blocking arteries is atherosclerosis, or "hardening of the arteries."

The term "arteriosclerosis" is often used synonymously with "atherosclerosis," but it is not really the same. "Arteriosclerosis" refers to a more general form of arterial disease that most often affects the elderly. Calcium deposits form in the

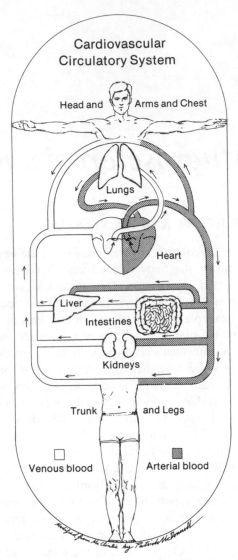

FIG. 2. The heart pumps oxygen-enriched blood from the lungs to all organs and tissues of the body through the system of vessels called arteries. When all of the blood's oxygen has been consumed by the body's tissues and the vital organs, the blood transports waste from the tissues and organs back to the heart through the network of vessels called veins. Arteries, through which life-giving blood flows, may become blocked as a consequence of the disease atherosclerosis.

arteries with the result that the arteries become less flexible.

Atherosclerosis, on the other hand, is a specific type of arteriosclerosis in which the initial injury begins in the innermost layer of the artery's wall. The surface of a normal artery is smooth and shiny. The contrast between the normal artery surface and the surface of an atherosclerotic artery is illustrated in Fig. 1.

HOW DOES ATHEROSCLEROSIS BEGIN?

No one knows precisely how atherosclerosis begins or what triggers the process. Most Americans, members of Western society, and to a varying extent members of other developed societies have some degree of atherosclerosis by the time they reach adulthood. In fact, autopsies performed on young American soldiers (in their twenties) killed in the Korean War revealed some degree of atherosclerosis in their arteries. By contrast, death due to atherosclerosis is uncommon in less developed societies.

The symptoms which signal atherosclerosis are related to a number of factors, including the site where the artery is narrowing, how much narrowing there is, and how fast it is developing. If the artery's passage is being filled in over a period of time, causing only minor slowing of the circulation, the body, by a remarkably adaptive mechanism, develops alternative channels of blood flow around the obstructed site. These channels, or new blood vessels, are called collateral vessels and can shunt blood around the obstructed area so it reaches the vital organs and tissues (Fig. 3).

Atherosclerosis was once thought to be a degenerative disorder, one in which the body's parts simply wore out. However, you have only to look at the age of those affected to realize this is not true. Heart attacks now represent one of the major causes of death in men under age 40 in the United States. Furthermore, when you look

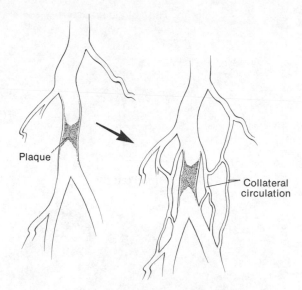

FIG. 3. In some individuals, plaque slowly forms over a long period of time, and as it blocks the flow of blood through the artery, new channels of blood flow may develop around the blockage. These new channels are referred to as collateral circulation.

at the arteries under a microscope, you find that the changes which occur in the wall of the artery initially are characterized by a growth of new cells, not by degeneration. (Degeneration may occur later, however, after the wall of the blood vessel has been severely damaged.)

Most researchers of atherosclerosis believe that something causes the protective lining of the innermost layer of the artery (the endothelium) to be damaged, thereby allowing toxic substances from the bloodstream to enter the artery wall. These substances then build up, eventually causing the artery to narrow and be blocked. The precise cause and nature of the original injury to the arterial lining is not known.

One of the potential sources of damage to the arterial wall lining is a high level of *cholesterol* and *triglycerides* in the blood (Fig. 4). These fats are transported in the blood by complex, spherical vehicles called lipoproteins. These fats have been proved dangerous in animal studies.

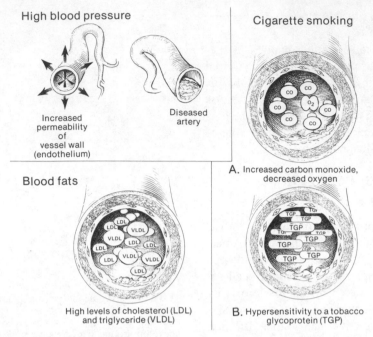

High blood pressure

Cigarette smoking

Increased
permeability
of
vessel wall
(endothelium)

Diseased
artery

A. Increased carbon monoxide,
decreased oxygen

Blood fats

High levels of cholesterol (LDL)
and triglyceride (VLDL)

B. Hypersensitivity to a tobacco
glycoprotein (TGP)

FIG. 4. Possible causes of injury to the endothelium are high blood pressure, high levels of blood fats, and cigarette smoking. High blood pressure may increase the ease with which substances pass through the endothelium thus causing damage to the arterial wall. High levels of the blood fats cholesterol (LDL) and triglycerides (VLDL) over a prolonged period of time are closely associated with injury to the endothelium. Cigarette smoking causes more carbon monoxide and less oxygen to be carried by the blood; consequently endothelial cells far from the heart may be deprived of oxygen, a condition which may encourage injury (A). Some individuals may be allergic to a substance in cigarette smoke, called tobacco glycoprotein (TGP), that causes a substance to be deposited on the arterial wall resulting in injury (B).

Another potential source of damage is *high blood pressure* (Fig. 4). This phenomenon may be explained by comparing the circulation in the human body to fluid in a pipe: If fluid is forced through a pipe at a high pressure over a period of time, there will be a greater degree of strain on the system of pipes (and on the pump) than if the liquid flowed through at a low pressure.

A third possible cause of injury to the arterial wall lining is *cigarette smoking* (Fig. 4). The smoker breathes in carbon monoxide with the cigarette smoke, which displaces some of the oxygen that should be carried in the blood. This, then, could result in the lining of the arteries some distance from the heart being deprived of oxygen as there would not be enough oxygen

left in the bloodstream to feed these distant arteries. In addition, the nicotine contained in cigarette smoke can directly damage the heart and blood vessels. And, as if these were not enough reasons not to smoke, some individuals are sensitive to tobacco smoke and have what appears to be an allergic reaction. The "invisible" damage that results, revealed only years later, is believed to be due to the formation of substances in the blood, called "immune complexes," that are provoked into existence by the tobacco smoke. These substances are then deposited onto the artery wall, subsequently causing injury to the cells that make up the wall's lining.

Once these cells are injured, they become dislodged from the artery wall, exposing the tissue

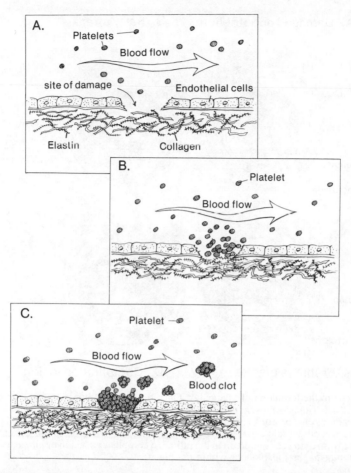

FIG. 5. Accumulation of platelets at the site of injury. A. When the endothelium in the artery is damaged, collagen from the connective tissue in the arterial wall becomes exposed to the blood. B. Blood platelets are attracted to the exposed collagen and collect at the site of damage. C. As large numbers of platelets collect on the injured endothelium, blood clots may form and may potentially cause a heart attack or stroke.

underneath. This tissue, called collagen, now has direct contact with the bloodstream. Collagen has a propensity for attracting and collecting certain cells from the blood, called platelets (Fig. 5). Platelets are intimately involved in the formation of blood clots, and under normal circumstances we need them to help us stop bleeding when we are cut or wounded. However, when platelets, which are sticky cells, collect in great numbers at a site where they are not wanted—in an artery—they may lead to the formation of

a clot that blocks the artery and stops the normal flow of blood. A blood clot in this way can cause a heart attack or stroke.

Other ways in which platelets may play a role in atherosclerosis are being explored. For example, it is known that platelets are involved in the formation of substances called prostaglandins, one of which may cause damage to the arteries. Platelets also contain a substance called "platelet growth factor" which can stimulate the growth of smooth-muscle cells. Although smooth-

A. Damaged endothelium   B. Fatty streak

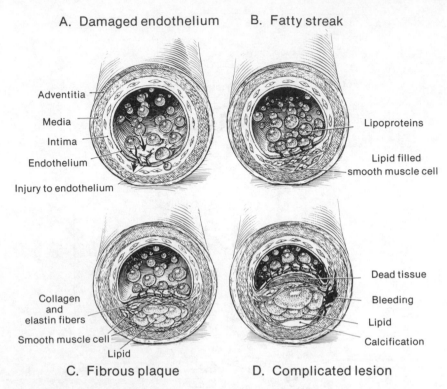

C. Fibrous plaque   D. Complicated lesion

FIG. 6. Progressive steps in the formation of plaque. A. Once the endothelium has been damaged, toxic substances may enter the arterial wall. B. Smooth muscle cells within the intima become filled with lipids thus forming a fatty streak. Lipoproteins containing cholesterol may be the source of these lipids. C. A fibrous plaque contains collagen and elastin (formed by the smooth muscle cells) and cholesterol (lipid). D. As smooth muscle cells, connective tissue, cholesterol and dead tissue from dying cells build up in the intima, a complicated lesion or plaque is formed. Calcification of tissue and bleeding (hemorrhaging) also occur within the plaque.

muscle cells are normally present in the artery wall, their growth and proliferation is believed to be one of the earliest events in the development of atherosclerosis (Fig. 6). The significance of platelet growth factor substance in the development of atherosclerosis in man remains to be established, but the pioneering work of Ross in Seattle has made this an attractive and exciting area of research.

Several drugs prevent platelet stickiness and so are being tested to determine if they have any potential for preventing heart attacks or for prolonging the lives of people who have already had one. Aspirin, dipyridamole, and sulfinpyrazone are among the drugs being investigated.

FORMATION OF PLAQUE AND ITS CONSEQUENCES

The precise factors which cause smooth-muscle cells to multiply and migrate into the innermost layer of the artery wall are not known. One theory, proposed by Benditt and Benditt in Seattle, is that the smooth-muscle cells undergo a mutation similar to that which happens to a malignant cell. Regardless of how it happens, these cells do indeed move into the artery wall, where they lay down a network of what is called connective tissue. This tissue network eventually becomes what is known as a *plaque*. This lesion, or plaque, comprises the basic injury to the artery wall during the development of atherosclerosis (Fig. 6). The plaque contains certain protein substances that are formed by the smooth-muscle cells. In addition, cholesterol is carried into the smooth-muscle cells by the lipoproteins from the blood and builds up within the plaque. A complex form of carbohydrate is also present and may help to entrap the cholesterol-carrying lipoproteins from the blood.

Over a period of time, smooth-muscle cells, connective tissue, cholesterol, and debris from damaged and dying cells accumulate within the artery wall. Because this material has nowhere else to go, it begins to protrude into the passageway of the artery. This atherosclerotic plaque may partially or totally obstruct the flow of blood through the artery before it is discovered. It is the plaque that eventually produces the symptoms which bring the patient to the attention of the physician. Several life-threatening situations may occur at the site of a plaque: Bleeding (hemorrhage) into the plaque may begin suddenly, or a blood clot (thrombus) may form on the plaque surface. If either of these possibilities occurs, the result may be a stroke or heart attack.

SYMPTOMS OF ATHEROSCLEROSIS

Plaques may occur in the coronary arteries, which carry blood (and thus oxygen) to the heart muscle. The first physical sign of coronary artery obstruction is often chest pain (angina pectoris). This pain occurs when too little blood and oxygen reach the heart muscle. Eventually a portion of the heart muscle dies from lack of oxygen and a heart attack (myocardial infarction) will probably result.

The arteries that supply oxygen to the brain may also be affected by plaques. Narrowing of these arteries may produce dizziness, transient weakness, or loss of speech. These changes can become permanent if a complete blockage occurs or if an artery is weakened sufficiently by the presence of a plaque to cause it to break, allow-

ing blood to hemorrhage into the brain. This situation—where too little oxygen reaches the cells of the brain—is called a stroke. Another type of stroke may occur if a blood clot (thrombus) breaks away from the surface of a plaque and is carried through the bloodstream to the brain, where it lodges in a small vessel and completely blocks the flow of blood (and hence the oxygen supply).

Plaques may appear in arteries that carry blood to the abdomen or the legs. The latter situation produces pain and tiredness in the legs or cramps when walking.

In some people, arteries are affected in more than one area of the body. The type of artery in which a plaque develops and the site of that buildup vary with the individual and of course influence the symptoms experienced (Fig. 7).

PROGRESSION OF ATHEROSCLEROSIS

Atherosclerosis may progress at a slow but steady pace for a period of time and then remain inactive for years. On the other hand, it is possible that the plaque may develop very rapidly. In the latter case the individual may die within months or only a few years after having the first symptoms. The presence of symptoms depends on the rate at which the disease progresses. For example, if an artery is narrowing slowly, over a long period of time, the body may compensate, developing other vessels to shunt blood around the blocked area. This new network of blood vessels around the blocked one, as mentioned earlier, is called collateral circulation (Fig. 3).

The damage produced by an atherosclerotic plaque most frequently manifests as a blocked artery. That is, the inner diameter of the artery, which carries the blood, becomes progressively smaller, much as the diameter of a water pipe is reduced as mineral deposits accumulate on its inner surface.

A different type of damage occurs when the muscular layer of the artery wall becomes weak-

Main Atherosclerotic Sites

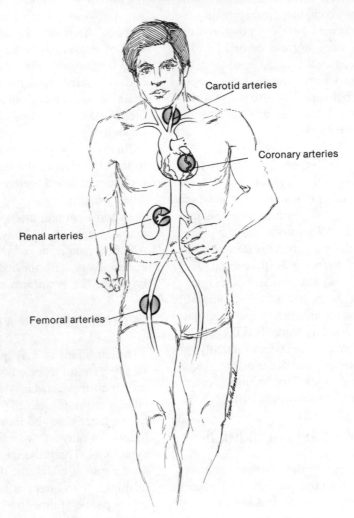

Carotid arteries

Coronary arteries

Renal arteries

Femoral arteries

FIG. 7.   Atherosclerosis may develop at different sites. Frequent areas of involvement are the carotid arteries in the neck, the coronary arteries in the heart, the renal arteries leading to the kidneys, or the femoral arteries in the legs. It is not known why atherosclerosis occurs at different sites in different people.

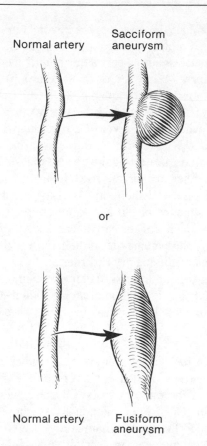

Normal artery   Sacciform aneurysm

or

Normal artery   Fusiform aneurysm

FIG. 8. Two types of aneurysms may occur when the arterial wall weakens as a result of atherosclerotic plaque inside the artery. The sacciform aneurysm is a ballooning out of one side of the artery while the fusiform aneurysm is a ballooning out of the entire arterial wall. An aneurysm of an artery is analogous to a weak point in the inner tube of a tire, which may balloon out and eventually burst.

ened and eventually balloons out. The weakened, ballooned-out segment of the artery is called an aneurysm (Fig. 8).

CORONARY ATHEROSCLEROSIS, ANGINA PECTORIS, AND HEART ATTACK

There are many questions and much confusion about the effects of coronary artery blockage. Therefore, we will give a more detailed expla-

nation of this potentially disastrous phenomenon. To begin with, a plaque builds up in one or more of the coronary arteries—the arteries which supply blood to the heart muscle cells. These cells together make up the muscle of the heart, which is called the myocardium. In someone with coronary artery disease, the amount of blood received by the heart may be sufficient to supply the needs of this muscle under resting conditions but insufficient when the individual is undergoing physical or emotional stress. When this occurs, he may feel a tightness or discomfort in the chest or base of the neck, and there may be a dull or squeezing pain that radiates from the chest and neck down into the left arm. The victim typically describes this pain, whose medical name is angina pectoris, graphically by clenching his fist.

A typical angina attack lasts for at least 2 minutes but not more than 10. An attack may be brought on by physical exertion (e.g., walking on a cold day after a heavy meal) or emotional excitement. In severe cases, angina pectoris may occur at rest and even awaken the victim at night.

Angina is usually a warning that one or more of the major coronary arteries are blocked. A person may have a stable pattern of mild angina for months or years and then suddenly the pain becomes more severe. If this happens, it should be reported to the physician, who will probably admit the individual to the hospital for observation and treatment.

For the individual with the stable, mild type of angina, rest may be enough to relieve the pain. If the anginal pain persists, nitroglycerin, in the form of a tablet that is placed under the tongue, may be prescribed. Nitroglycerin generally relieves anginal pain within a few minutes. (It is absorbed by the many small blood vessels under the tongue and is carried directly to the coronary arteries; in fact, it reaches the heart and begins acting within about 30 seconds.)

A heart attack and an anginal attack may be indistinguishable in the beginning. The heart attack lasts longer, however, and is not relieved by rest or nitroglycerin. The pain of a heart attack is usually more severe, requiring Demerol® (meperidine) or morphine sulfate to relieve it.

The terms "myocardial infarction" and "coronary thrombosis" are used interchangeably with "heart attack." Thrombosis refers to the formation of a blood clot, which has usually been regarded as the cause of the heart attack. Recently, though, studies have shown that sometimes the heart attack precedes the formation of the clot. In some cases, too, spasm of a coronary artery may be the cause of a heart attack. Spasm usually occurs at or near the site of an atherosclerotic plaque but has rarely been observed in normal coronary arteries.

The heart is essentially a muscle. When the blood supply to any part of this muscle is severely reduced or cut off because an artery is blocked, a heart attack will occur. That part of the heart muscle which has not received nutrients and oxygen will die if the deficiency is not rapidly reversed.

More than half of the deaths from heart attacks occur before the victim can get to a hospital. If a heart attack is suspected, it is critically important to call an ambulance that is outfitted especially for heart attack victims, if possible, and to go immediately to a hospital that has a coronary care unit.

RISK FACTORS

There is still no way to innoculate against heart attacks or stroke, although research suggests that this may some day be possible. There is hope, however, that we will be able to prevent or reverse atherosclerosis.

Roughly 50% of people in the United States today die of some form of cardiovascular disease, most commonly heart attacks and strokes. There are certain entities known as "risk factors" which, when present, increase the likelihood of a stroke or heart attack.

Some of these factors are beyond our control. For example, women appear to be somewhat protected against heart attacks until menopause (compared with men of that age group). We do not know the full explanation for this, although one of the reasons may be that women have a somewhat higher level of a particular fat in the blood (high density lipoproteins), and this fat appears to protect against heart attacks.

Another unalterable risk factor for cardiovascular disease is heredity. If both parents die in their nineties of old age, their children are less likely to die of an early heart attack or stroke than if the parents die in their forties, fifties, or sixties of circulatory disorders.

Age is another risk factor that cannot be controlled: The likelihood of an individual suffering a heart attack or stroke increases as he grows older.

The risk factors for coronary heart disease and stroke have been identified in studies of large populations carried out over periods of years. One of the most extensive of these studies was conducted in Framingham, Massachusetts, and is called the Framingham study (see *Glossary*). For the average 55-year-old man in the Framingham study, the likelihood of developing coronary heart disease within 6 years was 9.5%. This typical man did not fall into the highest risk category but, rather, had an average level of blood cholesterol, blood pressure, weight, and cigarette smoking habits. From the Framingham and other studies, at least three major factors have been identified as risks for early heart attacks (Table 1): 1) an elevation of cholesterol in the blood; 2) an elevation of blood pressure (hypertension); and 3) cigarette smoking. Other, less serious risk factors include diabetes mellitus, an elevated blood triglyceride (another type of blood fat) level, lack of exercise, obesity, excessive stress, and certain personality traits that together form the "Type A" personality. Although space does not permit a detailed discussion of all of these risk factors, we will talk about their rela-

TABLE 1. *Risk factors for coronary artery disease*

Major Risk Factors
  Elevated serum cholesterol
  Elevated blood pressure
  Cigarette smoking

Secondary Risk Factors
  Elevated serum triglycerides
  Heredity
  Diabetes
  Obesity
  Lack of physical exercise
  Type A personality
  Diet high in saturated fat
  Stressful environment

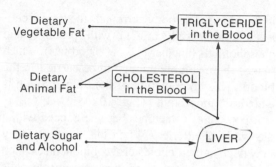

FIG. 9. How do cholesterol and triglycerides get into the blood stream? The two major sources are the diet and the liver. Triglycerides may originate from either animal or vegetable fat in the diet. Cholesterol may be consumed in the diet as animal fat and dairy products—it does not occur in vegetable fat. The liver, which produces 60 to 80% of the blood cholesterol, converts sugar and alcohol from the diet into both cholesterol and triglycerides.

tionship to diet and how best to reduce their importance through diet.

BLOOD FATS (LIPIDS): CHOLESTEROL AND TRIGLYCERIDES

The terms "fats" and "lipids" are synonymous. A lipid (or fat) is a substance that does not dissolve in water and which floats to the surface when it is poured into water. Although cholesterol and triglycerides are both lipids, they are different chemical entities and do not represent equal risks for coronary heart disease. The lipids cholesterol and triglycerides in the bloodstream have two origins: Some come from the diet, and the rest are made in the body. The liver produces most of the cholesterol and triglycerides in the body, and the intestine contributes the rest.

The cholesterol we consume is found exclusively in animal products. Our bodies need cholesterol for making cell membranes and as a building block for producing hormones in the adrenal glands and the sex glands. However, the average person in Western society has more cholesterol in the blood than is necessary because of our dietary habits. From three-fifths to four-fifths of our cholesterol is manufactured in the body; the remainder comes from the diet (Fig. 9). The amount of cholesterol manufactured by the body is closely regulated in the liver, and

when more cholesterol is consumed in the diet, less is manufactured by the liver. Because of this finely tuned regulatory mechanism, it is possible to lower the amount of cholesterol in the body through dietary measures.

Unlike cholesterol, triglycerides are found in animal *and* vegetable fats. Triglycerides from vegetable sources (e.g., corn oil or safflower oil) are liquid at room temperature because they contain polyunsaturated fats. In contrast, most triglycerides from animal fat (e.g., lard, bacon grease, or butter) are solid at room temperature because they are rich in saturated fats. Triglycerides may be either deposited in fat cells or broken down to produce energy. The liver converts excess calories and foods (e.g., fatty acids, sugar, and alcohol) into triglycerides, which are then transported to the blood. Triglycerides, then, represent a storage form of fat.

LIPOPROTEINS: THE CARRIERS OF CHOLESTEROL AND TRIGLYCERIDES IN THE BLOOD

As lipids do not dissolve in water (are not soluble), the body has devised a mechanism for keeping them in solution as they are transported in the blood. The body surrounds the lipids (cholesterol and triglycerides) with proteins and phospholipids (another class of blood fats), which makes them soluble enough to be carried in the blood. This combination of lipid plus protein is called a "lipoprotein" (Fig. 10).

Lipoproteins sometimes become trapped within the walls of arteries. When this happens, they may deposit their cholesterol components, which in turn may stimulate the smooth-muscle cells of the arterial wall to multiply. Or the buildup may damage cells or other structures in the arterial wall.

High concentrations of certain types of lipoproteins in the blood increase an individual's chances of developing atherosclerosis at an early age. In the Framingham study, 30- to 50-year-old men were three to five times more likely to have a heart attack within 5 years if their cholesterol level was 260 milligrams per deciliter (mg/dl) than men of the same age whose cholesterol level was under 220 milligrams of cholesterol per deciliter of blood plasma. (See Table 2 for normal cholesterol levels.)

When lipids or lipoproteins are present in too high a concentration, this condition is referred to as hyperlipidemia (*hyper* = too much, *lipid* = fat, *emia* = in the blood) or hyperlipoproteinemia. (These conditions are discussed in detail in the section beginning on page 16.)

THE FAMILIES OF LIPOPROTEINS

Some description of the various types of lipoproteins is helpful for explaining their relevance to coronary heart disease. The triglycerides ingested in the diet are taken up into large lipoprotein particles (chylomicrons) in the intestine. These chylomicrons then move from the intestine into the blood. They may be cleared from the blood of a normal individual if he fasts for 12 hours.

Triglycerides manufactured in the liver are carried through the blood by smaller particles, called very low density lipoproteins (VLDL).

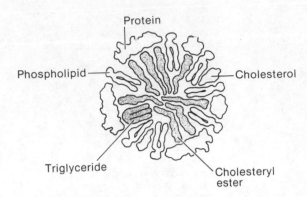

FIG. 10. Lipoproteins are round and contain the fats cholesteryl ester (a chemical variant of cholesterol) and triglycerides in their core. This cross section of a lipoprotein shows the core (shaded in grey) surrounded by phospholipids, protein, and some cholesterol particles, which keep the fats in the core.

TABLE 2. *Desirable levels of plasma lipid values*[a]

Age (years)	Cholesterol (mg/dl)	Triglycerides (mg/dl)
1–9	170	120
10–19	180	140
20–29	200	140
30–39	210	150
40–49	< 220	160
≥50	< 220	190

[a]These values should not necessarily be considered safe ones. Current knowledge does not allow us to state absolutely that a specific value of cholesterol or triglycerides is "normal" or "safe."

Like the chylomicrons, VLDL also transport triglycerides from the intestine into the bloodstream. VLDL may be broken down in the body, forming smaller particles, called the low density lipoproteins (LDL). During this breakdown, VLDL release their triglycerides. The new LDL particles transport mainly cholesterol. In fact, LDL are the major cholesterol carriers in the blood. There is still another type of lipoprotein, the smallest one, called the high density lipoproteins (HDL). These small HDL transport some of the cholesterol that has been made in the liver and the intestine.

All four types of lipoproteins—chylomicrons, VLDL, LDL, and HDL—may carry triglycer-

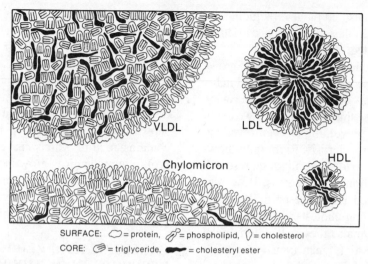

SURFACE: ◯ = protein, 🖋 = phospholipid, ◊ = cholesterol
CORE: ✐ = triglyceride, ➤ = cholesteryl ester

FIG. 11. Although all lipoproteins contain triglycerides and cholesterol, each carries a preponderance of one of these fats. Chylomicrons are the largest lipoprotein whose major component is triglycerides from the diet. VLDL are somewhat smaller and carry triglycerides made in the liver and the intestine. Chylomicrons and VLDL are broken down into smaller particles, LDL, which contain mainly cholesteryl ester, a chemical form to which cholesterol is converted while it is transported by lipoproteins. The LDL are highly atherogenic. The smallest lipoproteins, HDL, transport some of the cholesterol made by the liver and intestine.

ides, cholesterol, and cholesteryl ester (a chemical variant of cholesterol), although each lipoprotein type is known to prefer one lipid over the others (Fig. 11). For example, triglycerides are the main lipid in VLDL and chylomicrons, even though small amounts of cholesterol are also present. When VLDL break down to form LDL, the main lipid carried is cholesteryl ester. HDL contain mainly phospholipids and cholesterol.

When the physician requests that a cholesterol level be measured, it is actually the total amount of cholesterol in HDL, LDL, and VLDL that is measured. High levels of LDL are often present in persons with early heart attacks, whereas high levels of HDL are associated with a decreased risk of coronary heart disease.

The relationship between VLDL (containing triglycerides) and coronary heart disease is not as well defined as the one between cholesterol and coronary heart disease. Some researchers report that triglycerides are an important risk factor for coronary heart disease, whereas others

fail to confirm this relationship. We have found that triglycerides are more plentiful in persons with coronary heart disease than in normal individuals.

The level of triglycerides in the blood has an inverse relationship with the level of HDL (which carry mainly cholesterol). Thus individuals with the highest concentration of triglycerides have the lowest concentration of HDL and hence less protection against coronary heart disease. Long distance running and vigorous exercise have been reported to raise HDL levels. There is also some evidence that alcohol consumption may increase HDL, although the adverse effects of excessive alcohol consumption outweigh potential benefits of increasing HDL. Prior to menopause, women have higher concentrations of HDL than do men. Cigarette smoking, obesity, and diets high in carbohydrate, on the other hand, are associated with low HDL levels.

It is not known how HDL protect against atherosclerosis. One possibility is that they transport cholesterol out of cells and tissues, including the arterial wall. The cholesterol is then carried to the liver and excreted into the bile.

Under normal circumstances, as a person grows older he gradually accumulates cholesterol in his tissues, including his artery walls. If there were some way to decrease this accumulation, we might have a method for preventing or even reversing the ravages of atherosclerosis. Right now, however, there is no way to do it, although research aimed in this direction is in progress. Researchers have synthesized HDL-like particles which are capable of binding cholesterol. Through experiments with animals, they will determine if these HDL-like particles can transport cholesterol and subsequently reduce the amount of cholesterol that accumulates in the artery wall.

DISPOSING OF CHOLESTEROL

With the exception of the liver, most cells in the body cannot metabolize (break down) cholesterol. A small amount of cholesterol is used to produce hormones in the adrenal glands, ovaries, and testes, and some is converted into bile acids in the liver. Cholesterol and bile acids can be excreted via the bile into the intestine and then eliminated in the stool. This is the body's only mechanism for disposing of cholesterol.

HYPERLIPIDEMIA AND HYPERLIPOPROTEINEMIA

Hyperlipidemia is the name of a disorder in which the concentration of lipids (cholesterol and/or triglycerides) in the blood is too high. Hyperlipoproteinemia is a disorder in which the concentration of the lipoproteins LDL, VLDL, or chylomicrons—which carry cholesterol and triglycerides—in the blood is too high. We use these two names—hyperlipidemia and hyperlipoproteinemia—interchangeably in this book. Either condition is capable of contributing to the development of atherosclerotic plaque. There are several ways by which this can take place. For example, cholesterol is more rapidly deposited into the artery wall when high levels of cholesterol and LDL are present in the blood. When the hyperlipidemia persists, damage occurs to cells in the arterial wall, a phenomenon believed to be one of the mechanisms that triggers the development of atherosclerosis. Also, it has been shown that the blood of hyperlipidemic animals contains factors which cause arterial tissue to proliferate when it is grown experimentally outside the body. These mechanisms and others may be involved either in initiating the atherosclerotic plaque or in stimulating its growth.

CAUSES OF HYPERLIPIDEMIA AND A DESCRIPTION OF THE VARIOUS TYPES

There are many causes of too much cholesterol (hypercholesterolemia) and too much triglyceride (hypertriglyceridemia) in the blood. Sometimes the increase is due to an underlying disease (e.g., an underactive thyroid, liver disease with obstruction of the flow of bile, or a type of kidney disease in which there is a massive loss of protein in the urine or kidney failure). In others the disease is inherited.

There are several forms of inherited hypercholesterolemia. One, seen in about 1 out of every 500 people, is called "familial hypercholesterolemia" and may be inherited from either parent. Men with this inherited disorder usually suffer their first heart attack at about 40 years of age. On average, women develop coronary disease later than men, but we have seen women in their twenties and thirties with familial hypercholesterolemia who are disabled by coronary heart disease.

There are various types of hyperlipoproteinemia, which are characterized by specific patterns of elevations of cholesterol, triglycerides, or the various lipoproteins. Types I, IIa and IIb, III, IV, and V are discussed in detail in Chapter 4.

A study of inherited hyperlipidemia in Seattle revealed that about one-third of the relatives of survivors of heart attacks had some form of the inherited disease. The incidence of hyperlipidemia was even higher among young persons in the study. Elevated cholesterol plus triglycerides was the most common form, elevated triglycerides alone was second, and elevated cholesterol (familial hypercholesterolemia) was the third most frequent. Typically, though, only about 1 out of 10 persons with a high cholesterol level will have one of these forms of inherited hypercholesterolemia. Other studies have not found such an association between elevated triglycerides and coronary heart disease, although triglycerides are usually higher in groups with known coronary disease. It is generally agreed that high triglycerides represent a risk factor in diabetics, in patients with kidney failure, in individuals with high cholesterol, and in certain high-risk families.

The most common form of hyperlipidemia encountered in the United States is called Type IV hyperlipoproteinemia, in which the triglycerides are elevated due to their overproduction by the body. Although common, it is not known to what extent Type IV disease is responsible for coronary heart disease.

Because only 10% of people with hyperlipidemia have inherited it, the physician must search for other causes of the disorder before attributing it to inheritance. Once it is determined that the individual is healthy, except for high lipid levels, the physician can then begin to test other members of the family for a possible familial connection. Occasionally, despite very careful workups, no reason can be found for the hyperlipidemia, and it is then treated as an entity unto itself.

The diagnosis of hyperlipidemia is sometimes clearly indicated by yellowish or reddish raised areas on the skin or tendons. These are deposits of cholesterol or triglycerides that have accumulated to the point where they form nodules. They are referred to as xanthomas. Cholesterol deposits in familial hypercholesterolemia are especially common on the eyelids and are also found on tendons of the hands and on the Achilles tendons on the heel.

HOW DO HYPERLIPIDEMIA AND HYPERLIPOPROTEINEMIA RELATE TO DIET?

The role of diet in the management of hypercholesterolemia, hypertriglyceridemia, and hyperlipoproteinemia is discussed in detail in Chapter 4. It deserves brief treatment here, however.

Dietary saturated fat tends to raise the cholesterol and LDL concentrations in the blood, whereas polyunsaturated fat tends to lower them. Removing 1 gram of saturated fat from the diet lowers cholesterol to approximately the same extent as adding 2 grams of polyunsaturated fat. The amount of dietary cholesterol also influences the level of blood cholesterol; cholesterol consumed in the diet tends to increase the plasma cholesterol.

The triglyceride level is also increased by eating saturated fat and decreased by eating polyunsaturated fat. The simplest way of lowering triglycerides if you are overweight is to restrict calories. Some people seem to be sensitive to dietary sugar, and so if they have hypertriglyceridemia they should reduce the amount of sugar they eat. Alcohol may also increase the degree of hypertriglyceridemia. Obesity and alcohol consumption are the two major contributors to high levels of triglycerides in the American population.

There is not an absolute cutoff point where you can say that a high-cholesterol or a high-triglyceride condition exists. Sometimes arbitrary values are established as guidelines, however. We suggest those given in Table 2. It must be emphasized, however, that there are no single values for blood levels of cholesterol or triglycerides that separate those at risk for coronary disease from those who are not at risk. There is a continuous relationship between the concentration of cholesterol and the risk of coronary heart disease; that is, as the cholesterol level increases, so does the risk (Fig. 12). In parts of the world where the level of cholesterol is relatively low, there is considerably less atherosclerosis and coronary heart disease. It is seldom possible to achieve this degree of cholesterol lowering in most individuals with high cholesterol in our country. The average value of cholesterol in adults in the United States is about 210 mg/dl and it tends to rise with age. In general, the higher the level of cholesterol, and particularly of LDL, the greater is the risk of dying of an early heart attack.

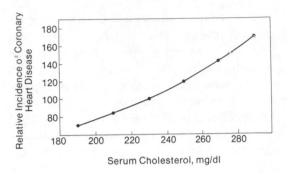

FIG. 12. A study of a large population has shown that as the level of cholesterol in the blood plasma increases, the incidence of coronary heart disease also increases. (Graph provided courtesy of Ancel Keys.)

HYPERTENSION

Hypertension is defined as increased blood pressure in the arteries. As the heart muscle contracts, it pushes blood into the major arteries and then on through the arteries and capillaries to the veins. It is the pressure within the arteries that is measured. The mean blood pressure in the arteries is calculated by multiplying the cardiac output by the resistance to flow through the arterial system.

In practice, blood pressure is expressed in millimeters of mercury (mm Hg), and two values are recorded. The first value, called the systolic pressure, is a measurement of the pressure in the arteries while the heart is contracting. This normally reaches a value of 110 to 130 mm Hg in young adults. The second reading—the diastolic pressure—is taken as the heart relaxes; this pressure is normally between 70 and 80 mm Hg. A normal blood pressure might be expressed as 110/70, or "110 over 70." The systolic and diastolic pressures usually increase with age, the systolic tending to rise more than the diastolic. Generally a systolic pressure of 140 and a diastolic pressure of 90 are used to define hypertension in adults.

According to life insurance statistics, the blood pressure is one of the single most important determinants of life expectancy. Metropolitan Life statistics predict that the life expectancy for a 35-year-old man is reduced by about 16 years if his blood pressure is greater than 150/100. In the Framingham study a diastolic blood pressure between 85 and 94 was associated with a 5-fold increase in heart attacks between ages 30 and 39. The likelihood of having a stroke was increased by an elevation of either systolic or diastolic pressure. For a young person or a child, a blood pressure of 140/90 is too high. It may also be too high for blacks, since their death rate from hypertension is 3 times greater than for whites. Normal and upper limits of normal blood pressure levels for different age groups are given in Fig. 13.

If the blood pressure is found to be elevated on several occasions, it should be treated. Treatment varies depending on the circumstances and age of the individual. For example, a condition known as labile hypertension, in which the pressure may be elevated during a period of acute stress but then returns to normal at other times, is treated differently from persistently high blood pressure.

When the blood pressure remains elevated, tests should be run to determine if there is an underlying cause. For example, a tumor of the adrenal glands or constriction of the aorta or of one of the arteries to the kidneys may cause hypertension, as may oral contraceptives.

If no underlying cause is found, a diagnosis of "essential hypertension" is made—meaning

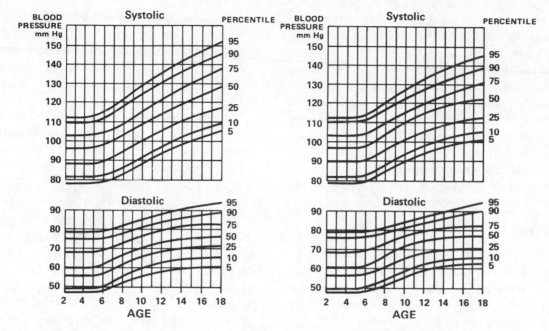

FIG. 13. **Left:** Percentiles of blood pressure measurement in boys (right arm, seated). **Right:** Percentiles of blood pressure measurement in girls (right arm, seated). From the Report of the NHLBI Task Force on Blood Pressure Control in Children (1977). *Pediatrics*, 59(Suppl.1):5:803.

simply that there is no identifiable cause of the hypertension. About 90% of hypertensive people fall into this category. Essential hypertension may be caused by the arteries and arterioles being constricted, by the volume within the arterial system being too great, or by both of these factors.

About 7 years ago it was estimated that there were approximately 23 million hypertensive Americans. Those same estimates showed that only half of the 23 million even knew about their hypertension and only about one in eight was being treated effectively. Since then, the statistics have improved. Extensive education and screening programs for hypertension have made a large number of people aware that they have the problem, and a greater proportion of hypertensives are now under effective treatment.

Hypertension may lead to early heart attacks, congestive heart failure, strokes, and kidney failure, so it is terribly important to control the dis-

order. It is one of the three major risk factors for heart attacks and is the single most important risk factor for stroke. Hypertension is particularly common among black Americans. High blood pressure (hypertension) should be better controlled among the population as its diagnosis is simple and its treatment readily available.

Although hypertension is a treatable disorder, treatment is usually a lifelong process. An elevated blood pressure (hypertension) is worsened by obesity and salt intake. Thus control of blood pressure begins with a reduction to ideal body weight and a decrease in dietary salt. In fact, these measures may be sufficient to control mild hypertension. If medication is required as an additional measure, it is still vitally important to continue a specified diet and to control body weight and salt intake. Blood pressure should be monitored frequently so as to be certain that the diet and/or medication are effective.

The greatest single problem in the treatment

of hypertension is the individual himself and his compliance with adhering to the diet and taking the prescribed medications. Quite obviously, the diet and drugs are effective only so long as the individual follows his physician's recommendations. It is very important also for the hypertensive to control his cholesterol level, to avoid cigarette smoking, and to follow a program of regular exercise.

In a later chapter of this book, we discuss in considerable detail a salt-restricted, low-calorie diet and how it affects health.

SMOKING

By 1964 the Surgeon General of the United States had seen enough evidence pointing to cigarette smoking as a culprit in lung cancer and chronic lung disease to issue a warning against smoking. Since that time there has been a significant decline in cigarette smoking among physicians and middle-aged men, although this has been offset by an increase in smoking by women and young people—so much so that there has actually been an overall yearly increase in cigarette consumption of 1 to 2%.

Since 1964 additional dangers associated with smoking have become apparent. The one we are most concerned with here is its danger to the heart. Smoking is one of the three major risk factors for heart attacks. Among the middle aged, the rate of heart attacks in smokers is twice that in nonsmokers. Atherosclerosis of the coronary arteries is accelerated by smoking. Moreover, cigarette smoking is undoubtedly one of the most important contributing causes to a syndrome called Buerger's disease, which causes severe damage to the arteries in the limbs of young men and often results in amputation at an early age.

Cigarette smoking may interact in a negative way with other risk factors as well. For instance, smoking is dangerous to diabetics, who from their diabetes alone suffer a high incidence of gangrene and arterial disease of the limbs and extremities. Smoking just adds to their problems.

Smoking should be particularly discouraged in hypertensives and in young women on birth control pills who have a history of thrombophlebitis, a disease in which the walls of the veins are inflamed and in which blood clots (thrombi) may form.

Cigarette smoking has been correlated with low levels of high density lipoproteins (HDL). As mentioned earlier, high levels of HDL appear to offer some protection against atherosclerosis.

We still do not know the precise manner in which cigarette smoking predisposes to atherosclerosis, although we can suggest some plausible hypotheses. One is that it increases the blood level of carbon monoxide, a gas also present in automobile exhaust fumes. Carbon monoxide then displaces some of the oxygen that is needed by the body's tissues, and so for a period of time the tissues do not receive sufficient oxygen, which could lead to damage.

Cigarette smoke also contains nicotine, and about 90% of this is absorbed into the bloodstream. Nicotine is a poison that is capable of damaging the blood vessels, heart, kidneys, and gastrointestinal tract. Various tars and arsenic are also present in cigarette smoke which may damage the lungs and lead to cancer.

We mentioned the particular risk of smoking in individuals who are susceptible to atherosclerosis of the limbs and extremities (peripheral vascular disease). Nicotine can cause constriction of blood vessels, which can be dangerous in diabetics and in those who already have a disease of the peripheral arteries.

Interestingly, damage to the small arteries in the hands and feet of persons with Buerger's disease may be arrested if the individual gives up smoking. In a study carried out at the Mayo Clinic, patients who had disease of the peripheral arteries showed improvement after they stopped smoking.

We are particularly concerned with smoking as it relates to diet. Cigarette smoking depresses the appetite. In fact, we have seen persons who stop smoking gain 15 to 20 pounds within the next 3 months; these individuals usually state that they never realized how good food tasted until they gave up smoking. For this reason it is not a good idea to stop smoking and start a diet at the same time. It is better to attempt one objective at a time; that is, either stop smoking or follow a diet, depending on the recommendation of your physician. We find that once weight is lost and a maintenance diet is well in hand, a program to stop smoking is more readily accepted.

There are a variety of techniques and programs aimed at eliminating the smoking habit. Some of the more popular ones are as follows:

Clinics. A number of organizations, public and private, hold clinics that treat smoking in a group format. The American Cancer Society and the Seventh Day Adventist Church, for example, offer periodic short-term programs, often without any charge to participants. Private clinics also offer treatment. There is little available information about the effectiveness of these clinics, although it is known that many people who begin treatment in a clinic drop out before completing the program.

Self-help. Despite the pessimistic results of research on giving up smoking, there is unquestionably a very large group of heavy smokers who have successfully quit without professional help of any kind. In fact, over 20 million people are estimated to have stopped smoking on their own. No one technique works for every person. We conducted a survey of former, long-term, severely dependent cigarette smokers who had quit on their own without professional help. They reported that they utilized many techniques for terminating their dependency. Motivation was highly important; those who quit successfully wanted to do so very badly. Motivation, which appears to develop in a highly idiosyncratic fashion, was reported to be the key element in almost half of the success stories. Some of the techniques they mentioned are as follows:

1. Challenging oneself: Putting cigarette packs in each room in one's home and refusing to smoke.
2. Having alternatives: Keeping hands busy with crocheting, painting, knitting. Chewing a sugarless gum.
3. Noticing the rewards of not smoking: Being aware of how much better one feels. Noticing the taste buds coming alive.
4. Challenges from others: Having a friend say that he would stop if the smoker would. Getting the spouse involved.
5. Delaying lighting up: Keeping track of how long it has been between cigarettes. Postponing lighting up for longer and longer periods.

One effective strategy is to choose a date a month or so in the future, and when that date arrives, go "cold turkey." The first 3 days are the most difficult. After that, the physiological and psychological needs gradually begin to lessen, although in some they persist for weeks or months. Various withdrawal effects have been described. Most people express an intense craving for cigarettes. Others report an increased appetite, nervousness, and periods of sweating and shakiness.

Our survey showed that some employ a step-by-step progression. That is, they use progressively stronger filters or graduate to brands of lower tar and nicotine content. Others adopt such measures as inhaling smoke fewer times, laying down the cigarette for certain lengths of time between puffs, and putting the cigarette out after smoking it for only a short time. Still others, in contrast, terminate the habit abruptly. Although no one technique guarantees success for everyone, heavy smokers who really want to quit are able to devise effective methods that suit them.

Drugs. Lobeline®, a substance extracted from the leaves of tobacco plants, is a nicotine substitute that may be taken in tablet form by smokers. Its usual side effect, though, is an irritation in the back of the throat. It is sold in drug stores under a variety of trade names. It is unfortunate, however, that most studies have shown it to be ineffective for most smokers trying to kick the habit.

Whatever the technique used to quit smoking, millions of adults in the United States have now given it up. Because of the great risk of heart attack and other forms of cardiovascular disease as well as the risk of chronic lung disease and cancer, we recommend that our people give up smoking subject to the conditions outlined above.

SECONDARY RISK FACTORS

Obesity

Obesity is a major problem of Western society. Despite its prevalence, it is not popular in our society to be fat. The media are filled with advertisements of slim, trim, young individuals offering a variety of methods for achieving a desirable degree of trimness. Whereas much of the advertising deals with obesity on the basis of aesthetics, we are concerned with its threat to health. Obesity in excess of 130% of ideal body weight is associated with a shortened life span. In the Framingham study (see *Glossary*), a correlation was established between obesity and angina pectoris, myocardial infarction, and sudden death. It is known from life insurance tables that markedly obese individuals have a greater chance of dying from cardiovascular disease than thin people.

Some researchers believe that one cause of obesity is an actual increase in the number of fat cells, a process that may begin early in life. For this reason, parents should make every effort to prevent obesity in their children by discussing eating habits and how they affect the body, by providing well-balanced, nutritious meals, and by encouraging appropriate exercise. Most adult obesity is characterized by an increase in the size of fat cells, where excess calories are stored in

the form of triglycerides. When the person loses weight, the fat cells shrink, with a loss of triglycerides.

Obesity has a bad effect on several other risk factors. It apparently is strongly associated with high blood pressure and worsens any hypertriglyceridemia that may be present. Obese individuals tend to have low HDL levels. Weight reduction in obese males (but not females) has been reported to decrease LDL, raise HDL, and improve the LDL to HDL ratio. Many individuals with mild forms of hypercholesterolemia also respond favorably to weight reduction. Obesity is also a very serious problem for diabetics or those with high blood sugar levels.

Adult-onset diabetes can often be controlled by diet and exercise. Whatever other treatment may be required, weight control is always very important in the treatment of diabetes and hypertriglyceridemia.

Individuals who are obese are most often those who engage in little physical activity. Obesity usually cannot be controlled by physical exercise alone, and so an exercise program should be used in conjunction with diet. Calorie restriction is the primary way of achieving weight reduction.

Although thyroid hormone is often prescribed for weight control in persons who do not actually have an underactive thyroid, it is not beneficial unless an actual deficiency exists. We do not advocate the use of drugs for treating obesity, as those drugs which diminish the appetite are potentially dangerous to the cardiovascular system. Moreover, once you go off the drug, its effect is usually quickly reversed and the lost weight is rapidly regained.

Our approach to weight control is simply to eat a balanced diet in which fewer calories are consumed than are burned up each day. This regimen results in a gradual weight loss of 1 to 2 pounds a week. It is not a miracle diet, but it can be easily learned and followed over a period of years. Because it is reasonable, most people do not have difficulty maintaining it. It is relatively easy to lose weight for short periods of time, but it is extremely difficult to maintain the weight loss over a period of months to years. *The Living Heart Diet* can be used as a lifelong guide to maintaining your ideal weight.

Exercise

Exercise must be included in daily activities along with a proper balance of work and relaxation in order to provide optimal physical and mental health. When muscles are not used, they become weak and begin to wither away, a process called "atrophy."

We do not yet know if exercise prevents heart attacks, although a number of studies suggest that it does in fact reduce the risk of dying of an early heart attack. Although there is evidence to suggest a protective effect of exercise against heart attacks, the Committee on Exercise of the American Heart Association states its current position on the subject as follows: "We do not consider it justifiable to advocate widespread adoption of vigorous exercise programs purely on the ground that exercise alone will prevent heart disease."

There has been an enormous upsurge in physical exercise in the United States during the past 5 years. As many as 20 million Americans now engage in some form of jogging or running, and it is estimated that there may be as many as 12 million people who run several miles a day.

The point made earlier deserves re-emphasis: that exercise without dieting does not adequately control weight in most individuals. In spite of the questions still unanswered about the value of exercise, however, an exercise program is a very helpful adjunct to diet. How much exercise is necessary and desirable is difficult to answer though. It is not our purpose here to give prescriptions for exercise—this should be done by your physician. We, however, certainly encourage people to exercise regularly, subject of course to approval of a personal physician. The pre-

scription for exercise must be given on an individual basis. For a person over age 35 or with suspected heart disease, we recommend that an exercise electrocardiogram or treadmill test be obtained prior to undertaking any new exercise program.

People recovering from an illness may greatly benefit from exercise as well. For example, exercise is a vital part of the rehabilitation of persons recovering from a stroke, a heart attack, or coronary bypass surgery. It is also good for those who have angina pectoris. In addition, exercise is often a useful adjunct in the control of obesity, hypertension, hyperlipidemia, and stress. Another benefit of exercise is that it can raise the concentration of the high density lipoproteins (HDL). (Remember that HDL appear to protect against heart attacks.) A relatively high level of physical activity is required to maintain an elevated concentration of HDL. Unfortunately, once the individual discontinues the exercise program, the HDL level tends to return to its original value. Long-distance runners are defined as running up to 70 kilometers (or about 43.4 miles) a week— the equivalent of running approximately 10 kilometers (or about 6.2 miles) daily for an hour. HDL levels are generally high in long-distance runners and cross-country skiers. Concentrations are higher in long-distance runners than in sprinters, and higher in sprinters than in physically inactive individuals.

Exercise should be tailored to your enjoyment and interests. A high level of exercise may be designed to achieve a given level of work at a low pulse rate. This is often referred to as the "aerobic effect." Simply achieving this goal provides enjoyment for some persons. Exercises may include stretching, jogging, swimming, tennis, jumping rope, and cycling. A very important aspect of exercise is to stretch and warm up before actually exercising and then cool down after vigorous exercise. "Pulling" or actual tearing of a muscle or tendon may result if there is not adequate warm up.

The exercise tolerance can certainly be increased in many people with coronary artery disease and angina pectoris. The effect of exercise can be measured by an exercise electrocardiogram. The individual session can range from a few minutes to 20 to 30 minutes daily and can be repeated three to five times per week, depending on your condition.

If you are unaccustomed to exercise, we cannot emphasize too strongly the importance of precautions. Have a complete physical evaluation that includes an exercise electrocardiogram as well as the approval and advice of your personal physician prior to undertaking a new program of physical activity. A few people die each year from heart irregularities during exercise, and although the risk is relatively small, you and your physician should be aware of it.

Diabetes

Diabetes mellitus, characterized by an elevated blood sugar, is a leading cause of death in the United States. Diabetes is usually defined in terms of a deficiency or inappropriate secretion of insulin by the pancreas in response to a particular amount of sugar. The body's organs, especially the brain, must burn sugar for their maintenance, and insulin is vital to the cells being able to take up the sugar.

The pancreas of the diabetic does not produce enough insulin, and so the blood sugar level is too high. This low insulin secretion alters the metabolism of carbohydrate, protein, and fat. In some diabetics the fat cells of the body are insensitive to insulin. Because of the deficient pancreas and/or the insensitive fat cells, carbohydrates and sugar are underutilized. Instead, protein and fat are broken down from the body's tissues. A similar phenomenon occurs during starvation or in persons on an extremely low carbohydrate diet.

Diabetes may be divided into two categories: Type I, which often begins in childhood and which requires insulin therapy, and Type II, which affects adults and does not require insulin. The most common type of diabetes is Type II, sometimes called maturity-onset, or non-insulin-dependent diabetes; this comprises about 90% of all diabetes. Usually Type II diabetes begins after age 40 or 50. A combination of diet (particularly weight control) and exercise can usually control this type of diabetes. Type I or insulin-dependent diabetes, on the other hand, cannot be controlled by diet and exercise alone.

There is a high percentage of deaths among diabetics due to the complications of the disease over the years. The most serious damage is to the blood vessels—the large arteries, small arteries, and capillaries. The kidneys and eyes are also frequently affected due to disease of the capillaries. Diabetes has been a leading cause of blindness. The nervous system is also affected by diabetes.

There are two main types of complication. One is the usual form of atherosclerosis, which leads to coronary artery disease and obstruction of the other "large" arteries. The atherosclerotic plaque in the diabetic is similar to that in nondiabetics but occurs at an earlier age. We believe that atherosclerotic complications in the diabetic can be reduced by close attention to risk factors and by controlling blood cholesterol, blood pressure, and weight.

A second type of diabetic complication involves the small blood vessels, mainly the capillaries. When these are affected there is damage to the retina, kidney, and probably the nerves. Atherosclerotic and small-vessel disease may interfere with blood circulation in the lower extremities and lead to gangrene. Small-vessel disease is probably not related to the same risk factors which predispose to the atherosclerotic disease of large arteries.

There are three cornerstones to the treatment of diabetes: insulin (if there is a deficiency), diet, and exercise. It has not been established unequivocally that tight control of the blood sugar reduces the damage to blood vessels but opinion is shifting in this direction. We believe that controlling the blood sugar might be more crucial to preventing damage to the small blood vessels than to the large ones, but this is just educated speculation.

Whichever form of diabetes is present, diet plays a central role in its management. For the Type II (non-insulin-dependent) diabetic, obesity is an important risk factor and must be controlled through diet and exercise. More than 80% of these diabetics are overweight. Exercise is especially important in controlling diabetes because the receptors on fat cells become more sensitized to insulin if the individual exercises regularly and is not overweight.

New Discoveries in Diabetes Research

Important advances in diabetes research may provide new methods of treatment, prevention, and eventually a cure of this disease. One of the most exciting developments has been the discovery of the interplay of genetics and viral infection in juvenile diabetes. Individuals with a certain type of genetic susceptibility may develop diabetes following viral infections.

Inheritance plays a role in both Type II (non-insulin-dependent) and Type I (insulin-dependent) forms of diabetes, although the pattern of inheritance differs. Very interesting studies have been carried out in identical twins in which one of the two had diabetes. In about 80% of Type II (non-insulin-dependent) diabetes, the second twin also develops diabetes, whereas in Type I (insulin-dependent), only about 50% of the second twins develop diabetes. In the Type I diabetic who has inherited specific genetic susceptibility, certain viruses may cause an inflammation of the insulin-producing cells in the pancreas, resulting in damage to those cells. Or the virus may induce immunological obstruction to the insulin-producing cells by causing the formation of antibodies to these cells.

Recently a virus was isolated from the pancreas of a young Type I diabetic who died suddenly. When injected into animals, this virus produced diabetes. These findings have significant implications concerning the origin of diabetes and suggest the necessity of developing a test to detect genetic susceptibility to diabetes in children. We need to find ways to protect these children against potentially dangerous viral infections.

Other important areas of progress in treating diabetes are transplantation of pancreatic insulin-producing cells and the use of artificial devices that will release insulin the same way the normal pancreas does.

At the present time, even with multiple daily injections of insulin, it is virtually impossible to control the blood sugar as closely as the normal body does. Insulin pumps for automatically administering insulin have been developed which permit a careful regulation of the blood-sugar level. Now that we are in a position to regulate the blood sugar and maintain it within a normal range, it should be possible to determine if such control will protect against the complications of diabetes involving the eye, kidney, nerves, heart, and cardiovascular system.

In another area of experimentation, pancreatic islet cells and whole pancreas have been successfully transplanted in diabetic animals. However, as with transplantation of other organs, the major problem is rejection because the transplanted organ is recognized as foreign protein. The usefulness of pancreatic cell transplantation may be studied in humans in the near future, although there is not a great deal of this tissue available for experimentation.

Stress and Behavior Patterns

Two major behavior patterns have been described by Friedman and Rosenman: Type A and Type B (Table 3). The Type A individual is hard-driving, very time-conscious, and extremely conscientious; he seldom takes off an afternoon or has a vacation. He probably has similar reactions in whatever environment he is placed, although the reactions may be magnified by stress.

TABLE 3.   *Type A and Type B behavior patterns*

Type A

Explosively accentuates important words in ordinary conversation even when unnecessary. Tends to utter the last few words of sentences far more rapidly than the opening words.

Moves, walks, and eats rapidly.

Feels impatient with the rate at which most events take place. For example, hurries the speech of others by saying "Yes, yes, yes" while someone talks or attempts to finish a sentence for them.

Indulges in polyphasic thought or performance, frequently striving to think of or do two or more things simultaneously.

Finds it difficult to refrain from talking about or bringing any conversation around to subjects which especially interest him; when unable to do this, pretends to listen while occupied with his own thoughts.

Almost always feels vaguely guilty when relaxing and doing absolutely nothing for several hours to several days.

No longer observes the more important or interesting or lovely objects that are encountered in his environment.

Does not have any time to spare to *become* the things worth being because he is preoccupied with getting the things worth *having.*

Attempts to schedule more and more in less and less time, thus making fewer allowances for unforeseen contingencies.

On meeting another severely afflicted Type A person, instead of feeling compassion for his affliction, finds himself compelled to "challenge" him.

Resorts to certain characteristic gestures or nervous tics.

Believes that whatever success he has enjoyed has been due in good part to his ability to get things done faster than his fellow men and is afraid to stop doing everything faster and faster.

Finds himself increasingly committed to translating and evaluating not only his own but also the activities of others in terms of "numbers."

Type B

Completely free of all the habits and exhibits none of the traits listed that harass the severely afflicted Type A person.

Never suffers from a sense of time urgency with its accompanying impatience.

Harbors no free-floating hostility, and feels no need to display or discuss his achievements or accomplishments unless such exposure is demanded by the situation.

When he plays, does so to find fun and relaxation, not to exhibit superiority at any cost.

Can relax without guilt, just as he can work without agitation.

Adapted from Friedman and Rosenman, 1974: *Type A Behavior and Your Heart.* A. A. Knopf, New York.

The Type B person, on the other hand, tends to be more low key and is less driven by time and deadlines.

"Stress" refers to the environment itself and a response of physical and/or mental tension to a stimulus from the environment. What is stress for one person may not be for another. People respond to stress by an increase in blood pressure and heart rate and a number of metabolic effects, including release of the hormones epinephrine (adrenaline) and norepinephrine (noradrenaline) and a rise in blood sugar. Because of the stress, the individual may stop eating or, as frequently happens, compensate by eating too much.

Altering Type A behavior, like other habit patterns, is difficult. Our society, with its emphasis on competitiveness, ambition, and achievement, encourages such behavior. Stress itself plays a major role in the lives of Type A people. The Type A individual constantly feels the pressure of meeting deadlines, is overcommitted to his work, or is driving himself very hard to be successful.

Reducing stress and altering Type A characteristics might be expected to reduce the risk of coronary heart disease. A major factor involves finding some method for relaxing. Sometimes the indirect approach (e.g., aerobic exercises, listening to music, or reading a good book) works, whereas in others, the more direct approach (e.g., physical massage, muscle tensing and relaxing exercises, or relaxation imagery; see Chapter 5 for details) is more helpful for reducing tenseness. The individual should use whichever methods work for him.

It is also important to identify environmental situations which tend to elicit stress. The individual might check himself periodically during the day for signs of stress, e.g., the feeling of "being under pressure" or a tightening of the neck or stomach muscles. Then if the signs are noted, he might try to discover what is causing the reaction. Daily records, similar to the food record discussed in Chapter 5, in which potential stressors are written down, are valuable for determining if there are any regular patterns to those feelings of stress.

Once the causes of the stress are identified, they can often be dealt with. For example, a relaxation technique may be helpful, or it may be possible to prevent the stressor from occurring in the first place by identifying the source of the problem and dealing with it directly.

In any case, the techniques to reduce stress should be implemented slowly and cautiously. Type A individuals in particular tend to feel challenged and may try to master their anti-stress techniques in a hurry. With practice, most people can learn to get control of themselves rather than allow themselves to be controlled by their environment. When they do indeed learn the control, their cardiovascular risk may also lessen because dangerous bodily reactions to the environment are avoided.

2

The Living Heart Diet

The Living Heart Diet provides a basis for developing new attitudes toward our daily eating patterns, attitudes that encourage general good health as well as a healthy heart. The Low-Calorie Diet (pages 30 to 31), which can be followed by diabetics as well as overweight individuals, and The Low-Sodium Diet (pages 52 to 56) are each modifications of the basic Living Heart Diet. All of these diets were designed to accomplish the following objectives:

1. Reduce the amount of fat consumed, especially saturated fat.
2. Substitute polyunsaturated fat for saturated fat in food preparation.
3. Decrease the amount of dietary cholesterol consumed.
4. Achieve and maintain ideal body weight.

One desired effect of The Living Heart Diet is to lower cholesterol and triglycerides in the blood. This is particularly desirable in those who have high levels of these two fats and who are at increased risk for developing atherosclerosis and coronary heart disease. The diet reduces the total number of calories derived from fat intake and balances the amount of polyunsaturated and saturated fat; this in turn lowers the cholesterol. Even for persons with average levels of cholesterol, the diet may reduce the risk of heart attack because the risk is reduced as the cholesterol level decreases.

Achieving and maintaining ideal body weight is a significant objective of this diet because obesity is a secondary risk factor for atherosclerosis. Among those who have tried numerous weight-reducing diets with varying degrees of success, many will agree that most diets, especially the so-called fad diets, are difficult to follow for any length of time. Weight may be lost initially, but when one finally gives up the diet out of frustration or boredom and reverts back to the previous diet, the weight is rapidly regained.

The Living Heart Diet is easy to follow because it is not drastically different from the average diet. A wide variety of well-balanced, nutritious, and desirable foods are allowed, with selections from all of the food groups: meat, fish, poultry, dairy products, fruits, vegetables, fats, bread, and cereal products. The diet is based on practical information about meal planning, shopping, food preparation, eating away from home, entertaining, and traveling. It is "portable" and can be used wherever you eat. Favorite recipes can be easily adapted, and special foods are not required. This diet can be incorporated into any lifestyle and, in fact, could easily become a way of life for people of all ages, especially children.

It is easier and more prudent to begin healthful dietary habits as a child than to change eating habits as an adult. For teenagers and adults who have tried dieting without success, a chapter is included on behavioral techniques (Chapter 5) which have proved highly successful.

The roles of dietary sodium and salt in hypertension, and of sugar in diabetes, are important considerations in The Living Heart Diet. Because hypertension (high blood pressure) is a major risk factor for atherosclerosis and coronary heart disease, special attention must be given to the salt- or sodium-restricted diet. Reducing sodium in the diet and losing weight (by the obese) will help lower blood pressure and may reduce the amount of medication necessary to control it. The Low-Sodium Diet is discussed in Chapter 3.

Diabetics require weight control, regular nutritious meals, and restriction of simple sugars and concentrated sweets, e.g., sugar, jelly, honey, and syrup. For this reason, diabetics will find the exchange list system used in the The Living Heart Diet a convenient method for controlling carbohydrate and total calorie intake. Diabetes is one of the most important risk factors for cardiovascular disease, and its control is essential. The Low-Calorie Living Heart Diet is the diet we recommend for diabetics: Concentrated sweets are eliminated, provisions are made for maintaining ideal body weight or for losing weight, and food exchanges are used to control the amount of carbohydrate, protein, fat, and calories eaten daily. A diabetic diet exchange system similar to the one prepared by the American Diabetes Association Inc. and The American Dietetic Association (1976) is used in The Low-Calorie Diet. The foods are all low in cholesterol and saturated fat.

The Living Heart Diet can be adjusted to various calorie levels. For simplicity, two calorie levels are utilized here: The Living Heart Diet and The Low-Calorie Living Heart Diet. The Living Heart Diet is for those who wish to maintain their present body weight while lowering their cholesterol level. The Low-Calorie Diet allows overweight persons to reduce to their ideal body weight. Table 1 in the *Appendix* can be

used for determining that weight. Individuals who need to lower their triglyceride levels should follow The Low-Calorie Diet, as triglyceride levels are often very sensitive to body weight, simple carbohydrates, and alcoholic beverages. If weight is not a problem but triglycerides are elevated, The Low-Calorie Diet should still be followed and the total calories adjusted to maintain weight.

The Living Heart Diet and The Low-Calorie Diet contain:

No more than 300 milligrams cholesterol
50% of the calories as carbohydrate
20% of the calories as protein
30% of the calories as fat with:
  Less than 10% of the fat calories from saturated fat
  Up to 10% of the fat calories from polyunsaturated fat
  The remaining fat from monounsaturated fat sources

The Living Heart Diet is discussed in detail according to food groups. A Low-Calorie Diet section follows each food group discussion, giving additional information about lowering weight and/or triglycerides.

Food groups in The Living Heart Diet are:

  Fats
  Meat, fish, and poultry
  Eggs
  Dairy products
  Dairy substitutes
  Bread and cereal products
  Vegetables
  Fruits
  Free/low-calorie foods

Food Guides on pages 317 to 335 list specific foods and quantities allowed in The Living Heart Diets. All the foods recommended are low in cholesterol and saturated fat. Foods are categorized as "Yes" or "No," and the quantity allowed in The Low-Calorie Diet is specified.

THE LOW-CALORIE LIVING HEART DIET

Weight reduction plans must be individualized and should produce a loss of 1 to 2 pounds a week. A pound of body fat is equivalent to 3,500 calories. Therefore, in order to lose 2 pounds per week, daily calorie intake must be reduced by 1,000 calories (1,000 calories × 7 days = 7,000 calories = 2 pounds per week). To most accurately determine your present daily calorie intake, keep a food record for 1 week, use a food composition table to tally the calories, and then average the daily calorie intake at the end of the week. Although calories must be restricted for weight loss, it is not necessary to count them. By using the food-exchange lists (described below) in The Low-Calorie Diet and eating the recommended number of servings from each food group, calorie control becomes easy.

Weight reduction is usually quite rapid at first due to fluid losses but quickly slows to a more gradual rate as body fat is utilized for energy. Exercise moderately increases calorie expenditure and is a valuable adjunct to any weight loss program, but reduced calorie intake is necessary as well. The key to losing weight is staying "full" on the *right kinds* of food. It is a good idea to fill up on "free" vegetables and other low-calorie foods.

Food-Exchange Lists

The Low-Calorie Diet uses food-exchange lists. The Food Guides on pages 317 to 335 categorize each food into a "Yes" or "No" column, and the amount allowed in The Low-Calorie Diet is specified. Food exchanges are used to specify the serving size of foods included in each of the food groups; the exchange simply indicates how large each serving may be. For example:

Bread and cereal products:
1 bread exchange = 1 slice bread *or*
             = ½ cup cooked cereal *or*
             = ½ cup cooked macaroni *or*
             = ⅓ cup corn *or*
             = ¼ cup sherbet

Meat group:
1 meat exchange = 1 ounce (30 grams) lean cooked meat *or*
             = ¼ cup flaked, cubed, or chopped meat

Dairy products:
1 dairy exchange = 1 cup skim milk *or*
             = ⅓ cup nonfat dry milk powder *or*
             = 1 cup reconstituted milk *or*
             = 1 cup buttermilk (made with skim milk) *or*
             = ½ cup canned evaporated skim milk (undiluted)

The exchanges are sometimes combined in one food, for example:
1 cup low-fat milk (1½ to 2% butterfat)
     = 1 dairy exchange + 1 fat exchange
½ cup creamed cottage cheese
     = 1 dairy exchange + 1 fat exchange

Some foods do not resemble the exchange which represents them. The calories from carbohydrates, protein, and fat are similar, for example:

1½ ounces of allowed coffee lightener
     = 1 bread exchange
5 ounces beer = 1 bread exchange
1 cup tomato sauce = 1 bread exchange
⅛ of a 4-inch avocado = 1 fat exchange
2 teaspoons peanut butter = 1 fat exchange

Some foods can be counted in either of two completely different food groups, depending on which works out best for the individual.

Counting foods in different food groups:

⅓ cup low-fat (2% butterfat) cottage cheese = 1 meat exchange *or* 1 dairy exchange

½ cup dried peas or beans = 1 meat exchange *or* 1 bread exchange

The exchanges can be used to estimate calorie intake. They represent the average calorie level for a group of similar foods. The calories of each food within a group vary according to the type of food.

Calorie content of one food exchange:

1 meat exchange (1 ounce)	= 59 calories
1 egg exchange	= 79 calories
1 dairy exchange	= 80 calories
1 bread exchange	= 68 calories
1 fruit exchange	= 40 calories
1 vegetable exchange	= 25 calories
1 fat exchange	= 45 calories

Some foods are very low in calories and *do not* need to be counted as an exchange, e.g., consommé, diet (sugar-free) carbonated beverages,[1] unflavored (unsweetened) gelatin, mustard, soy sauce, sugar substitutes, spices, and seasonings.

Table 1 shows how many exchanges are allowed from each food group for various calorie levels.

Food exchanges are given with each recipe in this book (except those very high in calories due to high sugar and/or fat content). For example, 1 serving of the recipe for Fish Fillets in Tomato Sauce on page 103 is equal to 4 food exchanges; however, these 4 exchanges are from three different exchange groups: 1 serving = 2½ meat exchanges, ½ bread exchange, and 1 vegetable exchange.

FAT IN THE LIVING HEART DIET

Fat is essential to the body for the transport of fat-soluble vitamins, and it supplies a concentrated source of calories. Fat makes food more palatable and gives the feeling of satisfaction after a meal. In addition, the amount and type of fat consumed affect the cholesterol level in the blood. For these reasons, fat deserves considerable attention when planning diets or when modifying eating habits.

The average American consumes about 40% of calories as fat; about 15% is saturated fat, 7% is polyunsaturated fat, and the remaining 18% is monounsaturated fat. The Living Heart Diet recommends that 30% of total calories come from fat, with less than 10% being saturated, up to 10% polyunsaturated, and the remainder monounsaturated.

Fat, although not readily visible, is present in most prepared, processed, and fried foods. In baked goods it may constitute almost 50% of the calories, in luncheon meat and sausage approximately 75% of the calories, and in fried foods 40 to 60% of the calories. For example:

Processed food	Total calories	% Calories from fat
1 piece frozen devil's food cake with chocolate icing	323	42
1 doughnut, yeast type	176	58
1 ounce salami	88	75
1 ounce bologna	74	71
1 piece custard pie	249	46

The amount and type of fat an individual eats plays an important role in reducing the risk of heart disease:

---

[1]Subject to current warning about saccharin.

TABLE 1. *Daily food plans for six calorie levels*

Amount	Food Group	Amount	Food Group
1,200-Calorie daily plan		**2,000-Calorie daily plan**	
6 Ounces	Meat, poultry, and seafood	6 Ounces	Meat, poultry, and seafood
2 Per week	Egg yolks	2 Per week	Egg yolks
2 Exchanges	Low-fat dairy products	2 Exchanges	Low-fat dairy products
3 Exchanges	Grains and starchy vegetables	12 Exchanges	Grains and starchy vegetables
As desired	Nonstarchy vegetables	As desired	Nonstarchy vegetables
5 Exchanges	Oils, margarines, and other fats	10 Exchanges	Oils, margarines, and other fats
3 Exchanges	Fruits	3 Exchanges	Fruits
1 Exchange	Extras (alcoholic beverages, sweets)	1 Exchange	Extras (alcoholic beverages, sweets)

Protein	= 24% of total calories	Protein	= 18% of total calories
Fat	= 29% of total calories	Fat	= 28% of total calories
Carbohydrate	= 47% of total calories	Carbohydrate	= 54% of total calories
P/S ratio	= 1.1	P/S ratio	= 1.5

Amount	Food Group	Amount	Food Group
1,500-Calorie daily plan		**2,200-Calorie daily plan**	
6 Ounces	Meat, poultry, and seafood	6 Ounces	Meat, poultry, and seafood
2 Per week	Egg yolks	2 Per week	Egg yolks
2 Exchanges	Low-fat dairy products	2 Exchanges	Low-fat dairy products
6 Exchanges	Grains and starchy vegetables	12 Exchanges	Grains and starchy vegetables
As desired	Nonstarchy vegetables	As desired	Nonstarchy vegetables
7 Exchanges	Oils, margarines, and other fats	12 Exchanges	Oils, margarines, and other fats
3 Exchanges	Fruits	4 Exchanges	Fruits
1 Exchange	Extras (alcoholic beverages, sweets)	1 Exchange	Extras (alcoholic beverages, sweets)

Protein	= 21% of total calories	Protein	= 19% of total calories
Fat	= 29% of total calories	Fat	= 29% of total calories
Carbohydrate	= 50% of total calories	Carbohydrate	= 52% of total calories
P/S ratio	= 1.3	P/S ratio	= 1.6

Amount	Food Group	Amount	Food Group
1,800-Calorie daily plan		**2,500-Calorie daily plan**	
6 Ounces	Meat, poultry, and seafood	6 Ounces	Meat, poultry, and seafood
2 Per week	Egg yolks	2 Per week	Egg yolks
2 Exchanges	Low-fat dairy products	2 Exchanges	Low-fat dairy products
9 Exchanges	Grains and starchy vegetables	15 Exchanges	Grains and starchy vegetables
As desired	Nonstarchy vegetables	As desired	Nonstarchy vegetables
9 Exchanges	Oils, margarines, and other fats	14 Exchanges	Oils, margarines and other fats
3 Exchanges	Fruits	4 Exchanges	Fruits
1 Exchange	Extras (alcoholic beverages, sweets)	1 Exchange	Extras (alcoholic beverages, sweets)

Protein	= 19% of total calories	Protein	= 17% of total calories
Fat	= 29% of total calories	Fat	= 29% of total calories
Carbohydrate	= 52% of total calories	Carbohydrate	= 54% of total calories
P/S ratio	= 1.4	P/S ratio	= 1.7

1. Excessive amounts of saturated fat in the diet tend to *increase* the level of cholesterol.

2. Polyunsaturated fat helps *reduce* cholesterol but has the same calorie content as saturated fat.

3. Monounsaturated fat has been thought to have had a neutral effect on cholesterol, neither raising nor lowering it. Recent evidence suggests that it may lower cholesterol, however. Monounsaturated fat has the same calorie count as saturated fat.

Fats and oils are a combination of glycerol (an alcohol) linked to three fatty acids. These compounds are classified according to their chemical structure. It is not necessary to understand the details of these structures. Suffice it to say that some fatty acids contain double bonds and are called "unsaturated," while others do not contain double bonds and are called "saturated." The unsaturated fatty acids are further subclassified as being monounsaturated and polyunsaturated. The latter two are found primarily in vegetable fats and fish oils. Examples of saturated, monounsaturated, and polyunsaturated fatty acids are shown in Fig. 1.

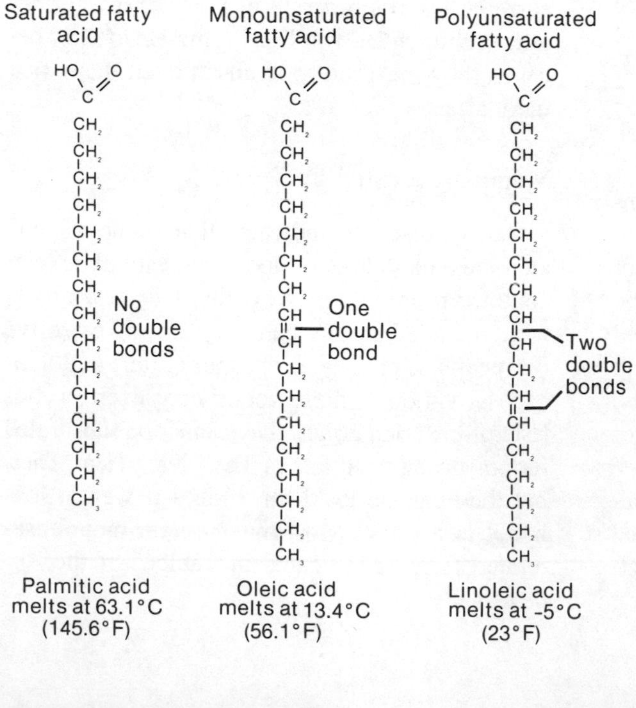

Saturated Fats

Saturated fats occur naturally in all foods of animal origin and in a few vegetable products. They are solid at room temperature. Table 2 in the *Appendix* shows the total fat content of some common foods and the amount of fat which is saturated, polyunsaturated, and monounsaturated. In butter, beef, cream, and whole milk, the majority of the fat is saturated, although a large amount of oleic acid, a monounsaturated fat, is present. Meats containing 10% or less total fat and dairy products with no more than 2% butterfat are considered low-fat foods and are allowed in The Living Heart Diet.

The few vegetable fats which are sources of saturated fat include coconut, palm, and palm kernel oil. The saturated fatty acids of these vegetable products and oils are uniquely stable. That is, they do not easily break down or become rancid. As a result, foods containing these oils have a longer shelf life than products prepared with other vegetable oils, e.g., corn, cottonseed, or soybean oil.

Cocoa butter is another saturated fat of veg-

FIG. 1. Saturated, polyunsaturated and monounsaturated fats differ only in the number of double bonds that occur in their fatty acid chain. Saturated fats have no double bonds; all the bonds are saturated, hence the name. Monounsaturated fats have one double bond in the fatty acid chain and polyunsaturated fats have more than one double bond. Polyunsaturated fats melt at low temperatures; for example, polyunsaturated corn oil and safflower oil are liquid at room temperature. In comparison, saturated bacon fat does not melt until very high temperatures are reached. C = Carbon; H = hydrogen; O = oxygen.

Saturated fatty acid — Palmitic acid melts at 63.1°C (145.6°F) — No double bonds

Monounsaturated fatty acid — Oleic acid melts at 13.4°C (56.1°F) — One double bond

Polyunsaturated fatty acid — Linoleic acid melts at −5°C (23°F) — Two double bonds

etable origin. Most of the fat in the form of cocoa butter is removed in making cocoa powder, so that the powder is low in fat and acceptable in moderate amounts on The Living Heart Diet.

Liquid vegetable oils can be converted to solid, saturated fats by the process called *hydrogenation*. This procedure hardens the fat, enhances its stability, and prolongs its shelf life. These hydrogenated, or partially hardened fats, are used commercially and in the home. The most common example is solid vegetable shortening, which should be avoided in The Living Heart Diet. However, small amounts of partially hydrogenated fat (e.g., those used in tub margarine to give it a solid consistency at room temperature) are acceptable in The Living Heart Diet.

Polyunsaturated Fats

Polyunsaturated fats are liquid at room temperature. They are predominantly vegetable in origin, although the fat from fish is also polyunsaturated. These oils, particularly safflower, sunflower, corn, soybean, and cottonseed oils, produce a cholesterol-lowering effect in the blood when included in the daily eating plan.

P/S Ratio

Vegetable oils differ in their degree of polyunsaturation. These variations are expressed as a ratio of polyunsaturated fat to saturated fat (P/S ratio). To determine this ratio the total polyunsaturated fat content is divided by the sum of the saturated fat content; monounsaturated fat is not included when determining the P/S ratio. The higher the P/S ratio, the more polyunsaturated the fat and the greater the cholesterol-lowering effect. The P/S ratios in commonly used oils, nuts, and animal fats are shown in Table 3 of the *Appendix*.

Some studies suggest that the long-term consumption of large amounts of polyunsaturated fat may present a potential risk for the development of cancer. However, this risk has not been substantiated in most studies. A high P/S ratio diet is achieved through the use of large amounts of highly polyunsaturated fat and is recommended only for the treatment of severe elevations of cholesterol. It is a therapeutic measure and therefore not recommended for general use. We suggest the use of polyunsaturated fat for food preparation and do not consider the amounts recommended in The Living Heart Diet to be excessive. As mentioned previously, the total fat content of The Living Heart Diet is only 30% of total calories.

Margarine

Margarines vary considerably in their degree of unsaturation. The manufacturer is required to list the ingredients on the label in the order of their preponderance. The Living Heart Diet recommends those which list liquid safflower oil, liquid corn oil, or liquid sunflower oil as the first ingredient on the label. The phrase "partially hydrogenated" or "partially hardened" oil may also appear among the ingredients but should not be listed first. A certain amount of hydrogenation is necessary to produce margarines which spread easily at room temperature. Soft tub margarines are recommended for The Living Heart Diet because they are more polyunsaturated than stick margarines.

Monounsaturated Fats

Recent research indicates that monounsaturated fats may lower blood cholesterol levels, contrary to an earlier view that they had no effect. Included in this category are olives, olive oil, peanuts, peanut oil, peanut butter, and avocados. Although these foods may exert a cholesterol-lowering effect, they cannot be substituted for polyunsaturated fats in The Living Heart Diet, but they can be used for variety if weight loss is not necessary. Most nuts contain monounsaturated fats, as indicated in Table 2 of the *Appendix*.

Fatty Acids

The fatty acid content of foods varies. In dairy products the fatty acid composition of milk is affected by the breed of the animal, what the animal eats, the stage of lactation, and the season. During the winter months, milk fat tends to be a little more saturated than during the summer months. The fatty acids in beef are affected by the age, sex, and diet of the animal. The fat content of beef tends to increase with age. The method of cooking beef—dry or moist heat—does not seem to affect the fatty acid composition, although frying does have some effect because of the fat added during preparation.

The diet of the pig apparently has a greater effect on the composition of pork products than the cow's diet has on beef products; for example, the pig's diet significantly affects the composition of the fatty acids in the meat. When unsaturated fat is fed to pigs, the result is an increase in the unsaturation of the meat. Pork typically has a higher percent of polyunsaturated fatty acids than beef if cuts with a comparable percentage of fat are compared; however, the total percentage of fat in pork is higher than that in a comparable grade of beef. Pork brains, heart, kidney, and liver have a higher percentage of polyunsaturated than saturated fatty acids when compared with the skeletal muscle or meat cuts of pork. This is offset, however, by the high cholesterol content of these organs; organ meat from pork as well as from beef should be avoided on The Living Heart Diet for this reason. Table 2 in the *Appendix* gives the amount of fat in pork products, as well as the distribution of fatty acids; this information is also given for beef, lamb, poultry, and fish.

The fat in eggs is found in the yolk. Large eggs contain more fatty acids per egg than small eggs, although small eggs contain more fat on a per-unit weight basis. One egg yolk weighing 17 grams contains about 5.5 grams of fat.

Fish provides a good source of protein and polyunsaturated fat. The fat in fish ranges from less than 1% to more than 20%. Examples of fish with less than 1% fat include Atlantic and Pacific cod, haddock, northern pike, lemon sole, and yellow fin tuna; this means that in 100 grams (about 3½ ounces) of fish there is less than 1 gram of fat. Bass, catfish, flounder, halibut, perch, and rainbow trout have less than 5% fat. Shellfish is very low in fat, ranging from less than 1% to about 3% fat, making it an excellent selection for low-calorie diets. The cholesterol content of fish and most shellfish is low (see Table 2 in the *Appendix*).

A recent study has indicated that persons who ate a diet rich in salmon for four weeks lowered their plasma cholesterol by 15% and triglyceride level by 38% even though they also ate 500 milligrams of cholesterol daily. Salmon contains ω-3 fatty acids, which appear to be anti-atherogenic (1).

The primary fatty acid in chicken and turkey is monounsaturated. Chicken and turkey are low in fat, especially when the skin is removed, and white meat contains less fat than dark meat.

In nuts, a monounsaturated acid is the primary source of fatty acid. The fat content for common nuts varies between 50 and 72%. Peanuts, although actually a legume, have about 50% fat and pecans about 70%. Walnuts have the highest polyunsaturated fat content, and black walnuts have a higher count than English walnuts.

Cereal products contain primarily a polyunsaturated fatty acid. The primary saturated fatty acid makes up only about 25% of the total fat in most grain products, and a monounsaturated acid makes up the remainder; however, the total is low.

Fat in the form of oil has increased in the American diet during the last 10 to 15 years because of availability. Fat (saturated and unsaturated) is widely used in many processed foods, e.g., salad dressings, sauces, cookies, candies, cheeses (special varieties), frozen desserts, cereals, meat products, meat substitutes, puddings, soups, and frozen vegetables with sauces. It is also used in the preparation of many home recipes, e.g., those in the recipe section beginning on page 77. Product labels are helpful for determining if the oil in the product is polyunsaturated. The most polyunsaturated oils are safflower oil, corn oil, soybean oil, cottonseed oil, and sunflower seed oil. Coconut oil contains almost 90% saturated fatty acids and is used in many baked goods. "Filled milk," which resembles milk, is a product made by removing the dairy fat from milk and replacing it with fat or oil from other sources. The fatty acids vary according to the type of fat added to these products. If coconut oil or palm kernel oil is added, it becomes quite saturated, whereas the addition of soybean oil or corn oil makes it a polyunsaturated product. Some varieties of canned milk are actually filled milk; the label will indicate if the product is filled milk and which type of oil has been added.

Fats in Common Foods

It is often difficult to detect the amount of fat in certain foods, especially when eating away from home. Even though these fats may not be visible, they add extra calories. For example, for each ounce of meat that is breaded and fried, 1 teaspoon (4 grams) of fat should be counted. In every 10 French fries there is approximately 1 teaspoon of fat. A typical white sauce has 1 teaspoon of fat in every 2 tablespoons of sauce. These equivalents apply to saturated and polyunsaturated fat. The guidelines given on pages 329–330 will help you count these hidden fats.

FATS IN THE LOW-CALORIE DIET

The Low-Calorie Diet limits the amount of saturated fat eaten daily and encourages the use of polyunsaturated fat. It is important to bear in mind, however, that polyunsaturated fats are not low in calories. Because all fats provide a concentrated source of calories—9 calories per gram—they must be used sparingly. Carbohydrate and protein each provide only about 4 calories per gram. To obtain the greatest cholesterol-lowering effect with the lowest fat intake, a small amount of polyunsaturated fat should be used when fat is needed in food preparation.

Saturated Fats

Foods rich in saturated fat (e.g., sour cream, whipping cream, and meat fat) are also high in calories and should be avoided. Even lean meats and low-fat dairy products contain some saturated fat and must be carefully controlled.

Polyunsaturated Fats

When it is necessary to use fat for food preparation in this book, safflower oil is recommended because it is more polyunsaturated than the other oils. However, all liquid oils have about the same number of calories; there is no low-calorie oil. Oils marketed in spray form, however, contain negligible calories and are useful for fat-free cooking.

The Low-Calorie Diet utilizes the same soft tub margarines as are used in The Living Heart Diet. Diet margarines generally have a lower P/S ratio than soft tub margarines, and water is usually listed as the first ingredient; a partially hydrogenated or hardened fat is generally the second ingredient. The calorie content of diet margarine is less than that of regular margarine because water replaces part of the fat, and often more of the diet margarine must be used to achieve the same flavor.

Monounsaturated Fats

Although monounsaturated fats may exert the cholesterol-lowering effect that polyunsaturated fats do, it is preferable to limit their use until your ideal weight is achieved. Although they are allowed on The Low-Calorie Diet, they add calories with no cholesterol-lowering benefit.

CHOLESTEROL IN THE LIVING HEART DIET

Cholesterol occurs in all animal tissues and fluids, and is essential for certain bodily functions. The human body manufactures cholesterol daily. Foods of animal origin (e.g., meats, dairy products, lard, butter, and meat fats) also supply cholesterol to the body. Egg yolks and organ meats are the most concentrated sources of cholesterol in the American diet. Fruits, vegetables, and grain products do not contain cholesterol. The cholesterol content of some common foods is shown in Table 2 of the *Appendix*.

People often think that fatty cuts of meat have a higher cholesterol content than lean cuts. In truth, the cholesterol content of meat is associated primarily with the lean tissue, not the fat. For example, fatty untrimmed beef has 94 milligrams of cholesterol in 3½ ounces (100 grams), whereas the same amount of lean well-trimmed beef has 91 milligrams of cholesterol. Thus equal weights of fatty and lean cuts of meat contain about equal amounts of cholesterol. Trimming meats is recommended not because it reduces cholesterol content but because it substantially reduces the saturated fat and calorie content.

MEAT, FISH, AND POULTRY IN THE LIVING HEART DIET

Requirements for protein vary with age (Table 2). The average adult needs 0.8 grams of protein per kilogram of body weight daily; that is, a man weighing 70 kilograms (154 pounds) requires 56 grams. Forty-six grams of protein satisfies the requirement of a 58-kilogram (128-pound) woman and can be provided by 4 ounces of meat and two glasses of milk daily. The meat group is not the only protein source in most diets. Dairy products (important for their calcium content) and grains (containing iron and B vitamins) supply protein as well.

Foods in the meat group contain saturated fat

TABLE 2. *Recommended daily dietary allowances of protein*[a]

Group	Protein
Infants, 0–1 year	2.0–2.2 times body weight (in kg)
Children	
1–3 years	23 g
4–6 years	30 g
7–10 years	34 g
Males	
11–14 years	45 g
15 years and older	56 g
Females	
11–18 years	46 g
19 years and older	44 g
Pregnant women	30 g (in addition to above value)
Nursing women	20 g (in addition to above value)

[a]Adapted from *Recommended Dietary Allowances*, Ninth Revised Edition, 1980, National Academy of Sciences, Washington, D.C.

and cholesterol as well as protein. Therefore The Living Heart Diet recommends that no more than 6 ounces of meat be eaten daily. The meat allowance includes fish, poultry, shellfish, beef, pork, and lamb, as well as certain game meats discussed on page 38. Poultry, fish, and shellfish (except shrimp) are lower in saturated fat than beef, pork, and lamb, and therefore should be selected as the meat allowance more often. Because liver is particularly high in cholesterol, it is limited to a maximum of 3 ounces per month. Shellfish are low in cholesterol and fat, and can be eaten as desired. By restricting intake of liver and egg yolks and limiting meat consumption to 6 ounces daily, The Living Heart Diet reduces cholesterol intake to no more than 300 milligrams per day.

When selecting meat *always* choose lean cuts with a minimum amount of marbling (the fat running through the lean tissue). All visible fat should be trimmed before cooking. A detailed list of lean cuts is given in the "Yes" column of the Meat, Fish, and Poultry Guide on pages 317 to 320.

Fish and Shellfish

Because fish contains polyunsaturated fat as well as γ-unsaturated fat, it is an excellent choice on a low-cholesterol eating plan. Most fish contain much less fat, and consequently fewer calories, than beef, pork, or lamb. Fish provides a quick, versatile entrée that can be prepared in many ways besides frying. The Recipe Section contains suggestions for baking, broiling, and poaching fish. Shellfish are also low in fat and cholesterol (Table 2 of the *Appendix*).

Poultry

The Living Heart Diet recommends eating poultry often because it contains less saturated fat than beef, lamb, or pork. Before cooking chicken at home, remove the skin because fat is stored beneath it and penetrates the lean tissue when cooked. When eating chicken away from home, the skin can be removed after it is cooked. This helps reduce the fat content, particularly if the chicken has been fried. By removing the skin, any fat absorbed by the batter will also be removed, which also helps reduce calories.

Turkey is recommended in The Living Heart Diet as well. The skin need not be removed prior to cooking as the fat does not seem to penetrate the lean meat of this fowl.

Veal and Calf

"Veal" refers to milk-fed beef slaughtered between the ages of 3 weeks and 3 months. "Calf" describes animals alaughtered at 14 to 52 weeks. Because veal and calf are young animals, they contain less fat than older ones are are recommended in The Living Heart Diet.

Beef

Beef is classified by the United States Drug Administration (USDA) according to its fat content. The five grades are prime, choice, good, standard, and utility. "Prime" beef contains the greatest amount of fat and "choice" is second, followed by "good," "standard," and "utility." Most beef packaged for commercial sale in supermarkets is "choice," which is acceptable in The Living Heart Diet, although "good" meat is lower in fat and is an even better selection. In supermarkets where meat is prepackaged, the butcher may be consulted to determine meat grades. When purchasing ground beef, select round steak or chuck with no more than 10% fat. Regular hamburger may contain up to 30% fat and should be avoided. Butchers are usually willing to trim off the visible fat on round steak or chuck roast and grind the lean portion separately. When browning ground meat, drain all the fat before adding other ingredients. The leanest and most fatty cuts of beef are listed in the Meat, Fish, and Poultry Guide on page 317 (lean cuts are listed in the "Yes" column and fatty cuts in the "No" column).

Lamb

Lean cuts of lamb, listed in the Meat, Fish, and Poultry Guide on page 318, can add variety to The Living Heart Diet. As with beef, select the leanest cuts and trim off all visible fat before cooking.

Pork

Pork contains about 25 milligrams of cholesterol per ounce and has more monounsaturated than saturated or polyunsaturated fat. Only lean, well-trimmed cuts with little or no marbling should be selected on The Living Heart Diet.

Game

Venison, rabbit, dove, quail, and squirrel are allowed in The Living Heart Diet. Recent studies have shown that the wild varieties of duck and goose have lower fat content and are preferable to domesticated varieties.

Meat Preparation in The Living Heart Diet

Before cooking any cut of meat, no matter what the grade, *always* trim away any visible fat. There are several low-fat methods for preparing meat:

Broiling is an excellent method as it allows the fat which cooks out of the meat to drip away. Placing water in the bottom of the broiler pan makes clean-up a lot easier. When broiling, aluminum foil should not be used to cover the pan or rack, as this prevents fat from dripping down.

Charcoal broiling is another form of cooking which allows the fat to drip away from the meat. A polyunsaturated oil or margarine seasoned with garlic powder, pepper, and other spices may be used for basting.

Roasting is a dry-heat method. A rack is used so meat will not reabsorb fat that cooks out.

Braising is a combination of dry- and moist-heat cooking in which meat is cooked in a *covered* pan on a rack. A polyunsaturated oil can be used for browning the meat.

Stewing means that water or some other liquid is used for cooking. It is important to remove the fat from the broth before using it to prepare sauce or gravy.

Crockpot cooking is similar to stewing, and care should be taken to remove the fat from the broth.

Grilling is a type of frying, and a polyunsaturated fat should be used if fat is required.

Frying adds unnecessary fat and calories to meat, fish, and poultry and should not be done frequently. When frying or sautéing, a polyunsaturated fat should be used.

Stocks and Gravies

When preparing meat in a liquid, such as water or tomato juice, part of the meat fat cooks out into the stock or broth. This fat must be removed from the meat drippings or stock *before* making gravy or sauce. Any of the following methods may be used to this end:

1. Cool the broth in the refrigerator. When the fat hardens, remove it with a spoon.
2. Add ice cubes to solidify the fat. The ice will slightly dilute the broth.
3. Use a gravy skimmer.
4. Use a paper towel or lettuce leaf to absorb the fat.

Estimating Meat Portions

Meat servings should always be determined *after* cooking. Meat shrinks during cooking because moisture evaporates and some fat cooks out. Lean beef, chicken, and fish normally lose approximately 25% of their raw weight when cooked. Fatty ground meat (e.g., sausage) may lose up to 50% of its raw weight. The estimated serving size of some typical cooked meat portions is given on page 320 in the Meat, Fish, and Poultry Guide.

MEAT, FISH, AND POULTRY IN THE LOW-CALORIE DIET

The following tips should be helpful:

1. Limit meat, fish, and poultry consumption to no more than 6 ounces daily. Carefully weigh meat portions *after* they are cooked. Remove bone, skin, and fat before weighing.
2. Select fish, shellfish, and poultry more frequently than beef and pork because they are lower in calories. Three ounces of cooked lean beef (chuck) has 183 calories; 3 ounces of fish (tuna) has 108 calories; and the same amount of chicken (white meat) has 141 calories.
3. Veal, calf, light beef, and baby beef are lower in calories than beef which has been aged.

Meat Preparation in The Low-Calorie Diet

Visible fat should always be trimmed away prior to cooking beef or pork, and the skin on chicken should be removed. Very little if any fat should be used in preparation. The methods described on page 39 are applicable for persons needing to lose weight, although frying meat should be avoided.

MEATLESS MEALS IN THE LIVING HEART DIET

Use of Vegetable Protein

Protein sources can be classified as "complete" or "incomplete" depending on their amino acid content. Amino acids are the building blocks of proteins, the raw material from which our bodies manufacture the proteins we need every day. Of the approximately 20 amino acids which have been identified in mammals, the human body can manufacture all but nine. These nine must be supplied by the diet and are thus referred to as "essential." Animal proteins (eggs, milk, cheese, and meat) are complete proteins because they supply all of the "essential" amino acids. Most plant proteins (dry beans and peas, lentils, and nuts) lack one or more of the "essential" amino acids and are thus incomplete. However, by combining two or more plant proteins, the amino acids lacking in one source may be supplied by another, depending on the combination. The practice of combining incomplete protein sources to achieve complete protein is known as "complementing proteins." Some examples of these patterns are as follows.

Grain products plus legumes (beans, peas, lentils):
  Bean and rice casserole
  Wheat bread with baked beans
  Corn tortillas and beans
  Legume soup with bread

Grain products plus seeds (sesame and sunflower):
  Rice with sesame seeds

Seeds (sesame and sunflower) plus legumes:
  Sunflower seeds and peanuts
  Sesame seeds in bean soup

Or an incomplete protein can be combined with a complete protein.

Seeds (sesame and sunflower) plus milk products:
  Sesame seeds and milk

Grain products plus milk products:
  Pasta with milk and low-fat cheese
  Cereal with skim or low-fat milk
  Low-fat cheese sandwich

Soybeans supply complete protein. Raw soybeans contain an enzyme called "trypsin inhibitor," which interferes with normal protein digestion and absorption; cooking the beans destroys this enzyme's activity. Because soybeans are bland in flavor, they combine well with other foods. Used as a meat extender, they reduce costs without significantly decreasing protein content. Soybeans also absorb and hold more than their weight in moisture. As a result of this characteristic, they should be mixed only with foods low in saturated fat. If soy meal (textured vegetable protein) is added to fatty ground beef, for example, the fat will be absorbed by the soy meal and does not cook out of the product.

When used as the sole source of dietary protein in an Italian study, soy protein produced a dramatic lowering of the plasma cholesterol concentration. A large number of recipes were devised in this study to allow the use of soy protein. In animal experiments, it has been shown that vegetable protein in the diet lowers plasma cholesterol and retards the development of atherosclerosis. On the other hand, casein, the protein from milk, and many meat proteins will raise the plasma cholesterol and accelerate atherosclerosis. It is also well-established that human vegetarians have lower levels of plasma cholesterol and less coronary heart disease than do other groups of the population who eat meat. The mechanism by which soy and other vegetable proteins reduce serum cholesterol is not known. The Italian studies used a "textured" protein while North American studies used an "isolated" soy protein that yielded less impressive results. Some investigators have suggested that the ratio of two of the amino acids in the protein (that is, the ratio of lysine to arginine) determines the effect of the protein on the concentration of plasma cholesterol.

Vegetables and grains contain no cholesterol and are typically low in fat. By substituting vegetable proteins for animal proteins, cholesterol and fat intake may be decreased. Because vegetable products are primarily carbohydrate and protein, and contain very little fat, their caloric and saturated fat content is usually lower than that of meat, fish, and poultry. Animal foods, on the other hand, contain considerable fat and protein. Gram for gram, fats provide more than twice as many calories as protein or carbohydrate.

Figure 2 dramatically illustrates the difference in saturated fat content between 1¼ cups each of beans and rice and 4 ounces of T-bone steak. The amount of protein in each is virtually the same.

FIBER

Dietary fiber is the part of food which is resistant to human digestive enzymes. At least five different components make up dietary fiber—cellulose, hemicelluloses, lignin, pectin, and gums. Cellulose and hemicelluloses are polysaccharides from the cell wall of plants. Lignin is a structural binding agent. Pectin and gums are water soluble non-structural polysaccharides.

Cellulose and hemicelluloses, e.g., wheat bran, act on the large bowel by increasing stool size and decreasing the amount of time food remains in the intestinal tract. The gums and pectins have

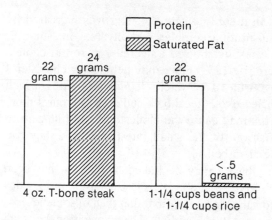

FIG. 2. The amount of protein in a portion of beans and rice is equivalent to that in a T-bone steak, however, there is a dramatic difference in the saturated fat content, which is much higher in the T-bone steak.

an effect on digestion and absorption in the stomach and small bowel. They hold water and delay the rate of emptying from the stomach.

Low-fiber diets have been associated with colon cancer, obesity, cardiovascular disease and diabetes. Fiber has been postulated to have a "protective" effect against atherosclerosis. This is based on evidence that Africans who often eat high-fiber diets do not have heart disease. Also vegetarians in this country who consume a high-fiber diet have lower cholesterol levels than Americans who eat less than 10 grams of fiber per day. There are undoubtedly other factors involved. High-fiber vegetarian diets are usually low in cholesterol and fat since they consist primarily of bread and cereal products, fruits and vegetables.

The effect of fiber on lipid metabolism is not clearly understood. It has been suggested that some types of fiber help lower cholesterol, but it is premature to rely on a high-fiber diet to lower cholesterol. Cellulose and bran have little or no effect on serum cholesterol. However, 6 to 36 grams of pectin help lower cholesterol by 9 to 15%. Pectin and gums inhibit cholesterol absorption by binding bile acids and bile salts, which are excreted in the feces, causing the liver to convert more cholesterol into bile salts.

In a study where the fiber was increased by substituting complex carbohydrate for sucrose, the results showed a decrease in serum cholesterol by 12%. Fiber may help lower cholesterol by virtue of its water retaining properties, which increase total fecal bulk and decrease transit time. This may cause the cholesterol and bile acid to rush out of the small intestine before they can be absorbed.

Obesity may be linked to fiber. It has been observed that obesity is less common in societies consuming a high-fiber diet than in societies eating a low-fiber diet. The connection between fiber and obesity may be due to the fact that low-fiber foods contain more calories than high-fiber foods. An increased amount of chewing is required for foods with high-fiber contents, which also slows down the rate of ingestion. Fiber-rich diets tend to be absorbed more slowly than fiber-poor diets, which make them more satisfying for a longer period of time.

The best way to increase fiber in the diet is to include good sources of fiber with each meal. These include whole grain breads and cereals, fruits and vegetables. Table 3 shows the dietary fiber content of some common foods. About 25 grams of dietary fiber per day are recommended.

When increasing the fiber content of the diet, it should be done gradually, since the side effect of increased fiber is flatulence. It usually subsides after a few weeks. Plenty of fluid should be consumed as fiber is increased.

EGGS IN THE LIVING HEART DIET

Egg yolk is the single most concentrated source of cholesterol in the average American diet. One yolk contains 274 milligrams of cholesterol. The yolk is also rich in the phospholipid lecithin. Adding one or more eggs to the diet does not have a great deal of influence on the total level of plasma cholesterol. Unless eggs are added to a diet in which the baseline contains no cholesterol, little change occurs in plasma cholesterol concentration. Consuming eggs in the diet may result in raising the concentration of a subfraction of HDL-cholesterol, the "good cholesterol," and perhaps also of LDL, the "bad cholesterol." It is not possible to determine at this time what these lipoprotein changes would mean in terms of risk of a heart attack. Eggs as well as any other food must be considered in terms of the overall diet, which must be balanced, nutritious, and appetizing. The Living Heart Diet recommends that egg yolks be limited to a maximum of two per week, including those used in cooking. Cholesterol-free egg substitutes can be used for cooking, as it is difficult to count yolks used in this manner. Egg whites contain no cholesterol and may be eaten freely. In many recipes, one whole egg may be replaced by two egg whites.

EGGS IN THE LOW-CALORIE DIET

Egg yolks (about 65 calories each) are limited to two per week in The Low-Calorie Diet. However, egg whites are low in calories (17 calories each) and cholesterol, and can be used freely without counting calories. Egg substitute can be used in The Low-Calorie Diet if the calories are accounted for, as shown in the Egg Guide ("Yes" column) on page 321. Some brands of egg substitute are lower in calories than others. This information is provided by the manufacturer in the nutrition labeling section on the container.

DAIRY PRODUCTS IN THE LIVING HEART DIET

Dairy products supply the richest sources of calcium, a nutrient that people of all ages require in varying amounts. The Living Heart Diet recommends the following amounts of low-fat milk to meet calcium requirements:

Adults	2 or more cups daily
Teenagers (15–18 years)	4 or more cups daily
Children (9–14 years)	3 or more cups daily
Children (under 9 years)	2 to 3 cups daily

TABLE 3. *Dietary fiber*[a]

	Unit	Dietary fiber (g)
Bread		
White bread	1 slice	0.76
Wholemeal bread	1 slice	2.38
Cereal		
All bran	½ cup	8.04
Cornflakes	½ cup	1.37
Puffed wheat	½ cup	1.15
Rice Krispies	½ cup	0.67
Shredded wheat	1 biscuit	3.06
Flour		
White flour	½ cup	1.97
Wholemeal flour	½ cup	5.73
Fruit		
Apple, 2½″ diam. (flesh only)	1 whole	1.63
Banana	½ whole	1.75
Cherries	½ cup	0.70
Peach	1 whole	2.62
Strawberries	½ cup	1.58
Nuts		
Brazil nuts	½ cup	5.44
Peanuts	½ cup	6.73
Vegetables		
Beans, baked (cooked)	½ cup	9.32
Beans, runner (cooked)	½ cup	2.18
Broccoli (cooked)	½ cup	3.15
Brussels sprouts (cooked)	½ cup	2.2
Cabbage (cooked)	½ cup	2.05
Carrots (cooked)	½ cup	2.85
Cauliflower (cooked)	½ cup	1.3
Corn (cooked)	½ cup	4.66
Lettuce (raw)	½ cup	0.42
Onion (raw)	½ cup	1.78
Peas (cooked)	½ cup	6.65
Potatoes (cooked)	½ cup	1.93

[a]Adapted from Southgate, D.A.T., Bailey, B., Collinson, E., and Walker, A.F. (1976): A guide to calculating intakes of dietary fiber. *J. Hum. Nutr.*, 30:303.

Pregnant women	3 or more cups daily
Nursing mothers	4 or more cups daily

The percentage of fat in milk varies according to the type, as shown below.

Fat Content of Milk

Type of Milk	Grams of fat per 1 cup milk
Whole (3.3% fat)	8.2
Low fat (2% fat)	4.7
Skim (<0.2% fat)	0.4
Buttermilk (1% fat)	2.2
Nonfat dry milk powder (¼ cup)	0.2
Condensed, sweetened	26.6
Evaporated milk, whole	19.1
Evaporated milk, skim	0.5

All dairy products, including low-fat cheese, provide important sources of calcium. Table 4 lists the calcium requirements for various age groups, and Table 5 shows the calcium content of some common dairy products.

Dairy products contain saturated fat in the form of butterfat; however, the concentration may vary from less than 1% to 80%, so it is important to read labels. Most cheese provides particularly concentrated sources of saturated fat (Table 2, *Appendix*).

The Living Heart Diet recommends only low-fat cheeses that contain no more than 12% butterfat or imitation cheese products made with skim milk and polyunsaturated oil. The Dairy Products Guide on pages 322 to 323 specifies the amount of low-fat cheese that may be used in The Living Heart Diet; even though the fat content is low, it must be restricted.

Calculating the Percentage of Fat in Cheese

Nutrients on a label are often listed as grams per serving. This can be confusing, especially when trying to choose dairy products that are low in fat. The following calculation converts grams of fat to percentage of fat using the nutrition information on the label.

Low-calorie cream cheese label: 1 serving (28 grams or about 1 ounce) = 80 calories, 3 grams protein, 7 grams fat, and 2 grams carbohydrate.

To find the percentage of fat, divide the amount of fat in 1 serving (in grams) by the total weight of 1 serving (in grams) and multiply by 100.

Example: 7 grams fat ÷ 28 grams
cheese = 0.25
0.25 × 100 = 25% fat content

This amount of fat is, of course, too high for
The Living Heart Diet.

Dairy Substitutes

Dairy substitutes (nondairy products) frequently contain saturated fat in the form of coconut oil, palm kernel oil, or hydrogenated fat
and should be avoided.

Certain dairy substitutes should be avoided:

Nondairy sour cream—tub, powdered, or
canned

Nondairy whipped toppings—tub, powdered,
aerosol, or frozen

Nondairy coffee creamers—liquid, powdered,
or frozen

"Filled milk" and "imitation milk" products
are generally not recommended. Vegetable fat
replaces butterfat in these products, and frequently the vegetable fat used is coconut oil. If
a filled milk or dairy substitute lists a polyunsaturated oil (e.g., safflower or corn oil) as the
source of fat, it can be included in The Living
Heart Diet. Be wary of the general term "vegetable oil," which is frequently used to avoid
listing the ingredients coconut or palm oil
(saturated fats).

DAIRY PRODUCTS IN THE LOW-CALORIE DIET

Individuals who need to lower their triglyceride level should follow the Dairy Products Guide
for The Living Heart Diet. Persons who need to
lose weight should choose dairy products with
1% or less butterfat because of the calories associated with the fat. Table 2 of the *Appendix*
shows that as the fat in dairy products is decreased, the calories are also reduced. Low-fat
cheeses can be included on this plan if the amounts

TABLE 4. *Recommended daily dietary allowance of calcium*

Group	Calcium (mg)
Infants	
Birth–6 months	360
6 months–1 year	540
Children, 1–10 years	800
Males	
11–18 years	1,200
19 years and older	800
Females	
11–18 years	1,200
19 years and older	800
Pregnant women	400 (in addition to above value)
Nursing women	400 (in addition to above value)

Adapted from *Recommended Dietary Allowances*, Ninth Revised Edition, 1980, National Academy of Sciences, Washington, D.C.

TABLE 5. *Calcium content of common dairy products*

Dairy product	Calcium (mg)
Cottage cheese (1 cup)	212
Whole milk (1 cup)	288
Skim milk (1 cup)	296
Low-fat milk with 2% nonfat milk, solids added (1 cup)	352

are carefully weighed according to the Dairy
Products Guide on pages 322 to 323.

BREAD AND CEREAL PRODUCTS IN THE LIVING HEART DIET

Because The Living Heart Diet contains less
meat and fat (to lower total fat in the diet), servings from the Bread and Cereal Group are increased. This includes grain and cereal products,
which provide protein, essential vitamins, minerals, energy, and fiber. The B vitamins, including thiamin (B_1), riboflavin (B_2), niacin,
pyridoxine (B_6), pantothenic acid, and folic acid,
are found in whole-grain cereal products. During

the milling process the vitamin and mineral contents are reduced and the fiber content is altered; hence whole-grain or "enriched" products are a preferable selection. The term "enriched" refers to federally regulated additions of certain nutrients to processed foods. Thiamin, riboflavin, niacin, and iron are commonly added during the enrichment process. During recent years consumption of high-fiber foods (e.g., whole-grain cereals, dried beans and peas, nuts, fruits, and vegetables) has increased. Fiber is discussed in greater detail on pages 41 to 42.

Cereal products, the cooked and dry varieties, may be included in The Living Heart Diet, except those which contain coconut. Commercial granola-type cereals often contain coconut or coconut oil and should be avoided. We have included several acceptable recipes for homemade granola in the Cereal section.

For simplicity, starchy vegetables are combined in the Bread and Cereal Group because they provide many of the same nutrients and are similar in calories. The starchy vegetables include potatoes, corn, lima beans, dried beans, and peas.

BREAD AND CEREAL PRODUCTS IN THE LOW-CALORIE DIET

People often think that bread is fattening, but this is not generally the case. A tablespoon of honey or preserves added to the bread, however, nearly doubles the calories. Therein lies the catch: *It is not the bread but the spread that contributes the excessive calories.*

Because the amounts of meat and fat are somewhat limited on The Low-Calorie Diet, servings of complex carbohydrate from the Bread and Cereal Group are increased. Although additional servings of carbohydrate-containing foods may seem like additional calories, the calorie plans in Table 1 were carefully calculated to control the amount of calories.

Breads, cereals, crackers, pastas, rice, fruits, starchy vegetables, legumes, sugars, syrup, molasses, honey, jams, and jellies all provide carbohydrate, either complex or simple. Foods that contain complex carbohydrates include grains, bread products, vegetables, and legumes, which contain starch. Simple carbohydrates are sugars such as those found in jam, jelly, syrup, and honey. Both types of carbohydrate supply energy (or calories), but complex carbohydrates also provide vitamins and minerals and only insignificant amounts of fat. Americans consume large amounts of refined sugar in the form of candy, jelly, syrup, and carbonated beverages. These foods provide little nutrition other than calories.

Foods other than bread and cereal products are included in the Bread and Cereal Guide on pages 324 to 325. This information allows persons who need to lose weight and/or control their triglycerides to include starchy vegetables, desserts, soups, and alcoholic beverages for greater variety. These foods may be eaten in specified amounts according to the serving sizes identified in the guide. However, they should always be substituted for bread servings; for example, ½ cup cooked rice = 1 slice bread.

ALCOHOLIC BEVERAGES

The Living Heart Diet recommends no more than 2 servings of alcohol daily because it tends to increase weight and triglyceride levels. Persons sensitive to alcohol may develop hypertriglyceridemia; alcohol appears to worsen already existing hypertriglyceridemia. For those who have this sensitivity, restricting alcohol intake to no more than 2 servings a day will usually reduce triglyceride levels. This effect may be due partly to a reduction in total body weight because of the decrease in calories from alcohol. Alcohol is often consumed in place of other, more nutritious foods.

A number of studies have reported that alcohol

TABLE 6. *Recommended daily dietary allowances of vitamin A[b]*

Group	Vitamin A (in retinol equivalents)[a]
Infants	
Birth–6 months	420
7 months–1 year	400
Children	
1–3 years	400
4–6 years	500
7–10 years	700
Males, 11 years and older	1,000
Females, 11 years and older	800
Pregnant women	200 (in addition to above value)
Nursing women	400 (in addition to above value)

[a]Retinol equivalents: 1 retinol equivalent = 1 mg retinol or 6 mg β-carotene.
[b]Adapted from *Recommended Dietary Allowances*, Ninth Revised Edition, 1980, National Academy of Sciences, Washington, D.C.

TABLE 7. *Recommended daily dietary allowances of vitamin C[a]*

Group	Vitamin C (mg)
Infants, Birth–1 year	35
Children, 1–10 years	45
Males	
11–14 years	50
15 years and older	60
Females	
11–14 years	50
15 years and older	60
Pregnant women	20 (in addition to above value)
Nursing women	40 (in addition to above value)

[a]Adapted from *Recommended Dietary Allowances*, Ninth Revised Edition, 1980, National Academy of Sciences, Washington, D.C.

consumption raises the level of the high density lipoproteins (HDL). In one study in which normal volunteers were given alcohol daily, levels of HDL were increased but toxic effects of alcohol on the liver were also observed. We do not recommend alcohol consumption as a therapeutic measure to raise HDL and prevent heart attack. The main reason is related to the dangers associated with an excessive consumption of alcohol. These diseases include cirrhosis of the liver, hypertension, cardiomyopathy (a form of heart failure), pancreatitis, psychosis, and alcoholism itself, the cause of untold social and personal distress and suffering. In our opinion, we do not yet know enough about the benefits of raising HDL by drinking small amounts of alcohol to recommend this as a public health measure. Drinking large amounts of alcohol is definitely associated with an increased morbidity and mortality. If drinking small amounts proves to be beneficial to the heart, drinking large amounts must cancel this benefit due to competing risks of the diseases caused by alcohol.

To determine the size of "1 serving" of alcohol, an exchange has been established for it as part of the Bread and Cereal Guide on page 327. It is part of this food group because of the carbohydrate it contributes to the diet. The exchange list illustrates that 1 serving of alcohol is equal to 1 exchange of bread, or can be used in place of 1 serving from the Bread and Cereal Group for up to 2 servings a day. For example, 1 ounce of gin, rum, vodka, or whiskey equals 1 exchange of bread, or a 10-ounce glass of beer is equal to 2 exchanges from the Bread and Cereal Group.

NONSTARCHY VEGETABLES IN THE LIVING HEART DIET

Vegetables are most nutritious when eaten raw or only lightly cooked. Spices and herbs add variety to cooked vegetables without adding calories. Sources of saturated fat (e.g., bacon, salt pork, ham hocks) should not be used to flavor the vegetables, although oil, tub margarine, and/or chopped lean meat are acceptable. On The Low-Calorie Diet, a fat exchange should be counted when fat is used for seasoning.

The nonstarchy vegetables provide vitamins and minerals, especially vitamins A and C. A vegetable that provides a rich source of each of the vitamins should be included daily. Table 6 shows the recommended amounts of vitamin A for various age groups, and Table 4 in the *Appendix* lists good sources of it. Recommendations for vitamin C are shown in Table 7, and the amounts provided by various foods are shown in Table 5 of the *Appendix*. The Vegetable Guide on pages 333 to 334 also identifies rich sources of vitamin A.

The nonstarchy vegetables are lower in calories than the other food groups, although some carbohydrate and a small amount of protein are present. Diabetics should carefully limit portions of nonstarchy vegetables according to their particular food plan in order to control carbohydrate and calories.

FRUITS IN THE LIVING HEART DIET

Fruits are an excellent source of vitamins A and C, and provide other important vitamins and minerals. A fruit rich in vitamin C should be included daily. Choose fresh, frozen, or canned fruits, preferably without added sugar. Rich sources of vitamins A and C are indicated with letters "A" and "C" in the Fruit Guide on pages 331 to 332.

FRUITS IN THE LOW-CALORIE DIET

Vitamin-rich fruits are an essential part of any diet, especially for the person who needs to lose weight. It is a naturally sweet food that can be used as a dessert, salad, or part of the entrée. Fresh, unsweetened, frozen, or water-packed canned fruits are the best selections because they contain about half the calories of fruit packed in

TABLE 8. *Calories in different preparations of the same fruit*

Fruit[a]	Weight (gm)[b]	Cal
Pineapple		
Raw, fresh	155	81
Candied	227	717
Canned, water-packed, no sweetener	246	96
Canned, heavy syrup	255	189
Canned, extra heavy syrup	260	234
Frozen, sweetened	245	208
Apple		
Raw, fresh (1 whole, 2½″ diam.)	115	59
Fresh, chopped	125	73
Dehydrated, uncooked	100	353[c]
Dried, uncooked	85	234[c]
Dried, cooked without sugar	255	199[c]
Apple butter	282	525
Apple juice	248	118
Applesauce, unsweetened	244	100
Applesauce, sweetened	255	232

[a]In each case, the calories and weight are those contained in 1 cup of fruit.
[b]Approximately 28 g = 1 ounce.
[c]Dehydrated and dried fruit account for more calories than fresh fruit in the same volume because the water has been removed. Caution should be used when eating fruits in these forms, i.e., 2 dried apple halves = 1 whole fresh apple.

syrup (Table 8). Fruit canned in its own juice has about the same calorie content as fresh fruit. If the natural juice is eaten with the fruit, however, it should be counted as an exchange from the Fruit Group.

MISCELLANEOUS FOODS

The Living Heart Diet encourages variety and allows for flexibility in order to accommodate different life styles. Seasonings may be used creatively to please your taste, add interest, or complement foreign cuisine. Foods recommended on this diet can be combined in an infinite variety of appetizers, soups, salads, entrées, casseroles, desserts, dips, snacks, and party foods.

Some foods have an insignificant number of calories and can be used *ad lib*. These include coffee, tea, sugar-free drinks,[2] spices, and herbs.

[2]Subject to current warnings about saccharin.

A list of other low-calorie foods is given in the Miscellaneous Food Guide on page 335.

MEALS AWAY FROM HOME

Almost every restaurant offers food choices that are low in cholesterol and saturated fat. When dining out, select a restaurant, cafeteria, or sandwich shop, rather than a "fast-food" establishment, which may serve only fried foods. The following suggestions will allow wise selections to be made.

When ordering:
Ask how foods are prepared if you are not sure.
Request margarine rather than butter.
If margarine is not available, eat bread or potato plain.
Order your entrée broiled or baked without butter.
Request that foods high in saturated fat (e.g., cheese and butter) be removed from your table.

When served:
Trim fat from meat.
Remove skin from poultry.

If your choice is limited:
Remove breading from meat.
Remove fried batter from fish.
Eat as little as possible of the sauce served on vegetables.
Push gravy aside.

When eating out, good selections are[3]:

Appetizers	Fruit compote
	Raw vegetable tray
	Crab fingers
Entrées	Fish, chicken or beef—
	broiled or baked

---

[3]These are not universal diets, and individuals with special health problems such as diabetes and hypertension (sodium-restricted diet) will require other modifications.

	Sliced turkey, veal, or ham
	Lean pork chop or lamb chop—broiled or baked
	London broil (flank steak)
	Crab, lobster, oysters—broiled or boiled
	Tuna, salmon, or other fish salad
	Cottage cheese and fruit plate
Salads	Tossed salad
	Coleslaw
	Carrot and raisin salad
	Waldorf salad
	Fruit salad
	Relish tray
Salad dressings	Vinegar and oil
	Italian
	French
	Thousand Island
	Mayonnaise
Vegetables	Baked potato with margarine and chives
	Any vegetable without butter or sauce
Breads	Sliced bread
	Hard roll
	Bread sticks
	Saltines
	Melba toast
	English muffin
	French bread
Desserts	Fruit
	Fruit ice
	Sherbet
	Gelatin dessert
	Unfrosted angel food cake

Avoid these menu items because they are high in fat and calories:

Fried meat	French fries
Pizza	Gravy

Casseroles	Butter
Bacon	Cheese
Sausage	Sour cream
Whole milk	Pie
Cream soups	Cake
Cheese dressings	Ice cream
Creamed vegetables	Pudding
Fried vegetables	Whipped cream

When traveling by airplane, you may request low-cholesterol or low-calorie meals when you make reservations. Then, when you board, tell the flight attendant you have ordered a special meal.

EATING ON THE RUN

Too busy to eat? Often daily schedules do not permit the time to eat regularly or properly. To fully enjoy an active life, however, you must feel good and have plenty of energy. This takes a careful selection of foods so that the body gets the calories and nutrients it needs each day. *It is possible to eat on the run and still follow The Living Heart Diet.*

We recommend beginning the day with breakfast, the meal most often neglected. Why all the emphasis on breakfast? Our bodies need certain amounts of calories and nutrients within a 24-hour period. Eating only two meals a day or less makes it difficult to satisfy these needs. Consistently operating at such a nutritional deficit takes its toll on the body in many ways: irritability, weariness, and midmorning or afternoon slump. Adequately fulfilling daily nutrient needs is important to people of all ages.

Eating before the activities of the day are begun breaks an 8- to 12-hour fast. By prolonging the fast until noon, you may experience certain physical reactions. Your blood glucose level may drop below normal, causing weakness, concentration difficulties, malaise, headache, or even nausea.

The human body is an intricate machine which operates 24 hours a day and needs a constant supply of energy. It functions most efficiently when it receives fuel in moderate amounts at regular intervals. Some people may not feel hungry in the morning because they eat more than they need at dinner or before bed. Others skip breakfast, planning to control their weight, but end up indulging in a sweet roll midmorning or overeating at lunch.

The foods eaten for breakfast determine how long you will feel satisfied through the morning. A breakfast high in simple carbohydrate enters the blood rapidly with the result that you feel hungry as soon as 2 hours later. Adding protein (e.g., skim milk or low-fat cheese) to the meal prolongs absorption and increases the duration of satisfaction. Fat is absorbed even more slowly than protein or carbohydrate and can postpone the "empty" feeling up to 6 hours. A breakfast that includes some protein, carbohydrate, and fat is the best combination. Breakfast does not have to be routine or boring. Many foods take on a new dimension when served in the morning. Adding a hot beverage such as coffee or even spiced tea will certainly complete a well-balanced breakfast.

LOW-CALORIE BREAKFAST IDEAS

⅓ cup apple juice	½ cup orange juice
½ cup cooked hot cereal with 8 ounces skim milk and 1 teaspoon margarine	1 English muffin toasted with 1 ounce Canadian bacon
	1 tomato slice
	1 ounce low-fat cheese
¼ fresh cantaloupe	½ grapefruit
2 slices French toast (made with skim milk, egg substitute, and margarine)	1 slice whole wheat toast with 1 ounce low-fat cheese
	8 ounces skim milk

Orange slices
Egg-substitute omelet with 1 ounce low-fat cheese
1 slice toast with 1 teaspoon margarine

½ cup tomato juice
¾ cup dry cereal with 8 ounces skim milk and ½ banana

Brown Bag Breakfasts

When you do not have enough time to make breakfast in the morning, prepare one the night before to take with you to work.

1 small apple
1 ounce low-fat cheese
4 pieces of Melba toast

1 orange
Peanut butter sandwich
Thermos of skim milk (8 ounces)

Fruit shake (blend ½ banana or other fresh fruit with 8 ounces skim milk and carry in thermos; spice with nutmeg, vanilla, or cinnamon)
1 homemade bran muffin

½ cup plain low-fat yogurt with ½ cup strawberries
1 homemade spice muffin

LUNCH BOX IDEAS

Bringing lunch from home is economical and places you in control of the food choices available for your noon meal. Use your creativity and try some of the following ideas to perk up your homemade lunch.

Sandwiches

Try a new bread: French, whole grain, rye, pumpernickel, raisin, oatmeal, soy-wheat. For even more variety, use buns, rolls, English muffins, bagels, tortillas, or pita bread.

Spread with mustard, catsup, mayonnaise, margarine, or tahini.

Fillings:
Chicken
Ham salad
Crab salad
Lean slice of roast beef or ham
Low-fat cheese (add pimentos for variety)
Peanut butter—try combined with either bell pepper, pickle, lettuce, or fruit slices (banana and apple are especially good)
Thin-sliced luncheon meats
Tuna salad
Turkey pastrami
Turkey salad
Avocado

Combinations:
Tomato and cucumber
Add a garnish—lettuce, tomato, pickle, fresh mushrooms, sunflower seeds, roasted sesame seeds, bean sprouts, alfalfa sprouts

Be imaginative with your sandwich fillings and try new combinations every week. An unlimited variety of delicacies is waiting to be discovered.

Other Lunch Ideas

Pack fresh vegetables and relishes: Artichoke hearts, broccoli pieces, carrot sticks, cauliflowerettes, celery sticks, cherry tomatoes, cucumber slices, dill pickles, fresh mushrooms, green pepper rings, yellow squash slices, zucchini sticks.

Salads should be creative and can provide endless variety: Greens and vegetables (try different varieties of lettuce and spinach); Chef's salad with turkey, roast beef, chicken, ham, or tuna and low-fat cheese (add imitation bacon bits or soy-based croutons found in the fresh produce sections of grocery stores for variety); low-fat cottage cheese and fruit combinations.

Fresh fruits: Apple, banana, dried fruits (apricots, raisins, apples, pears), grapefruit, melon, orange, peach, pear, plums, strawberries.

Soups (keep cold or hot in a thermos): Tomato,

bouillon, gazpacho (omit fat), hot soups (check soup list on page 327).

Desserts: Plain low-fat yogurt (add artificial sweetener,[4] cinnamon, vanilla, or almond extract); plain low-fat yogurt with fresh fruit or canned unsweetened fruits (e.g., pineapple, applesauce); low-fat cottage cheese with fruits (add cinnamon and artificial sweetener[4]); homemade muffins (check allowed list on page 324).

Beverages: (You may want to carry a thermos of skim milk or low-fat milk with your lunch if it is not available when or where you eat.) Sugar-free canned drinks,[4] sugar-free hot cocoa, fruit juices, herb teas, bouillon.

REFERENCE

1. Harris, W. S., Connor, W. F., and McMurry, M. P. (1983): The comparative reductions of the plasma lipids and lipoproteins by dietary polyunsaturated fats. *Metabolism*, 32(2):179–184.

[4]Subject to current warnings about saccharin.

3

The Low-Sodium Diet

Sodium is a mineral necessary for the growth, development, and maintenance of many of the body's functions. Most Americans consume more sodium than their bodies need. Under certain medical conditions, excess sodium cannot be properly excreted by the body and results in fluid retention (edema), which places a strain on the kidneys, heart, and blood vessels.

To prevent the accumulation of sodium and water in your body, your physician may prescribe a low-sodium diet. Sodium restriction is recommended in individuals with heart failure, elevated blood pressure, or fluid accumulation due to kidney or liver insufficiency. When it is necessary to follow a low-sodium diet, it is important to evaluate all sources from which a person may be receiving sodium, including food, salt added to food, water, medicines, and dentifrices. All foods of plant and animal origin contain sodium in varying degrees. Table 2 in the *Appendix* shows the sodium content of many common foods.

RESTRICTING SODIUM

Sodium in the American diet ranges from 1,600 to 10,000 milligrams per day. Sodium can be restricted to as low as 200 milligrams per day. However, the development of effective diuretic drugs, and the unpalatability of and difficulty in following a severely sodium restricted diet have made the use of such diets less common in the practice of medicine.

The most common sodium-restricted diets are the "Low-Salt Diet," which contains about 3,000 milligrams sodium, and the 2,000 milligram diet. On the "Low-Salt Diet" food can be salted in ordinary amounts during cooking, but the use of highly salted foods and additional salt at the table is eliminated.

SODIUM IN FOOD

A physician determines the level of sodium necessary for the treatment of hypertension or other disorders. The prescribed sodium level can then be translated into a practical eating pattern by one of three methods:

1. Point system for calculating sodium
2. Calculating milligrams of sodium
3. Restricting high-sodium foods (used only for a mildly restricted sodium intake)

The Point System

The point system has been developed as a means of calculating sodium intake for a day. By simply adding up points for each day, the sodium content can easily be determined. One point is equal to 1 milliequivalent (23 milligrams) of sodium. Point values for various sodium levels are given below (some of the point values have been rounded off).

Sodium (milligrams)	Points
250	11
500	22
1,000	43
1,500	65
2,000	87
2,500	109
3,000	130
3,500	152
4,000	174
4,500	196
5,000	217
5,500	239
6,000	261
6,500	283
7,000	304

Table 7 in the *Appendix* gives the point values for sodium in common foods. They were determined by dividing the milligrams of sodium by 23 and rounding off. For example, there are 126 milligrams of sodium in 1 cup of skim milk, which is equivalent to 5 points.

$$126 \div 23 = 5.48, \text{ or } 5 \text{ points}$$

All recipes in this book give the milligrams of sodium per serving. By dividing the number of milligrams by 23, you can convert this number to the point system.

The point system allows a person on a low-sodium diet to include a high-sodium food in his diet by carefully selecting other low-sodium foods for that particular day. Thus a high-sodium food need not be totally avoided.

Calculating Milligrams of Sodium

Milligrams of sodium may be calculated simply by adding the total number of milligrams contained in each serving of food eaten during the entire day. Table 2 in the *Appendix* gives the milligrams of sodium for most common foods.

Food tables usually give the sodium content of food in milligrams per serving. It may be necessary to convert other units of measure into milligrams as follows:

1 milliequivalent sodium = 23 milligrams sodium
1 gram sodium = 1,000 milligrams sodium
1 gram salt = 400 milligrams sodium (plus 600 milligrams chloride)
¼ teaspoon salt = 533 milligrams sodium

Other helpful conversions:

500 milligrams sodium = 1.25 grams salt
2 grams sodium = 5 grams salt
3 grams sodium = 7.5 grams salt
5 grams sodium = 12.5 grams salt

Restricting High-Sodium Foods

The high-sodium foods listed on page 55 may be avoided in order to restrict sodium in the diet. However, it is difficult to accurately determine the level of sodium a person is consuming by simply avoiding or restricting high-sodium foods. Consequently this system is recommended only if you are following a moderate sodium restriction.

The low-sodium recipes given later in this book can be used on any sodium-restricted diet; the sodium per serving is listed. Generally, if your physician has ordered a 2-gram sodium diet (or higher), regular bread, soft tub margarine, and canned vegetables can be used in place of the low-sodium varieties. By using the recipe for Stuffed Onions, let us illustrate how the sodium content for the low-sodium recipes can be increased:

Stuffed Onions

6 medium onions, peeled
1 tablespoon low-sodium corn oil margarine, melted
3 tablespoons low-sodium corn oil margarine
¼ cup chopped celery
¼ cup chopped green pepper
¼ teaspoon ground sage
1 clove garlic, minced
⅛ teaspoon pepper
1 tablespoon chopped fresh parsley
1 cup fine, dry low-sodium bread crumbs
¼ cup chopped unsalted walnuts
¼ cup cubed low-sodium low-fat cheese

See page 247 for recipe directions.
Yield: 6 servings

1 serving contains[1]:

Cal	Prot	Fat	Carb	Sat	Mono	Poly	Chol	Na
202	5	12.9	18	2.0	4.4	5.5	0	49

To increase the sodium in the Stuffed Onions recipe, change the low-sodium corn oil margarine and the low-sodium bread crumbs to regular products, which results in 142 milligrams sodium per serving. This value is derived as follows: 140 milligrams sodium per tablespoon of margarine × 4 (tablespoons of margarine in recipe) = 560 milligrams sodium per recipe. Divide 560 by 6 servings = 93 milligrams sodium per serving from margarine. Add 49 milligrams sodium from other ingredients. Hence the total sodium per serving of Stuffed Onions is 142 milligrams.

---

[1]*Abbreviations:* **Cal,** calories; **Prot,** protein; **Carb,** carbohydrate; **Sat,** saturated fat; **Mono,** monounsaturated fat; **Poly,** polyunsaturated fat; **Chol,** cholesterol; **Na,** sodium. Protein, fat, carbohydrate, saturated fat, monounsaturated fat, and polyunsaturated fat are expressed in *grams*. Cholesterol and sodium are expressed in *milligrams*.

FOOD LABELS

Low-sodium dietetic foods may be used on most low-sodium diets. Note, however, that the terms "dietetic" and "low-sodium" are not synonymous. Always read the label of any food product you purchase and select only foods that are identified as being low in sodium or which do not have sources of sodium listed on the label.

COMPOUNDS CONTAINING SODIUM

The words "salt" and "sodium" should not be confused, even though they are related. Sodium is not salt, but salt (sodium chloride) contains about 40% sodium. With careful planning, small amounts of salt can be included on moderately restricted sodium diets (¼ teaspoon salt contains 533 milligrams sodium). Read labels and be aware of certain compounds which provide sodium to the diet (sodium additives), such as those listed below.

Sodium Additives

Monosodium glutamate (MSG), sold under several trade names: A seasoning used in foods prepared at home and in restaurants, and in many prepared and frozen foods.

Sodium benzoate: A preservative in many condiments, sauces and salad dressings.

Brine (salt and water): Used in processing foods to inhibit the growth of bacteria and in foods such as corned beef, sauerkraut, and pickles.

Sodium propionate: Used to inhibit the growth of bacteria in processed cheese and some baked products.

Sodium sulfite: Used as a preservative in some dried fruits and in foods which are artificially colored (e.g., maraschino cherries).

Disodium phosphate: Used in processed cheese and some quick-cooking cereals.

Sodium hydroxide: Used in food processing to soften and loosen skins of fruits, hominy, and olives.

Sodium alginate: Used in ice cream and chocolate milk to ensure a smooth texture.

SALT SUBSTITUTES

Salt substitutes can be used to add a salt-like flavor to food if your physician approves. The main ingredient of most salt substitutes is potassium chloride, which may be harmful to certain people. You must therefore always check with your physician before using a salt substitute. This applies to low-sodium meat tenderizers and seasoned salt substitutes as well.

SODIUM IN THE WATER SUPPLY

All natural water supplies contain sodium, although the concentration varies depending on the source. Even rain water contains a very small amount of sodium (1 milligram per liter), and water from brackish or saline wells may contain several thousand milligrams of sodium per liter. The sodium content of drinking water is not of great concern unless you are trying to follow a very low sodium (500 milligrams or lower) diet or the water is from brackish wells. The average person consumes 2 to 2 ½ quarts (8 to 10 glasses) of water a day, including coffee and tea as well as cooked foods. To find out the sodium content of your local water supply, call the local health department or water department. In addition, be aware that any water softeners you may use increase the sodium content of the water by exchanging sodium for calcium.

HIGH-SODIUM FOODS

Foods differ greatly in their natural sodium content. The following foods and seasonings are high in sodium and should be avoided if your physician recommends sodium restriction. If he has recommended a diet containing less than 3,000 to 4,500 milligrams of sodium, you will need to avoid additional foods.

Avoid these foods on a sodium-restricted diet:

Anchovies	Nuts, salted
Bacon	Olives
Barbecue sauce	Pastrami
Bologna	Pepperoni
Bouillon cubes	Pickles
Buttermilk	Pizza
Catsup	Salami
Celery salt	Salt
Cheese, except cottage	Sauerkraut
Chips, potato and corn	Sausage
Crackers	Seasoned salt
Cured meat	Seeds, salted
Diet soft drinks in excess of 2 per day	Soup, canned
	Soy sauce
Frankfurters	Steak sauce
Garlic salt	Tomato juice
Ham, cured	Vegetable juice
Meat, canned or frozen in sauce	Weiners, beef, pork, and turkey
Monosodium glutamate (MSG)	Worcestershire sauce
Mustard	

SEASONING LOW-SODIUM FOODS

Foods do not have to taste flat on a low-sodium diet. Be creative and enjoy fresh and dried spices, herbs, and flavorings to enhance the flavor of recipes for meat, fish, and poultry. Natural low-sodium vegetable seasonings do not contain potassium chloride. They are blends of herbs, spices, and dried vegetables, which can be used to add flavor and zest to low-sodium foods.

Add spice to meat, fish, and poultry:

Beef—bay leaf, dry mustard, green pepper, sage, marjoram, fresh mushrooms, nutmeg, onion, pepper, thyme

Chicken—cranberries, fresh mushrooms, paprika, parsley, poultry seasoning, rosemary, thyme, sage

Lamb—curry, garlic, mint, pineapple,[2] rosemary

Pork—apples,[2] applesauce,[2] garlic, onion, sage

Veal—apricots,[2] bay leaf, curry, ginger, marjoram, oregano

Fish—bay leaf, curry, dry mustard, green peppers, lemon juice, marjoram, fresh mushrooms, paprika

EATING AWAY FROM HOME ON A LOW-SODIUM DIET

It is possible to eat out while following a low-sodium diet, although a great deal of consideration must be given to food selection. Food may contain a large amount of sodium without tasting salty, so be careful. Certain types of food (e.g., Oriental and Mexican cuisine) are particularly high in sodium. The best choice of entrée when eating out is a broiled piece of meat; ask the waiter to have it prepared without salt or sauce. Other alternatives include an inside cut of roast or poultry without skin or gravy. A plain vegetable (e.g., a baked potato) and a vegetable salad with oil and vinegar or lemon juice may be ordered to accompany the entrée. Fruit and fruit juice add little sodium to the diet. Often restaurants and airlines will provide special low-sodium meals if you let them know in advance.

---

[2]If fruit is eaten with meat, count it as a serving from the fruit group. Serving sizes and the equivalent exchange are given in the Fruit Guide for The Low-Calorie Diet.

4

Dietary Treatment of Hyperlipidemia

LOWERING PLASMA LIPID LEVELS

Elevated levels of cholesterol or triglycerides are often reduced to normal by simply making certain changes in the diet. The effects of diet should be observed for at least 4 to 6 weeks before taking any type of medication. If medication is then deemed necessary, it should be used in conjunction with the diet.

Several dietary factors affect cholesterol and triglyceride levels: total calories; percent of calories from carbohydrate, protein, and fat; type of fat (saturated, polyunsaturated, or monounsaturated); and the ratio of polyunsaturated to saturated fat (P/S ratio). Other factors include dietary cholesterol, sugar, and alcohol. Any one or a combination of these components of the diet can have an influence on cholesterol or triglyceride metabolism if consumed in excessive or unbalanced amounts.

The precise effect of factors such as total calories, type of fat, or percent of calories from fat or protein on the metabolism of cholesterol and triglycerides is not clearly understood. However, there are several facts which are known, and these are discussed in greater depth in Chapter 2. Table 1 notes the effects of the fats on the lipid levels in the blood.

A modest reduction in cholesterol results when concentrated sources of dietary cholesterol (e.g., egg yolk and organ meat) are restricted.

Excessive amounts of alcohol and foods rich

TABLE 1. *Effects of fat on cholesterol and triglycerides in the blood*

Fats	Effect
Saturated fats (e.g., meat fat, cream, butter, and whole milk cheese)	Elevate cholesterol
Polyunsaturated fats (e.g., vegetable oil and margarine)	Reduce cholesterol
Monounsaturated fats (e.g., olives, olive oil, peanuts, peanut oil, and avocados)	Do not significantly affect cholesterol

in sugar (e.g., jelly, honey, candy, and desserts) tend to increase triglyceride levels (measured after fasting).

Weight loss is the key to lowering triglycerides, but restriction of desserts and alcohol is also generally recommended.

TRADITIONAL DIETARY RECOMMENDATIONS FOR THE TREATMENT OF HYPERLIPIDEMIA

Traditionally, specific diets were prescribed according to the type of hyperlipidemia that had been diagnosed, as outlined in Table 2. These diets have many similarities, which are discussed on the following pages. Each of the diets is low in cholesterol and saturated fat [diets for Types IIa and IIb hyperlipoproteinemia (hyperlipidemia) are the lowest]; most restrict simple carbohydrate (except Types I and IIa); all promote the use of polyunsaturated fat in place of satu-

TABLE 2. *Comparison of diets for treating hyperlipidemia*

Parameter	The Living Heart Diet	The Low-Calorie Living Heart Diet	Type I Diet	Type IIa Diet	Types IIb and III Diet	Type IV Diet	Type V Diet
Calories	Controlled[a]	Controlled[b]	Not limited	Controlled[a]	Controlled[b]	Controlled[b]	Controlled[b]
Carbohydrate	50% (of total calories)	50% (of total calories)	High because of fat restriction	Not limited	50% (of total calories)	45% (of total calories)	50% (of total calories)
Protein	20% (of total calories)	20% (of total calories)	Not limited[c]	Not limited[d]	20% (of total calories)	Not limited except to control weight	20% (of total calories)
Fat	30% (of total calories)	30% (of total calories)	25–35 grams; supplement with MCT oil[e]	↓ Saturated fat ↑ Polyunsaturated fat (High P/S)	30% (of total calories)	Substitute polyunsaturated fat for saturated fat	30% (of total calories)
Cholesterol	<300 mg	<300 mg	Not limited[c]	Low as possible	Low as possible	No more than 300 mg	No more than 300 mg
Alcohol	No more than 2 servings per day	No more than 2 servings per day	Not recommended	Allowed with discretion	No more than 2 servings per day	No more than 2 servings per day	Not recommended

[a]Controlled to maintain ideal body weight.
[b]Controlled to attain and maintain ideal body weight.
[c]Consumption of animal products will be low due to fat restriction.
[d]Consumption of animal products will be low due to cholesterol restriction.
[e]MCT oil = medium-chain triglyceride oil.

rated fat; and all are designed to control weight. By using The Living Heart Diet for the treatment of hyperlipidemia (discussed on pages 61 to 62), we have incorporated all of the similarities in the diets for Types I through V and have attempted to simplify the approach to treating hyperlipidemia by proposing one general diet for all types.

Type I Hyperlipoproteinemia

A deficiency or absence of the enzyme that breaks down the chylomicrons and very low density lipoproteins (VLDL) occurs in Type I hyperlipoproteinemia. As a result, triglycerides from the diet cannot be cleared from the blood. This very rare inherited disorder is diagnosed during early childhood and is characterized by severe abdominal pain following a meal containing fat.

The diet of an adult with Type I should allow no more than 25 to 35 grams of fat daily; children under 12 are allowed 10 to 15 grams daily. Because this fat allowance is so low, the primary source of calories is carbohydrate. The amount of cholesterol consumed in such a diet is very low because of the limited fat consumption. Meat is limited to 5 ounces daily for adults and only 2 to 3 ounces for children. Alcohol is not recommended on the Type I Diet. Preparation of food and seasonings for food is difficult because of the severe fat restriction. Therefore medium-chain triglyceride (MCT) oil, which does not have to be incorporated into the chylomicrons or VLDL to be absorbed into the blood, provides an ideal dietary supplement. This oil is available at most pharmacies. As there are no drugs that can successfully control Type I hyperlipoproteinemia, it is very important to closely adhere to the diet even though it is quite restrictive. The diet tends to be low in iron, vitamin E, and the essential fatty acids. It is therefore important that a person following this diet be closely monitored by a physician. Supplementation with the fat-soluble vitamins A, D, E, and K may be desirable.

Type IIa Hyperlipoproteinemia

Type IIa hyperlipoproteinemia is characterized by an increase in low density lipoproteins (LDL) with normal concentrations of VLDL. It is often caused by an inherited disease called familial hypercholesterolemia, and people with this disorder usually develop premature atherosclerosis. The first heart attack in men with familial hypercholesterolemia generally occurs at about age 40. There are several common manifestations: premature corneal arcus (a white arc which appears on the cornea of the eye), xanthomas (fat deposits which form large lumps on the skin), and early blood vessel disease. Xanthomas may occur on the tendons of the hands and elbows or the Achilles tendons.

The Type IIa Diet requires limiting cholesterol intake to less than 300 milligrams per day. Preferably, no more than 200 milligrams should be ingested daily, with the polyunsaturated to saturated fat (P/S) ratio increased to 2. Protein, alcohol, sugar, and calories may not need to be limited unless one is overweight. The triglyceride levels are not elevated in Type IIa.

The Type IIa Diet is similar to The Living Heart Diet discussed in Chapter 2 with the following exceptions:

1. Use only skim milk dairy products (those containing no more than 1% butterfat).

2. Limit beef, pork, and lamb intake to a 3-ounce portion three times a week. This will help reduce the intake of total saturated fat.

3. Unless calorie restriction is required, an effort should be made to increase the P/S ratio to as high as 2. This should be viewed as a therapeutic measure for this potentially dangerous disorder and is analogous to using a drug.

4. Use vegetable oil and margarine with a very high P/S ratio in order to increase the total P/S ratio of the diet. Margarines listing liquid safflower oil, liquid corn oil, or liquid sunflower oil as the first ingredient should be selected.

5. Use at least 1 teaspoon of polyunsaturated

fat daily for each ounce of meat consumed as a means of increasing the P/S ratio.

6. Avoid all high-cholesterol foods, e.g., egg yolk and organ meat (liver and brains). Cholesterol-free egg substitutes may be used as desired.

The Type IIa Diet will effectively reduce cholesterol by 10 to 15%, and it meets the Recommended Daily Dietary Allowances of the National Research Council in all nutrients except possibly iron. Careful planning to include a wide variety of foods, especially meat, iron-fortified foods, and citrus fruit (to aid iron absorption), can provide a diet adequate in iron.

Types IIb and III Hyperlipoproteinemia

Type IIb is characterized by elevated levels of LDL, VLDL, cholesterol, and triglycerides.

Type III is characterized by an elevation of VLDL, and some of the VLDL are abnormal. In Type III, xanthomas (skin lesions containing fat) often occur in the creases of the palm of the hand. The risk of coronary and peripheral atherosclerosis is greatly increased.

The diet for treating Types IIb and III is the same and initially focuses on weight loss. Because triglycerides are elevated, calorie restriction to achieve and maintain ideal body weight is mandatory. Dietary cholesterol and saturated fat are restricted in an effort to reduce the elevated cholesterol level. During the weight loss phase, principles of a weight maintenance diet can be learned and then continued after the weight is lost. Cholesterol is limited to less than 300 milligrams daily, and ideally should be limited to about 200 milligrams daily. Because total fat is limited, it is important to use a polyunsaturated fat (e.g., safflower oil) for food preparation.

In some individuals with Type IIb or III, alcohol stimulates the liver to produce excessive triglycerides. To control this effect, intake of alcoholic beverages should be limited to two servings a day (see the Bread and Cereal Guide, "Alcohol," on page 327).

The Type IIb and III Diet is similar to The Low-Calorie Diet described in Chapter 2. The only exception is the amount of cholesterol allowed. The cholesterol restriction is more severe in the Type IIb and III Diet than in The Living Heart Diet. Eggs and organ meats should be avoided on this diet. Oils and margarines with the highest P/S ratio should be used.

Type IV Hyperlipoproteinemia

The Type IV pattern is very common and is often normalized by weight reduction and limiting alcohol intake. This pattern of hyperlipoproteinemia is characterized by an elevation of VLDL levels, which represent triglycerides manufactured in the body. Some individuals with Type IV have an increased sensitivity to carbohydrate, but we do not recommend restriction of complex carbohydrates, such as starch; we do advise, however, limiting sugar and concentrated sweets. The VLDL concentration is influenced by obesity and alcohol ingestion.

The Type IV Diet is essentially the same as The Low-Calorie Living Heart Diet. If a maintenance diet is needed after ideal weight is attained, or if weight is not a problem, The Living Heart Diet can be followed as discussed in Chapter 2.

Type V Hyperlipoproteinemia

In Type V hyperlipoproteinemia, triglycerides consumed in the diet and manufactured by the body accumulate in the blood. Triglyceride levels are very high, and the cholesterol level is elevated as well. Abdominal pain occurs frequently after a meal containing fat. This pain may or may not be associated with pancreatitis (inflammation of the pancreas), which occurs in 40 to 50% of those with Type V.

The diet for Type V focuses on weight reduction and control of alcohol. Initially, alcohol consumption should be eliminated and a fat-restricted weight control diet, such as The Living

Heart Diet, should be followed. The frequent attacks of abdominal pain are usually eliminated when fat intake is reduced. Cholesterol is moderately restricted, as in The Living Heart Diet. Polyunsaturated fat is substituted for saturated fat whenever possible, although the *total* fat consumption should be restricted (saturated, polyunsaturated, and monounsaturated). The Type V Diet resembles The Low-Calorie Diet, except that the fat content is lower. As fat is contained in so many naturally occurring foods (e.g., meat and even the low-fat dairy products), it is important to read food labels and eliminate excessive fats. Table 2 shows similarities and differences between The Living Heart Diet, The Low-Calorie Living Heart Diet, and the specific diets for hyperlipoproteinemia.

THE LIVING HEART DIET FOR TREATMENT OF HYPERLIPIDEMIA

The Living Heart Diet for the treatment of hyperlipidemia is basically a stepwise, progressive approach, based on the idea that an individual's diet should not be restricted more than necessary. If cholesterol and triglyceride levels are reduced to normal by following The Living Heart Diet (Step 1), then this diet should be continued. If these lipids remain elevated, however, a more restricted diet (Step 2 or 3) should be tried, as judged by the physician. Step 2 and 3 Diets are progressively lower in fat and cholesterol.

In the treatment of hyperlipidemia, The Living Heart Diet can be modified to a low-calorie or low-sodium diet or to one suitable for the diabetic. The Low-Calorie Living Heart Diet can be followed by those needing to lose weight and by diabetics. The Low-Sodium Diet is designed for persons who must restrict their sodium consumption. Hyperlipidemic women who are pregnant or nursing should be certain that all of their calorie and protein needs are met while restricting cholesterol and saturated fat. Vegetarians with

hyperlipidemia should be advised to pay particular attention to complementing proteins. The Type I person, who requires a very low fat diet, should consult a dietitian who will calculate dietary needs (personalized to the individual's specific likes and dislikes) because achieving the very restricted low-fat content required for the Type I person is exceptionally difficult.

Step 1 Diet

The Living Heart Diet is the Step 1 Diet for treatment of hyperlipidemia, i.e., 300 milligrams of cholesterol, 20% of calories as protein, 30% calories as fat, and 50% calories as carbohydrate. All of the recipes in this book are low in cholesterol and saturated fat, and may be used in the Step 1 Diet. Following The Living Heart Diet will reduce cholesterol and triglyceride levels in most individuals. Persons with severe hyperlipidemia should begin their dietary treatment with Step 1 and progress gradually to Steps 2 and 3 as recommended by their physician.

Step 2 Diet

Progressing to Step 2 entails reducing fat to 25–30% of total calories and reducing cholesterol intake to 200–250 milligrams by eating less meat; meatless entrées should be eaten several times each week. What meat is eaten should be very lean, and fish and poultry should be selected frequently. Low-fat dairy products and less total fat (oil, margarine, salad dressing, and nuts) help reduce total fat intake. High-cholesterol foods (egg yolk, organ meat, and shrimp) should be avoided.

Step 3 Diet: Very Low Fat Diet

As mentioned previously, we do not recommend that the Step 3 Diet be used immediately, even in persons with severe hyperlipidemia, as abrupt changes in dietary habits are undesirable. Step 1 should be followed initially with a gradual progression to Step 3 as recommended by your physician.

For the person who is not responding adequately to diet, the Step 3 Diet can then be ordered by the physician. In this diet, fat comprises only 20 to 25% of the total calories, and cholesterol is decreased to 100 milligrams daily. Great care is required in selecting foods for preparation at home, and label reading is essential. Most commercial foods with fat appearing among the first three or four ingredients on the label will be too high in fat, e.g., salad dressings, most baked goods, canned meat products, cheese, and frozen desserts. This is also true of foods with large amounts of naturally occurring fat, e.g., nuts, avocados, cream, whole milk, and fatty meat.

Because fat is the most concentrated source of calories, it is essential to replace the fat calories with carbohydrate calories, preferably complex carbohydrate; more legumes, cereal products, grains, and bread products should be included in the diet. These foods increase the bulk beyond that which the average American consumes. Therefore, it may be more satisfying to eat five or six small meals daily. If meatless meals are eaten frequently, the diet will be lower in fat content (see recipe section on Meatless Entrées). All meat contains fat, and the leanest cuts of meat are water-packed tuna, fish, and chicken and turkey without skin (Table 2 in the *Appendix*). Fruit and vegetables will give a full, satisfied feeling as well as provide essential vitamins and minerals.

This diet requires special consideration when eating away from home. Fruit plates served with sherbet or low-fat cottage cheese, vegetable plates which do not have sauce or fat added to the vegetables, or broiled poultry or fish are good selections. Fresh fruit, hard rolls, melba toast, and tossed salad with vinegar or lemon juice as dressing are always good choices on the Step 3 Diet.

The Step 3 Diet is not recommended for everyone. A great deal of dedication and determination is required to follow this diet over a period of time. It should be prescribed by a physician, and the individual should have intensive instructions and follow-up by a dietitian. To ensure adequate amounts of nutrients, vitamins, and minerals, careful planning is necessary and supplements may be needed.

Table 3 lists all of the recipes in this book that are acceptable in the Step 3 Diet when sodium is not restricted. Table 4 lists recipes that are low in sodium and acceptable in the Step 3 Diet.

TABLE 3. *Recipes acceptable for Step 3 in the stepwise approach to treating hyperlipidemia*[a]

[a]These recipes are very low in fat and are identified as "recommended for Type V" in the recipe.

TABLE 3. *(continued)*

TABLE 4. *Low-sodium recipes acceptable in Step 3 of the stepwise approach to treating hyperlipidemia[a]*

[a]These recipes are very low in fat and are identified as "recommended for Type V" in the recipe.

5

Losing Weight and Keeping It Off

Harold Thomas is a 45-year-old Houston attorney: hard-working, busy, successful. When he walked into The Methodist Hospital's Diet Modification Clinic, he weighed 285 pounds. He had tried everything to reduce, losing and regaining hundreds and hundreds of pounds during the past 20 years.

Exactly 1 year later, Thomas weighed 181 pounds. His 6'3" frame was slim and fit. With great relish he reported that a judge had taken to calling him "Skinny." Now, more than 2 years since beginning the program, he still weighs 181 pounds. How did he do it? How did he lose 104 pounds this time without putting it right back on again?

"The food record," Thomas said. "That's the key. It helped me lose weight and is helping me keep it off." Figure 1 presents Thomas' weight loss over a 2-year period. He reached his ideal weight, 181 pounds, at week 52, and has maintained that ideal weight for another year. The food record is one part of a total behavioral treatment program that Thomas completed during his successful attempt to lose over 100 pounds.

BEHAVIORAL APPROACH TO WEIGHT LOSS

The premise underlying behavioral treatment is that for weight loss to occur and be maintained a person must make substantial changes in eating *behavior*. Obesity is believed to result from en-

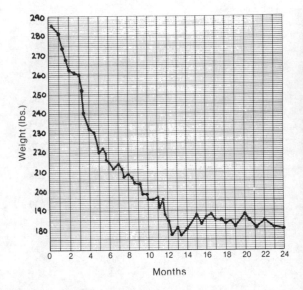

FIG. 1. The behavior modification approach to weight loss requires that a weight loss chart be kept. This chart was kept over a 2-year period by an individual who is following The Living Heart Diet. Ideal weight was attained gradually during the first 12 months and was then maintained during the second year.

vironmental factors, leading to increased calorie intake and/or decreased activity level, not from underlying disease.

Prior to the development of behavioral treatment techniques, most people tried to lose excess weight by dieting alone. Others tried dieting in combination with exercise or medication. A few have even tried fasting, hypnosis, psychotherapy, ear staples, wired jaws, or the potentially dangerous ileal bypass operation. Attempts at weight reduction with these techniques usually involved a frustrating cycle of losing and regaining a few pounds at a time. Unfortunately, for most people, dieting, exercise, medication, or combinations of these are usually unsuccessful over the long term. Doctors who rely on these treatments see little sustained weight loss. Many studies have shown clearly that dieting, exercise, medication, fasting, hypnosis, psychotherapy, ear staples, or wired jaws do not result in any significant long-term success for the great majority of overweight adults.

It is easy to see why these techniques do not work very well. A "diet" is something to do for a while to lose weight. Once the weight is lost, the "diet" is over. If there are no accompanying changes in *behavior*, individuals go back to their old ways and the weight returns. The same holds true for exercise, medication, and other techniques. Only by changing habits can individuals expect any permanent changes in weight. This chapter describes a behavioral treatment program aimed at doing just that: changing weight permanently.

Before making any attempt to lose weight, you must first consult your physician. Then, set a goal weight. Desirable weights for adults are listed in Table 1 in the *Appendix*.

After setting your goal, begin the following program. It consists of 11 steps. The first four steps are the most important: food record, daily weight chart, limiting at-home eating to one place, and slowing down eating. The other seven steps will give you some further helpful tips, but remember that the first four are the critical ones.

After you have followed the four steps for a month, begin the fifth step, which discusses self-rewards. Read the suggestions several times and try to follow them. Add one new step each week, and continue following the suggestions from the previous steps. They are not easy and will require perseverance. Ask your family or

friends to help you. Check off each item after you have done it.

Continue keeping the daily food and weight records until you have reached your goal and have maintained it for a month. You may then discontinue recording and charting, but if your weight creeps up 5 pounds, start again. The same holds true for the other behavioral steps, although we hope that by repeatedly practicing the suggestions many of the steps will become habits that remain with you. Remember, only by developing good habits will you be successful in maintaining your goal weight.

These techniques have worked for others. Give them a chance, and you will be pleasantly surprised with the results.

STEP 1: THE FOOD RECORD

The food record is a simple technique to learn. It is based on the idea that obesity often results from poor eating habits. Until those habits are recognized and changed, weight control will continue to be an unending struggle. *Habit change* is the key to weight loss and proper weight maintenance.

The first step in altering poor eating habits is recognizing them. Recording daily food intake makes you aware of *when*, *where*, and *how much* you eat. Buy yourself a small notebook and mark each page like the food record in Fig. 2. Write your name and the date at the top of the food record. In the first column, TIME, record the exact time you consume any food or beverage except plain water. If you eat breakfast at 8:17 a.m., write "8:17 a.m." In the PLACE column, record where you ate or drank. "Home" is not specific enough. Write "kitchen table" or "couch in den" or "rocker in living room." If you ate in a restaurant, include the name, e.g., "Main Café." In the third column, list the amounts of *all foods and beverages* consumed, e.g., "4 ounces orange juice, 1 egg fried in bacon grease, 2 slices bacon, 2 slices toast, 2 teaspoons margarine, 2 tea-

FOOD RECORD

Name _Harold Thomas_

Date _May 14_

Time	Place	Food: Amount and How Prepared
8:17a N	kitchen table alone	4 ounce glass orange juice 1 egg fried in bacon grease 2 slices bacon 2 slices toast 2 teaspoons stick margarine 2 teaspoons jelly 2-6 ounce cups coffee with sugar (2 teaspoons each) and non-dairy creamer (1 teaspoon each)
10:00a B	living room friend	1 donut 6 ounce cup coffee, black
1:25p N	kitchen table alone	1 ounce bologna 1 ounce American cheese 2 slices bread 1 tablespoon mayonnaise 10 potato chips 12 ounce can coke
4:32p F	couch in den alone	chocolate candy bar 12 ounce can coke
6:35p N	kitchen table alone	1 chicken breast - fried in shortening 1/2 cup mashed potatoes 2 tablespoons cream gravy 1 ear corn-on-cob with 2 teaspoons margarine 2 biscuits 2 teaspoons margarine 8 ounce glass whole milk
10:14p A	couch in den alone	3 x 3 inch square chocolate cake 8 ounce glass whole milk

FIG. 2.   Keeping a food record allows you to observe when, where and how much is eaten. To change undesirable eating habits, you must first become aware of your habits; thus, the time, place and amount of food and how it is prepared must be precisely recorded. In the TIME column, feelings prior to eating are recorded by using the first letter of one of the following adjectives: angry, bored, depressed, fatigued, hungry, starved, tense or neutral.

spoons jelly, 2 cups coffee with 2 teaspoons sugar and 1 teaspoon non-dairy creamer in each." Be specific about how foods are prepared. Remember, everything except plain water must be recorded. Be sure to include coffee, tea, diet drinks, and snacks. Do not forget the sugar and cream in the coffee, the margarine on the bread, or the dressing on the salad. The best time to record your food intake is just before or just after you eat. Be accurate—even when you overeat.

It is also helpful to become aware of your feelings just prior to eating, so under the TIME column write the first letter of the adjective that best describes your mood each time you eat:

Angry	Hungry
Bored	Starved
Depressed	Tense
Fatigued	Neutral

Under the PLACE column, indicate whether you ate alone or with someone, e.g., spouse, child, or neighbor. Your daily food record should resemble Fig. 2.

FOOD RECORD

Name _Harold Thomas_

Date _May 24_

Daily Food Exchanges

Meat	_6 ounces_
Dairy	_2 exchanges_
Fat	_5 exchanges_
Fruit	_3 exchanges_
Bread	_4 exchanges_

Time	Place	Food: Amount and How Prepared	Food Exchanges
8:15a N	kitchen table alone	1 small orange 1 slice toast 2 teaspoons tub margarine 8 ounce glass skim milk 6 ounce cup coffee, black	1 fruit 1 bread 2 fat 1 dairy free
1:25p H	kitchen table alone	tuna salad sandwich 1/2 cup tuna 1/2 stalk celery 1/2 dill pickle 2 teaspoons mayonnaise 2 slices toast 1 leaf lettuce 1 small apple 8 ounce glass iced tea	 2 ounces meat free free 1 fat 2 bread free 1 fruit free
6:05p H	dining room table friend	4 ounce lean ground beef pattie, broiled 1/2 cup rice, boiled in beef bouillon 1 cup broccoli tossed salad (lettuce, tomato, cucumber, green pepper) 4 teaspoons vinegar & oil dressing 3/4 cup strawberries 8 ounce glass iced tea	4 ounces meat 1 bread free free 2 fat 1 fruit free
10:15p N	den couch alone	8 ounce glass skim milk	1 dairy

FIG. 3. In recording food exchanges in the daily food record, you can keep track of food intake without counting calories. The Food Guides at the end of the book (pages 317 to 335) list equivalent food exchanges for almost every type of food and drink. For example, 1 ounce of meat is 1 meat exchange, so a 4-ounce broiled lean ground beef pattie is 4 meat exchanges; 8 ounces of skim milk is 1 dairy exchange.

Food Record with Food Exchanges

After filling out the food record for a week begin recording food exchanges in the fourth column. Use the Food Guides beginning on page 317 to convert your food and drink intake into exchanges. (Refer to Chapter 2, page 30, for a detailed explanation of the food exchange system.) For example, as indicated on page 327, a 1-ounce shot of bourbon is categorized in the bread group and provides about as many calories as 1 bread exchange, so write "1 bread." An 8-ounce glass of skim milk is considered 1 dairy exchange; write in "1 dairy." An ounce of lean meat is 1 meat exchange, so 4 ounces of broiled steak equals "4 meats." The food exchange system is a convenient way to keep track of food intake without counting calories. After you have added the food exchanges, your food record should resemble Fig. 3.

Recording what you eat accomplishes two things: It makes you more aware of how much you are eating, and it reveals your eating habits, some of which will need to be changed if you are to lose weight permanently. It may seem like a chore at first but do not give up. You will soon

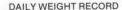

DAILY WEIGHT RECORD

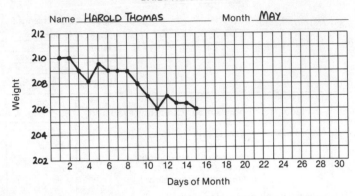

FIG. 4. A daily weight record chart not only helps you keep track of the weight you are losing but it is a source of encouragement to revise bad eating habits and to maintain your diet plan. It should be displayed in a prominent place.

recognize how valuable it is in changing your habits. Continue keeping an accurate record until you reach your goal weight.

STEP 2: DAILY WEIGHT CHART

The second step in changing eating habits is becoming aware of your weight through the use of a Daily Weight Record similar to the one in Fig. 4. Make a weight record for yourself using graph paper. Along the left column, enter your present weight two spaces below the top, giving yourself a maximum weight fluctuation of 2 pounds. Then list 1-pound weight differences on each line below your present weight. Next, across the bottom of the chart, write today's date under the first line, followed by tomorrow's date, and so on, until the chart is filled with days of the month. Use Fig. 4 as your guide. Circle the point that intersects your present weight and today's date.

Weigh yourself daily at the same time, preferably before you dress and have breakfast in the morning, and record your weight on the chart. Connect each day's weight with a straight line so you can monitor gains and losses easily. Do not be concerned about daily fluctuations of a

pound or two as this is normal. Your goal is to see a downward trend.

Hang the chart on the bathroom door near your scale, on your bedroom door, or on your refrigerator. It is important that it hang in a prominent place. *Do not* hide it in a drawer or under a pile of socks. It must be in a place where others can see it. Hanging it within easy view will not only remind you to weigh each day but will also prompt encouragement from family and friends. Think how good you will feel as you see the line moving downward.

STEP 3: LIMIT AT-HOME EATING TO ONE PLACE

After you have filled out the food and weight record for 2 weeks, begin the third step. Your food record may indicate that you are eating in several places in your home. You may be nibbling peanuts while sitting on the sofa watching television or eating your morning cereal standing over the kitchen sink. You may have a late-night sandwich in bed watching Johnny Carson or sample your food while preparing it in the kitchen. For step three, you limit all at-home eating to one place, preferably sitting down at the dining room table. Never eat standing up. If you sometimes eat at the kitchen table and sometimes at the dining room table, it is usually better to get out of the kitchen and limit all eating to the dining room. The only exceptions to the rule are drinking black coffee, plain tea, water, or diet carbonated beverages, which may be consumed anywhere in the home.

In addition to *sitting* at the dining room table whenever you eat or drink, it is also important to eliminate distractions. Turn off the television and the radio. Soft dinner music is acceptable, but save the rock, jazz, or country music and the news or talk shows until after your meal. Reading is not allowed either—and that includes newspapers, magazines, books, and cereal boxes.

What can you do? Enjoy your food! Talk with other people. But above all, pay attention to the act of eating, so that you will feel more satisfied when you finish.

STEP 4: SLOW DOWN

The fourth step, our last major technique, will help you eat more slowly. Many people with a weight problem eat rapidly. It takes about 20 minutes for the brain to receive a signal from the stomach indicating that you are satisfied, so it is important to spend at least that long enjoying your meal. The easiest way to slow the rate of eating is to lay down utensils between bites. That is, take a bite of food, lay your utensils on the table, put your hands in your lap, chew thoroughly, and swallow before taking the next bite. The swallow becomes your cue to pick up the utensils for another bite. If you are eating a food that does not require utensils (e.g., a sandwich), use the same principle: Take a bite, put the food down, place your hands in your lap, chew thoroughly, and swallow. Then pick up the food again for another bite. After finishing a third to a half of your portion, stop for a minute or more before finishing the rest.

If you have trouble remembering to do this,

make a small sign on a folded-over index card saying: *lay down utensils between bites*. Place it by your plate at each meal. The longer you stretch a meal, the less food it will take to feel full.

STEP 5: REWARDING YOURSELF

Losing weight is hard work. We know of no easy way to do it. You can, however, make the task a little less difficult by rewarding yourself for following the eating plan and doing the behavioral assignments. If a person is rewarded for a particular behavior, then that behavior will tend to be repeated. Rewards come from supervisors, spouses, parents, children, or friends and neighbors—or from you. By systematically rewarding yourself for improving your eating behavior, you increase the probability that you will lose weight.

The first step is to identify exactly what is rewarding to you. If someone offered you a lot of money for losing 30 pounds, would you do it? Of course. The principle behind the self-reward technique is similar, except most of us do not have a lot of money to use as a reward. Instead, we use smaller rewards for smaller behavioral changes.

Pleasure connotes different things for different people. Fill out The Living Heart Pleasure Questionnaire (Table 1): Simply put an "X" in the column that indicates how much pleasure each item gives you. For example, the first item listed is "sleeping late." If you do not enjoy sleeping late, put an "X" in the NONE column. If you get A LITTLE pleasure from sleeping late, mark that column. What you are looking for are those activities which give you VERY MUCH pleasure in your daily living. These are the rewards you will program into your weight reduction plan.

After you have filled out the questionnaire, record the activities you rated as most pleasurable in a notebook. Select one of these items each week to reward yourself for completing your behavioral assignments. For example, if you keep a food record listing all food and drink you con-

TABLE 1. *The Living Heart Pleasure Questionnaire*

Activity	None	A little	Much	Very much
Sleeping late	—	—	—	—
Telephoning a friend long distance	—	—	—	—
Watching television	—	—	—	—
Listening to radio	—	—	—	—
Listening to records or tapes	—	—	—	—
Playing cards	—	—	—	—
Doing crossword puzzles	—	—	—	—
Reading books or magazines	—	—	—	—
Dancing	—	—	—	—
Shopping	—	—	—	—
Buying new clothes	—	—	—	—
Buying kitchen appliances	—	—	—	—
Buying records	—	—	—	—
Visiting friends	—	—	—	—
Taking a relaxing bath or shower	—	—	—	—
Attending plays or concerts	—	—	—	—
Attending movies	—	—	—	—
Attending sporting events	—	—	—	—
Golfing	—	—	—	—
Bowling	—	—	—	—
Bicycling	—	—	—	—
Playing tennis	—	—	—	—
Participating in team sports	—	—	—	—
Camping	—	—	—	—
Traveling	—	—	—	—
Gardening	—	—	—	—
Peace and quiet	—	—	—	—
Other activities	—	—	—	—

sume during the week, reward yourself. If "watching television" gives you very much pleasure, then allow time for your favorite show. Tell yourself and others close to you that you are watching the show because you completed your weight loss assignment. If you do not complete the assignment, do not allow yourself to watch the show.

Reward yourself as soon as possible after you have done the required behavior. The only reward you should never use in a weight control program is food. *Never* reward yourself with a hot fudge sundae!

With a little practice, you will find that the reward system encourages you to follow your program, helps you feel good about yourself, and makes the job of losing weight easier.

The Living Heart Pleasure Questionnaire

The Pleasure Questionnaire (Table 1) will help you identify various activities that give you pleasure. Check the column that best describes the amount of pleasure each item gives you. Omit any which do not apply to you. At the end of the questionnaire, add any other activities that give you pleasure.

STEP 6: CONTROL AND CHANGE OF FOOD CONSUMPTION

1. Serve yourself your allotted portion once. To avoid seconds, serve your plate in the kitchen before the meal and keep it warm in the oven while you put any extra food away. You will be less likely to nibble after the meal if leftovers are out of sight when you clean up the dishes.

But I have to have seconds! If one portion is an absolute impossibility for you, divide your allotted portion in half and eat only half at a time. You may have second helpings of vegetables or other "free" foods.

What about my family? Either serve their food in the kitchen too, or keep serving plates as far away from you as possible on the table.

2. Use a slightly smaller plate and spread the food out on the plate. This makes your measured food portions look larger.

But won't a smaller plate look conspicuous on the table? No. People are usually too engrossed in their meal and conversations to notice.

STEP 7: CONTROL OF OBTAINING FOOD

1. Prepare a menu plan for the week with a

regular meal pattern of at least three meals distributed throughout the day. It is best to accustom your body to a regular schedule of eating either medium meals or small meals, if you prefer.

Why can't I have all my calorie allowance once a day at a large meal? Your body is like a machine. It needs "fuel" regularly to function at an optimum level. By eating everything at one time you overload the digestive system. Also, you are more likely to overeat or to indulge in high-calorie snacks if you have deprived yourself of food until dinner. Besides, you enjoy eating—why not engage in this activity three times a day instead of just once?

2. Make a shopping list from your menu plan. Check your refrigerator and pantry to see what you have on hand before making the list. Read newspaper ads and incorporate weekly specials into your meal plan.

3. Do all your grocery shopping after a meal when you are not hungry—never before. It is surprising what extra items you may be tempted to nibble or buy if you go to the store with an empty stomach. Remember, use your list, not your memory!

But I always stop at the store on my way home from work. Try buying food on a regular schedule, e.g., once a week after your evening meal. You will soon find that you are buying less "junk" food and staying within your food budget.

4. Put the grocery bags in the trunk for the ride home to avoid any temptations to snack. Remember, eating in the car is very hazardous and should be avoided.

STEP 8: CONTROL OF EATING CUES

1. Store all food out of sight. You are less likely to snack if you do not see any food on the counter or in glass jars as you walk into the kitchen.

What about foods that are in the house for other members of the family? Store "problem" foods in inaccessible places (e.g., in the freezer or on the back of a top shelf) where you cannot easily reach them. Remember, out of sight, out of mind.

2. Store refrigerated foods (except "free" foods) in opaque containers. When you open the refrigerator, you should see only "free" items, e.g., sliced raw vegetables or low-calorie beverages. Store leftovers in opaque containers and use foil rather than clear plastic for wrapping and covering foods. Removing the light bulb from the refrigerator also discourages between-meal browsing.

3. If you find yourself nibbling while you cook, try brushing your teeth before preparing the food, chewing gum, or if necessary wearing a surgical mask. Try to do as much food preparation as possible when you are not hungry. For example, pack lunches after dinner rather than before breakfast.

4. If possible have someone else scrape the dishes and put away any leftovers. This technique will prevent you from eating foods left on plates, taking one last bite of the mashed potatoes in the pan, or licking the serving utensils.

But I live alone. Reread the techniques suggested in Step 3. Serve your plate and place it in the oven to keep it warm while you store the leftovers in opaque containers. Let the pans soak while you enjoy your dinner. As soon as you finish, scrape your plate directly into the garbage or the disposal and clean up the dishes.

STEP 9: CONTROL OF INDISCRIMINATE EATING

1. *I always want to eat when I'm tired, bored, angry, frustrated, etc. What can I do to avoid a food binge?* First of all, make a list of alternative activities in which you can engage when you feel the urge to eat. These activities may be either enjoyable—a specific hobby, reading, music, sports, a movie—or necessary—cleaning a closet, running an errand, paying bills, doing the laundry. Keep the list in plain view, if possible.

Second, eliminate any "junk" or high-calorie foods from your environment. If you must eat, a lettuce, celery, or cucumber binge is relatively harmless, calorie-wise. Try practicing relaxation techniques at this time. If you are just plain tired, take a short nap.

2. Relaxation. Many of us overeat when we are anxious, tense, angry, lonely, bored, or depressed. We eat as a result of these feelings, not in response to physiological hunger. Relaxation is one way to deal with this tendency—it is not possible to feel anxious and relaxed simultaneously.

Can I teach myself to relax? Most likely you can, and it is not as difficult as you might think. The techniques are presented in many popular books; group classes that teach relaxation are offered in many communities. The techniques take some practice, but most people can actually teach themselves to relax in about 3 weeks if they practice 15 minutes twice a day.

Here is one way: Find a comfortable chair in a quiet room in your home, away from the children, television, and dog. Dress in loosely fitting clothes. Turn down the lights, settle back, close your eyes. For a few minutes, block out all the cares of the day.

Keep your eyes closed and try to imagine yourself standing on a bridge looking down on a black stream of water that is flowing away from you rather slowly. Sitting very brightly, very clearly on top of this black stream of water is a white light. Imagine yourself looking at this white light. As you watch it, it begins to move downstream, and as it goes downstream it becomes smaller and smaller. As it gets smaller it seems brighter, and then it starts to turn. Brighter . . . whiter . . . smaller . . . farther and farther away. You can hardly continue to watch it. Your eyelids are so heavy, your arms so limp. You feel very calm, very relaxed. Begin to count to five, slowly.

One, you are starting to relax. You are going to feel very calm, very relaxed, very good.

Two, you are going into a dream-like state, becoming more relaxed.

Three, you feel calm, relaxed, peaceful.

Four, you are very calm, beginning to drift.

Five, you are slowly drifting off.

You are so calm, secure, peaceful. This is complete relaxation. Linger for about 5 minutes. Then count backward from three to one:

Three, you are waking up. You will feel relaxed when you wake and not at all tired.

Two, you are waking. You will feel refreshed, relaxed, and able to go about your daily chores serenely.

One, open your eyes, move your arms and legs. You feel relaxed, refreshed.

Practice this technique twice a day for 3 weeks. Choose times when you are away from the family, e.g., just before falling asleep at night or after lunch each day. Try to follow a regular practice schedule.

After 3 weeks of practice you should be able to relax yourself fairly rapidly. Use the technique when you catch yourself thinking about food at inappropriate times. For example, when you are watching television and that "psychological hunger" hits, relax yourself instead of wandering into the kitchen for a snack. The feelings of psychological hunger will diminish. Bring yourself out of the relaxed state by counting from three to one and telling yourself you are going to be refreshed and awake.

Does the technique work? The answer is unquestionably "yes" for many people who eat in response to anxiety and stress. Relaxation can help reduce psychological hunger and break the reflexive eating chain. Try it for a few weeks and see if it works for you.

STEP 10: CONTROL WHEN EATING AWAY FROM HOME

1. If you eat out often, it is wise to select a particular restaurant as some of your food requires special attention. A "regular" customer is more likely to get this attention.

2. Be familiar with your eating plan and keep it in mind as you order from the menu, being careful to limit the amount from each food group according to your particular diet plan.

Meat: Ask that all fat be trimmed. The safest choice is a chop, steak, chicken, or fish. Request that the meat be broiled without fat.

Vegetables: Most vegetables are not limited on your eating plan; however, avoid those that are buttered, creamed, or prepared in a sauce containing fat, whole milk, or cheese. Ask that your serving of vegetables be prepared without fat.

Salad: Most salad ingredients are allowed. A vegetable salad is the best choice. A gelatin or fruit salad is also a good selection. Avoid cheese, cream cheese, and dressings prepared from sweet or sour cream.

Fat: Margarine and salad dressings may be selected according to the limitations of your eating plan.

Bread: Saltines, sliced bread, and hard rolls are usually available in restaurants. Avoid hot rolls, biscuits, cornbread, and muffins as these may contain too much saturated fat.

Beverage: Skim milk, vegetable juice, or fruit juice may be selected. You may also wish to have just coffee or tea.

Dessert: Your best choice is fresh or unsweetened fruit. Sherbet, fruit ice, or gelatin is also permissible.

3. *If I am going to an unfamiliar restaurant, what should I do?* Call ahead. Tell the *maître d'* that you follow a special diet and ask his suggestions in ordering.

4. *How about airplanes?* When booked on a meal flight, call your airline at least 24 hours in advance and request a low-calorie meal. Then, when boarding the plane, tell a flight attendant that you called ahead and ordered the meal.

5. *What do I do at a party?* First of all, eat something before going to the party. Do not expect yourself to maintain control when you are hungry. Hopefully, the hostess will provide some "legal" nibbles: fresh vegetables, low-calorie beverages, or plain popcorn. If you suspect the contrary, bring a plate of vegetables with a low-calorie dip. Your hostess will appreciate your thoughtfulness, and you will have something safe to eat. At a dinner party, eat small amounts of the rich foods and fill up on vegetables and salad. Passing up a rich dessert is rarely questioned after a large meal. Just say the meal was delicious, and you are full.

6. *What should I do when the hostess starts serving generous portions of a rich dessert?* Keep your eyes away from the dessert. Explain to the hostess that you have eaten too much and want to limit dessert to "just coffee" after such a delicious meal. If temptation intervenes, ask for a small serving and eat only half.

7. *What about buffet tables laden with food?* STOP! Take a step backward and survey the table first. Decide exactly what you will eat and have small servings. Carry your plate to an area where you can be seated to eat. Avoid "grazing" beside the buffet table. Converse elsewhere. Limit second helpings to low-calorie foods.

8. *I am sitting next to a bowl of peanuts, my favorite snack. Help!* Either move yourself or the bowl of peanuts to another area of the room. Holding your drink with both hands will also help.

9. *The host keeps pushing drinks. How do I refuse?* Sip slowly. After one alcoholic beverage, switch to club soda, diet soda, tomato juice, or water with a wedge of lemon. Or say, "I'm skipping this round."

10. *What about when I am on the convention or banquet circuit?* Talk more, eat less.

STEP 11: MAINTAINING GOAL WEIGHT

How can I maintain my weight once I reach my goal?

1. Continue to keep your food record for 1 month after you have reached your goal weight.

This acts as a safeguard against regaining any weight as you gradually add foods to your eating plan.

2. Always maintain awareness of your weight by weighing daily and continuing to graph the pounds.

3. Set a 5-pound weight gain limit for yourself. If you exceed the limit, review the steps and begin to follow them again.

4. Continue to use those new eating habits you have developed. By doing so, your weight should not fluctuate more than 5 pounds. Guard against redeveloping poor eating habits by occasionally reading through the behavior modification steps.

5. There may be times (i.e., vacation) when you will be prone to gain. Remember to lose weight before you go. If you do not lose the pounds, do not allow yourself to splurge. The old saw of "eating today and dieting tomorrow" will lead only to weight gain.

6. If you hit a period in your life when problems stack up, do not add to them by trying to lose weight; just "aim to maintain."

7. Give away or tailor the clothes that are now "too large." The excess seam allowances should be cut off. Purchase some new attractive clothes that fit well. Do not allow any "big" clothes to occupy space in your closet as a temptation to return to your old size.

8. If you are at goal weight, you will look and feel good. Enjoy.

Recipes

The recipes in this section comply with The Living Heart Diet. Each is prepared with ingredients low in cholesterol and saturated fat. Many recipes are designed for individuals who need to lose weight, control diabetes, restrict sodium, or who have elevated levels of cholesterol or triglycerides. Foods which should be restricted, limited, or avoided—butter, sour cream, whole milk, or high-fat cheese—are not used in the recipes. Each recipe is analyzed for its nutrients, and the diets for which the recipe is recommended are noted. This information is particularly helpful to those of you who will be using the exchange system or who need to calculate calories, carbohydrate, protein, fat, or sodium.

The recipes are divided into two sections:

1. *Living Heart Diet Recipes,* and
2. *Low-Sodium Living Heart Diet Recipes*.

Each of these sections includes:

1. low-calorie recipes;
2. recipes for diabetics;
3. recipes for persons with Type I, IIa, IIb, III, IV, or V hyperlipidemia; and
4. very low fat recipes to accommodate Step 3 treatment of hyperlipidemia (identified in the recipe as "recommended for Type V diets").

Section I.
The Living Heart Diet: Recipes

LIVING HEART DIET RECIPES

Although recipes for this diet are low in cholesterol and saturated fat, some contain concentrated sources of calories—sugar, honey, oil—and should be used in moderation.

LOW-CALORIE RECIPES

Some of the recipes are designated "low-calorie," and the exchanges for meat, bread, dairy products, fat, fruit, and vegetables are given. Individuals who want to lose weight or control their triglycerides may not need to use the "vegetable" exchange. Usually nonstarchy vegetables can be used freely on low-calorie diets. However, those of you who are diabetics or have difficulty controlling your weight should take into account the carbohydrate and protein calories contained in them. These exchanges correspond to amounts listed in the food groups on pages 317 to 335.

DIABETIC DIET

The recipes for diabetics have exchanges similar to those in the diabetic booklet entitled *Ex-*

change Lists for Meal Planning distributed by the American Dietetic Association and the American Diabetes Association, Inc. (1976).

TYPE I HYPERLIPIDEMIA DIET

Only recipes containing very little or no fat per serving are recommended for the Type I hyperlipidemia individual, as fat is almost totally restricted on this diet.

TYPE IIA HYPERLIPIDEMIA DIET

Persons following this diet may use any recipe in this book. A word of caution, however: All of our nutrient analyses are based on the use of corn oil, and because a high P/S ratio is an important aspect of the Type IIa diet, safflower oil should be used in place of corn oil in the recipes. This simple modification is a means of increasing the P/S ratio.

TYPES IIB, III, IV, AND V HYPERLIPIDEMIA DIETS

The recipes for the hyperlipidemia types have a controlled number of calories. That is, the concentrated sources of carbohydrate, fat, and alcohol are limited. The exchanges can be used to determine portion size and to control calories and carbohydrate. For the Type V person, recipes that are not designated "recommended for the Type V diet" can be used, but only by carefully counting the fat exchanges.

VERY LOW FAT RECIPES

Persons who must progress to Step 2 or 3 of The Living Heart Diet for treatment of hyperlipidemia may use the same recipes that are used in the Type V diet.

SPECIAL INGREDIENTS

Some of the ingredients used for the preparation and analysis of recipes in The Living Heart Diet are:
Corn oil
Corn oil tub margarine
Skim milk yogurt made at home
Very lean ground meat—round steak trimmed and ground
Low-fat cheese—any cheese containing 8% fat or less, or one of the special cheeses containing polyunsaturated fat
Imitation bacon bits
Egg substitute—cholesterol-free
Cornbread mix—any brand that does not contain shortening or eggs

Appetizers

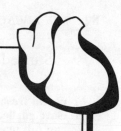

VEGETABLE APPETIZERS

Relish Stuffed Tomatoes

3 jalapeño peppers, seeded and finely chopped
½ cup finely chopped celery
3 tablespoons finely chopped green onion, including tops
2 tablespoons wine vinegar
1 teaspoon sugar
¼ teaspoon salt
40 cherry tomatoes

1. Combine jalapeños, celery, onion, vinegar, sugar, and salt.
2. Slice top off each tomato and scoop out insides.
3. Mix tomato insides with relish mixture and fill tomatoes.

Yield: 40 tomatoes

1 tomato contains:

Cal	Prot	Fat	Carb	Sat	Mono	Poly	Chol	Na
6	0	0.1	1	0	0	0.1	0	17

Exchanges: 1–4 tomatoes = free; 5 tomatoes = ½ bread
Recommended for: The Living Heart; Low Calorie; Diabetic; Types I, IIa, IIb, III, IV, and V Diets

Pickled Beet Relish

¼ cup water
½ cup white vinegar
¼ cup brown sugar, firmly packed
¼ teaspoon salt
½ teaspoon ground cinnamon
¼ teaspoon ground cloves
1 can (16 ounces) beets, drained and chopped

1. Bring water and spices to a boil in a saucepan. Pour over beets and let stand at least 8 hours.
2. Store in covered jar in refrigerator.

Yield: 2 cups

1 tablespoon contains:

Cal	Prot	Fat	Carb	Sat	Mono	Poly	Chol	Na
11	0	0	3	0	0	0	0	43

Exchanges: 1–2 tablespoons = free; 3 tablespoons = ½ bread
Recommended for: The Living Heart; Low Calorie; Types I, IIa, IIb, III, IV, and V Diets

Abbreviations: **Cal,** calories; **Prot,** protein; **Carb,** carbohydrate; **Sat,** saturated fat; **Mono,** monounsaturated fat; **Poly,** polyunsaturated fat; **Chol,** cholesterol; **Na,** sodium. Protein, fat, carbohydrate, saturated fat, monounsaturated fat, and polyunsaturated fat are expressed in *grams.* Cholesterol and sodium are expressed in *milligrams.*

Stuffed Mushroom Caps

½ **pound fresh mushrooms**
1 **clove garlic, minced**
¼ **cup tub magarine**
¼ **teaspoon salt**
⅛ **teaspoon pepper**
2 **tablespoons chopped, fresh parsley**
2 **tablespoons minced onion**
¼ **cup fine dry bread crumbs**

1. Preheat oven to 350°F.
2. Clean mushrooms, removing stems.
3. Chop stems finely and sauté with garlic in margarine.
4. Add salt, pepper, parsley, and onion. Remove from heat and add bread crumbs.
5. Fill each mushroom cap with stuffing and place in a shallow baking dish.
6. Bake 10–15 minutes.

Yield: about 20

1 mushroom cap contains:

Cal	Prot	Fat	Carb	Sat	Mono	Poly	Chol	Na
27	0	2.4	1	0.4	0.8	1.0	0	66

Exchanges: 1 mushroom cap = free; 2 mushroom caps = ½ fat
Recommended for: The Living Heart; Low Calorie; Diabetic; Types IIa, IIb, III, and IV Diets

Tangy Italian Mushrooms

½ **pound fresh mushrooms, sliced**
¾ **cup low-calorie Italian dressing**
1 **tablespoon tub margarine**

1. To marinate mushrooms, place in Italian dressing for at least 1 hour or overnight.
2. Drain mushrooms and sauté in margarine in skillet or chafing dish for 5 minutes.
3. Serve warm using either toothpicks or relish forks.

Yield: 2 cups

⅓ cup contains:

Cal	Prot	Fat	Carb	Sat	Mono	Poly	Chol	Na
28	1	2.0	2	0.4	0.7	0.9	0	29

Exchanges: ⅓ cup = 1 vegetable
Recommended for: The Living Heart; Low Calorie; Diabetic; Types IIa, IIb, III, and IV Diets

Relish Tray Ideas

Arrange a combination of the following vegetables on a tray or dish to use as dippers:

Cucumber Flowers
1. Run the tines of a fork down the length of an unpeeled cucumber.
2. Cut thin slices crosswise.

Carrot or Celery Curls
1. Slice carrots or celery lengthwise in paper-thin slices.
2. Chill in ice water until curled.

Pickle Fans
1. Make four lengthwise cuts almost to the ends of small gherkins.
2. Spread open gently as a fan.

Cauliflowerettes or Broccoli Flowerettes
1. Break off small buds from head of cauliflower or spear of broccoli.

You may also use green pepper strips or rings, mushroom caps, radish buds, summer squash slices or strips, turnip slices, cherry tomatoes, olives, or cocktail onions.

Seaside Cherry Tomatoes

40 **cherry tomatoes**
 salt
 pepper
1 **can (3 ounces) tiny smoked oysters, drained**

1. Slice down through center of each tomato almost to base.
2. Lightly season tomato inside with salt and pepper and slip an oyster into each tomato.

Yield: 40 tomatoes

1 tomato contains:

Cal	Prot	Fat	Carb	Sat	Mono	Poly	Chol	Na
6	0	0.1	1	0	0	0.1	1	30

Exchanges: 1–4 tomatoes = free; 5 tomatoes = ½ bread
Recommended for: The Living Heart; Low Calorie; Diabetic; Types I, IIa, IIb, III, IV, and V Diets

Cherry Tomato Stars

1 cup low-fat cottage cheese
2 tablespoons finely chopped green pepper
2 tablespoons finely chopped celery
3 tablespoons finely chopped green onion
¼ cup mayonnaise
30 cherry tomatoes
paprika

1. Mix together cottage cheese, green pepper, celery, onion, and mayonnaise.
2. Cut each cherry tomato into fourths almost to the base. Do not cut completely through the tomato.
3. Fill with cottage cheese mixture and sprinkle with paprika.

Yield: 30 tomatoes

1 cherry tomato contains:

Cal	Prot	Fat	Carb	Sat	Mono	Poly	Chol	Na
26	1	1.7	2	0.4	0.4	0.8	2	43

Exchanges: 1 cherry tomato = free; 2 cherry tomatoes = 1 fat
Recommended for: The Living Heart; Low Calorie; Diabetic; Types IIa, IIb, III, and IV Diets

Variation:

Fill four small regular tomatoes and serve as salad.

1 regular tomato contains:

Cal	Prot	Fat	Carb	Sat	Mono	Poly	Chol	Na
194	10	12.5	12	2.7	2.7	6.0	14	322

Exchanges: 1 regular tomato = 1 dairy, 2½ fats
Recommended for: The Living Heart; Low Calorie; Diabetic; Types IIa, IIb, III, and IV Diets

FRUIT APPETIZERS

Fresh Fruit Kabobs

1 fresh pineapple peeled and cubed
1 pint fresh strawberries
10 dried pitted prunes

1. Alternate chilled fruits on small skewers.
2. To serve, arrange kabobs on platter or stick skewers into a whole pineapple.

Yield: 10 servings

Variation:

Use canned, fresh, or frozen fruits of choice. If fresh bananas or apples are used, dip in lemon or orange juice to prevent discoloration.

1 serving contains:

Cal	Prot	Fat	Carb	Sat	Mono	Poly	Chol	Na
61	1	0.3	16	0	0	0.3	0	2

Exchanges: 1 serving = 1½ fruits
Recommended for: The Living Heart; Low Calorie; Diabetic; Types I, IIa, IIb, III, IV, and V Diets

Abbreviations: **Cal,** calories; **Prot,** protein; **Carb,** carbohydrate; **Sat,** saturated fat; **Mono,** monounsaturated fat; **Poly,** polyunsaturated fat; **Chol,** cholesterol; **Na,** sodium. Protein, fat, carbohydrate, saturated fat, monounsaturated fat, and polyunsaturated fat are expressed in *grams*. Cholesterol and sodium are expressed in *milligrams*.

Spicy Pineapple Pickups

1 **can (16 ounces) pineapple chunks, packed in own juice, drained, reserving liquid**
⅓ **cup vinegar**
½ **cup sugar**
2 **whole cloves**
1 **cinnamon stick**

1. To ⅓ cup of pineapple juice, add vinegar, sugar, and spices. Simmer for 8 minutes.
2. Add pineapple chunks and heat until just boiling. Remove from heat.
3. Chill 1–2 days.
4. Drain and serve speared with toothpicks.

Yield: 2 cups

¼ cup contains:

Cal	Prot	Fat	Carb	Sat	Mono	Poly	Chol	Na
49	0	0.1	13	0	0	0.1	0	1

Exchanges: ¼ cup = 1 fruit
Recommended for: The Living Heart; Low Calorie; Types I, IIa, IIb, III, IV, and V Diets

CRISPY APPETIZERS

Guacamole Nachos

12 **soft corn tortillas**
12 **ounces low-fat cheese**
12 **jalapeño peppers, seeded**
1 **cup Guacamole (see recipe, page 158)**

1. Preheat oven to 400°F.
2. Cut each tortilla into six wedges, place on an ungreased baking sheet, and heat 8–10 minutes or until crisp.
3. Reduce oven temperature to 350°F.
4. Cut cheese into small pieces and place a piece on each toasted chip.
5. Slice each jalapeño into six pieces and place on top of cheese.

6. Heat in oven until cheese melts.
7. Remove from oven and top with Guacamole.

Yield: 72 nachos

1 nacho contains:

Cal	Prot	Fat	Carb	Sat	Mono	Poly	Chol	Na
26	1	0.9	3	0.3	0.3	0.1	2	88

Exchanges: 1 nacho = free; 2 nachos = ½ bread, ½ fat
Recommended for: The Living Heart; Diabetic; Types IIa, IIb, III, and IV Diets

Nippy Nachos

12 **soft corn tortillas**
12 **ounces low-fat cheese**
12 **jalapeño peppers, seeded**

1. Preheat oven to 400°F.
2. Cut each tortilla into six wedges, place on an ungreased baking sheet, and heat 8–10 minutes or until crisp.
3. Reduce oven temperature to 350°F.
4. Cut cheese into small pieces and place a piece on each toasted chip.
5. Slice each jalapeno into six pieces and place on top of cheese.
6. Heat in oven until cheese is melted.

Yield: 72 nachos

Variations:
Add 1 cup refried beans or ¾ cup onion slices with cheese.

1 nacho contains:

Cal	Prot	Fat	Carb	Sat	Mono	Poly	Chol	Na
21	1	0.4	3	0.2	0.1	0	2	83

Exchanges: 1 nacho = free; 2 nachos = ½ bread
Recommended for: The Living Heart; Low Calorie; Diabetic; Types IIa, IIb, III, IV, and V Diets

Toasted Tortilla Chips

1 **package (9 ounces) soft corn tortillas**
  salt *or* garlic salt *or* taco seasoning mix

1. Preheat oven to 400°F.
2. Cut each tortilla into six wedges and sprinkle with desired seasoning.
3. Toast 8–10 minutes or until crisp.

Yield: 6 dozen chips

1 chip contains:

Cal	Prot	Fat	Carb	Sat	Mono	Poly	Chol	Na
12	0	0.1	2	0	0	0	0	17

Exchanges: 6 chips = 1 bread
Recommended for: The Living Heart; Low Calorie; Diabetic; Types I, IIa, IIb, III, IV, and V Diets

Texas Scramble

5 **cups pretzel sticks**
5 **cups small, round oat cereal**
5 **cups small, square cereal**
2 **cups walnut pieces**
⅔ **cup oil**
½ **tablespoon garlic salt**
½ **tablespoon onion salt**
½ **tablespoon celery salt**
1 **tablespoon Worcestershire sauce**

1. Preheat oven to 250°F.
2. Place pretzels, cereals, and nuts in small roasting pan or 9 × 13-inch baking pan.
3. Mix the oil, seasonings, and Worcestershire sauce, sprinkle over top of cereal mixture and toss well.
4. Bake 60 minutes, stirring occasionally.

Yield: 17 cups

½ cup contains:

Cal	Prot	Fat	Carb	Sat	Mono	Poly	Chol	Na
139	2	9.3	13	1.1	2.0	5.6	0	249

Exchanges: ½ cup = 1 bread, 1½ fats
Recommended for: The Living Heart; Diabetic; Types IIa, IIb, III, and IV Diets

Pastry Cheese Puffs

½ **cup shredded low-fat cheese**
2 **tablespoons tub margarine**
5 **tablespoons flour**
⅛ **teaspoon salt**
¼ **teaspoon paprika**
12 **walnut halves, cocktail onions, olives, or pickled vegetables**

1. Preheat oven to 400°F.
2. Blend cheese with margarine. Mix in flour, salt, and paprika.
3. Wrap 1–2 teaspoons dough around each walnut or vegetable and place on ungreased baking sheet.
4. Bake 15 minutes.

Yield: 12 puffs

Note: Puffs can be frozen on sheet before baking. When frozen, transfer to plastic bag. Remove from freezer and bake according to directions.

1 puff with walnut contains:

Cal	Prot	Fat	Carb	Sat	Mono	Poly	Chol	Na
50	2	3.5	3	0.7	1.0	1.7	2	117

Exchanges: 2 puffs with walnut = ½ bread, 1½ fats;
2 puffs with onion, olive, or vegetables = ½ bread, 1 fat
Recommended for: The Living Heart; Diabetic; Types IIa, IIb, III, and IV Diets

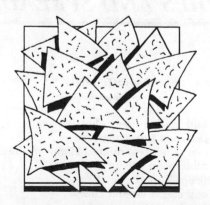

Abbreviations: **Cal,** calories; **Prot,** protein; **Carb,** carbohydrate; **Sat,** saturated fat; **Mono,** monounsaturated fat; **Poly,** polyunsaturated fat; **Chol,** cholesterol; **Na,** sodium. Protein, fat, carbohydrate, saturated fat, monounsaturated fat, and polyunsaturated fat are expressed in *grams.* Cholesterol and sodium are expressed in *milligrams.*

Quick Pizza Snacks

1 **can (10¾ ounces) condensed tomato soup, undiluted**
1 **clove garlic, minced**
¼ **teaspoon dried oregano**
50 **saltines or other low-fat crackers**
¾ **pound low-fat cheese, sliced**
6 **fresh mushrooms, sliced**
1 **green pepper, cut into small slices**

1. Preheat oven to 400°F.
2. Combine soup, garlic, and oregano. Let stand 20–30 minutes.
3. Top each cracker with 1 teaspoon sauce, a slice of cheese, and a mushroom or green pepper slice.
4. Bake until cheese melts, about 10 minutes.

Yield: 50 pizzas

1 snack contains:

Cal	Prot	Fat	Carb	Sat	Mono	Poly	Chol	Na
22	1	0.6	3	0.2	0.2	0.1	2	118

Exchanges: 3 snacks = ½ bread, ½ fat
Recommended for: The Living Heart; Low Calorie; Diabetic; Types IIa, IIb, III, IV, and V Diets

DIPS AND SPREADS

Clam Dip

2 **tablespoons finely chopped onion**
1 **teaspoon tub margarine**
1 **can (7 ounces) minced clams, drained**
1 **tablespoon catsup**
2–3 **drops Tabasco**
1 **cup cubed low-fat cheese**
1 **teaspoon Worcestershire sauce**

1. Sauté onion in margarine.
2. Add remaining ingredients and heat, stirring constantly, until cheese melts.

3. Serve with fresh vegetables or Toasted Tortilla Chips (see recipe, page 85).

Yield: 2 cups

1 tablespoon contains:

Cal	Prot	Fat	Carb	Sat	Mono	Poly	Chol	Na
15	2	0.5	6	0.2	0.1	0.1	6	84

Exchanges: 1 tablespoon = free; 2 tablespoons = ½ meat
Recommended for: The Living Heart; Low Calorie; Diabetic; Types IIa, IIb, III, IV, and V Diets

Chili Con Queso

2 **pounds low-fat cheese**
1 **can (10 ounces) Italian style tomatoes with green chilies**

1. Melt cheese slowly in saucepan or fondue pot.
2. Stir in tomatoes.
3. Dip using fresh vegetables or Toasted Tortilla Chips (see recipe, page 85).

Yield: about 3 cups

1 tablespoon contains:

Cal	Prot	Fat	Carb	Sat	Mono	Poly	Chol	Na
35	4	1.1	2	0.7	0.3	0	7	298

Exchanges: 1 tablespoon = ½ dairy
Recommended for: The Living Heart; Diabetic; Types IIa, IIb, III, and IV Diets

Broccoli Cheese Dip

¾ **cup chopped celery**
1 **small onion, chopped**
¼ **pound fresh mushrooms, chopped**
¼ **cup plus 1 tablespoon tub margarine**
¼ **cup flour**
2 **cups skim milk**
1 **pound low-fat cheese, cubed**
2 **cloves garlic, minced**
1 **package (10 ounces) frozen chopped broccoli, cooked and drained**

2 drops Tabasco
⅛ teaspoon red pepper
⅛ teaspoon Worcestershire sauce
⅛ teaspoon salt
⅛ teaspoon pepper

1. Sauté celery, onion, and mushrooms in 1 tablespoon margarine. Set aside.
2. Melt ¼ cup margarine in a separate saucepan. Remove from heat.
3. Stir in flour until smooth.
4. Add milk all at once and heat, stirring constantly, until sauce is thick.
5. Add cubed low-fat cheese to white sauce a little at a time, stirring until thoroughly melted.
6. Stir in remaining ingredients.
7. Pour into a chafing dish to serve hot, or refrigerate and serve cold.
8. Serve with fresh vegetables or Toasted Tortilla Chips (see recipe, page 85).

Yield: 6 cups

1 tablespoon contains:

Cal	Prot	Fat	Carb	Sat	Mono	Poly	Chol	Na
18	1	0.9	1	0.3	0.3	0.3	2	86

Exchanges: 1 tablespoon = free; 2 tablespoons = ½ dairy
Recommended for: The Living Heart; Low Calorie; Diabetic; Types IIa, IIb, III, IV, and V Diets

Chip and Vegetable Dip

½ bouillon cube
¼ cup hot water
2 cups low-fat cottage cheese
½ teaspoon onion salt

1. Dissolve bouillon cube in hot water.
2. Mix all ingredients in blender until smooth.
3. Dip with fresh vegetables.

Yield: 2¼ cups

Variations:

Add one of the following: ⅛ teaspoon garlic powder or 2 tablespoons chopped chives.

1 tablespoon contains:

Cal	Prot	Fat	Carb	Sat	Mono	Poly	Chol	Na
11	2	0.2	0	0.2	0.1	0	1	87

Exchanges: 2 tablespoons = free; 3 tablespoons = ½ dairy
Recommended for: The Living Heart; Low Calorie; Diabetic; Types IIa, IIb, III, IV, and V Diets

Guacamole Dip

3 avocados, peeled and mashed
1 tomato, chopped
1 onion, chopped
1 jalapeño pepper, seeded
¼ teaspoon salt
¼ teaspoon pepper
½ teaspoon sugar
¼ cup mayonnaise
¼ cup lemon juice

1. Combine all ingredients with electric mixer or blender until smooth.
2. Store in covered container with avocado seed in center.
3. Dip using fresh vegetables or Toasted Tortilla Chips (see recipe, page 85).

Yield: approximately 2 cups

1 tablespoon contains:

Cal	Prot	Fat	Carb	Sat	Mono	Poly	Chol	Na
50	1	4.8	0.2	0.9	1.8	1.2	1	29

Exchanges: 1 tablespoon = 1 fat
Recommended for: The Living Heart; Diabetic; Types IIa, IIb, III, and IV Diets

Abbreviations: **Cal,** calories; **Prot,** protein; **Carb,** carbohydrate; **Sat,** saturated fat; **Mono,** monounsaturated fat; **Poly,** polyunsaturated fat; **Chol,** cholesterol; **Na,** sodium. Protein, fat, carbohydrate, saturated fat, monounsaturated fat, and polyunsaturated fat are expressed in *grams.* Cholesterol and sodium are expressed in *milligrams.*

Hearty Cheese Fondue

1½ **cups buttermilk**
  3 **tablespoons flour**
  1 **pound low-fat cheese, cubed**
  ½ **teaspoon dry mustard**
  ⅛ **teaspoon garlic powder**

1. Combine buttermilk and flour in a saucepan.
2. Heat to a simmer but do not boil.
3. Gradually add cheese, stirring well, until cheese is melted.
4. Add seasonings and place in fondue pot over low flame.
5. Dip using bread cubes, cherry tomatoes, raw cauliflowerettes, or other vegetables.

Yield: 3 cups

Variation:
Decrease buttermilk to 1¼ cups and add ¼ cup dry sherry.

1 tablespoon contains:

Cal	Prot	Fat	Carb	Sat	Mono	Poly	Chol	Na
22	2	0.6	2	0.4	0.2	0	4	151

Exchanges: 1 tablespoon = free; 2 tablespoons = ½ meat
Recommended for: The Living Heart; Low Calorie; Diabetic; Types IIa, IIb, III, IV, and V Diets

Taco Dip

  ½ **cup low-fat cottage cheese**
  ¼ **cup catsup**
  1 **tablespoon taco seasoning mix**
  1 **teaspoon horseradish**
  ½ **teaspoon salt**
  ½ **cup skim milk yogurt**

1. Combine cottage cheese and catsup in blender until smooth.
2. Add taco mix, horseradish, and salt.
3. Place in a bowl, fold in yogurt, cover, and chill.
4. Serve with fresh vegetables or Toasted Tortilla Chips (see recipe, page 85).

Yield: 1¼ cups

1 tablespoon contains:

Cal	Prot	Fat	Carb	Sat	Mono	Poly	Chol	Na
12	1	0.1	2	0.1	0	0	1	313

Exchanges: 1–2 tablespoons = free; 3 tablespoons = ½ meat
Recommended for: The Living Heart; Low Calorie; Diabetic; Types IIa, IIb, III, IV, and V Diets

Onion Dip

  2 **cups low-fat cottage cheese**
  1 **tablespoon lemon juice**
  ¼ **teaspoon salt**
2–4 **tablespoons skim milk**
  1 **envelope dehydrated onion soup mix**

1. Mix cottage cheese, lemon juice, and salt in blender. Add skim milk.
2. Place in bowl and stir in soup mix.
3. Chill at least 15 minutes before serving, with fresh vegetables.

Yield: 2 cups

1 tablespoon contains:

Cal	Prot	Fat	Carb	Sat	Mono	Poly	Chol	Na
13	2	0.3	1	0.2	0.1	0	1	98

Exchanges: 1–2 tablespoons = free; 3 tablespoons = ½ meat
Recommended for: The Living Heart; Low Calorie; Diabetic; Types IIa, IIb, III, IV, and V Diets

Cheese Spread

  2 **cups Mock Cream Cheese (see recipe, page 90)**
  ½ **pound low-fat cheese, cubed**
  1 **tablespoon chopped pimento**
  1 **tablespoon chopped green pepper**
  1 **tablespoon finely chopped onion**
  2 **teaspoons Worcestershire sauce**
  1 **teaspoon lemon juice**
  ⅛ **teaspoon red pepper**
  ⅛ **teaspoon salt**
  1 **cup finely chopped pecans**

1. Combine cheeses.
2. Mix in remaining ingredients except pecans and form into log or ball.
3. Press pecans over surface and chill.

Yield: about 3 cups

1 tablespoon contains:

Cal	Prot	Fat	Carb	Sat	Mono	Poly	Chol	Na
51	3	4.1	1	0.8	1.9	1.3	2	143

Exchanges: 1 tablespoon = ½ meat, ½ fat
Recommended for: The Living Heart; Diabetic; Types IIa, IIb, III, and IV Diets

Pimento Cheese Spread

1 pound low-fat cheese, cubed
1 jar (3 ounces) pimentos, drained
½ cup mayonnaise

1. Blend half of the cheese cubes, the pimentos, and the mayonnaise in blender or mash thoroughly using a fork.
2. Blend in remaining cheese cubes and chill.

Yield: about 2 cups

1 tablespoon contains:

Cal	Prot	Fat	Carb	Sat	Mono	Poly	Chol	Na
51	3	3.6	2	1.0	0.8	1.4	7	245

Exchanges: 1 tablespoon = ½ meat, ½ fat
Recommended for: The Living Heart; Diabetic; Types IIa, IIb, III, and IV Diets

Variation:

Place Pimento Cheese Spread in 4 celery ribs and cut into 2-inch chunks.

Yield: about 20 pieces

1 piece contains:

Cal	Prot	Fat	Carb	Sat	Mono	Poly	Chol	Na
42	2	2.9	2	0.8	0.7	1.1	6	209

Exchanges: 1 piece = ½ dairy
Recommended for: The Living Heart; Diabetic; Types IIa, IIb, III, and IV Diets

Tropical Cheese Spread

½ cup low-fat cottage cheese
¼ cup crushed pineapple, drained
1 teaspoon lemon juice

1. Combine all ingredients thoroughly in blender or with electric mixer.
2. Serve as a sandwich filling or spread on toast or allowed crackers.

Yield: ¾ cup

1 tablespoon contains:

Cal	Prot	Fat	Carb	Sat	Mono	Poly	Chol	Na
12	1	0.2	1	0.1	0.1	0	1	38

Exchanges: 1–2 tablespoons = free; 3 tablespoons = ½ meat
Recommended for: The Living Heart; Low Calorie; Diabetic; Types IIa, IIb, III, IV, and V Diets

"Help Your Heart" Sour Cream

1 cup low-fat cottage cheese
2 teaspoons lemon juice

1. Place ingredients in blender and blend 20 seconds.
2. Use in any recipe that calls for sour cream. This may be added to hot dishes at the last moment.

Yield: 1 cup

1 tablespoon contains:

Cal	Prot	Fat	Carb	Sat	Mono	Poly	Chol	Na
13	2	0.3	1	0.2	0.1	0	1	57

Exchanges: 1–2 tablespoons = free; 3 tablespoons = ½ meat
Recommended for: The Living Heart; Low Calorie; Diabetic; Types IIa, IIb, III, IV, and V Diets

Abbreviations: **Cal,** calories; **Prot,** protein; **Carb,** carbohydrate; **Sat,** saturated fat; **Mono,** monounsaturated fat; **Poly,** polyunsaturated fat; **Chol,** cholesterol; **Na,** sodium. Protein, fat, carbohydrate, saturated fat, monounsaturated fat, and polyunsaturated fat are expressed in *grams.* Cholesterol and sodium are expressed in *milligrams.*

Mock Cream Cheese

1 cup low-fat cottage cheese
¼ cup tub margarine

1. Rinse cottage cheese with cold water.
2. Drain well, pressing with fork to squeeze all water out.
3. Mix drained cottage cheese and margarine in blender, using spatula to scrape sides of container.
4. Refrigerate in a covered container. Consistency will be slightly softer than regular cream cheese.
5. Use in any recipe that calls for cream cheese.

Yield: about 1 cup

1 tablespoon contains:

Cal	Prot	Fat	Carb	Sat	Mono	Poly	Chol	Na
38	2	3.1	1	0.7	1.1	1.3	1	92

Exchanges: 1 tablespoon = 1 fat
Recommended for: The Living Heart; Low Calorie; Diabetic; Types IIa, IIb, III, IV, and V Diets

Herb Spread

1 cup dry garbanzo beans (2 cups cooked)
⅓ cup Brazil nuts, chopped
¼ teaspoon garlic powder
¼ teaspoon dried oregano
¼ teaspoon mustard powder
2 tablespoons chopped chives
¼ teaspoon dried sage

1. Soak beans overnight in water.
2. Drain beans and combine with remaining ingredients in blender until smooth.
3. Place in double boiler over boiling water.
4. Cover and cook 30 minutes, stirring occasionally.
5. Mold in small loaf pans rinsed with cold water and refrigerate overnight.
6. Serve with cucumber slices.

Yield: 2 pounds

¼ cup contains:

Cal	Prot	Fat	Carb	Sat	Mono	Poly	Chol	Na
105	5	4.2	13	1.0	1.3	1.6	0	2

Exchanges: ¼ cup = 1 meat, ½ bread
Recommended for: The Living Heart; Low Calorie; Diabetic; Types IIa, IIb, III, IV, and V Diets

Garbanzo Spread

2⅓ cups cooked garbanzo beans, drained, reserve liquid
¼ cup chopped onion
½ cup thinly sliced celery
¼ package (0.6 ounce) Italian salad dressing seasoning
2–3 drops Tabasco
½ teaspoon dry mustard
2 tablespoons chopped, fresh parsley
½ teaspoon salt

1. Combine all ingredients in blender container and blend until smooth, adding liquid from garbanzo beans as needed.
2. Serve as dip or spread for vegetables or allowed crackers.

Yield: 2½ cups

¼ cup contains:

Cal	Prot	Fat	Carb	Sat	Mono	Poly	Chol	Na
56	4	0.2	10	0	0	0.1	0	331

Exchanges: ¼ cup = 1 meat
Recommended for: The Living Heart; Low Calorie; Diabetic; Types I, IIa, IIb, III, IV, and V Diets

Garbanzo Pimento Spread

1 cup dried garbanzo beans (2 cups cooked)
⅓ cup Brazil nuts, chopped
1 jar (4 ounces) pimentos
⅛ teaspoon garlic powder
½ teaspoon onion powder
¼ cup lemon juice
1¼ cups water
1 teaspoon salt

1. Soak beans overnight in water.
2. Drain beans and combine with nuts, ¾ of pimentos and remaining ingredients in blender until smooth.
3. Place mixture in double boiler over boiling water.
4. Cover and cook 30 minutes, stirring occasionally.
5. Stir in remaining pimentos. Mold in small loaf pans rinsed with cold water and refrigerate overnight.
6. Serve with vegetables or allowed crackers.

Yield: 2 pounds

¼ cup contains:

Cal	Prot	Fat	Carb	Sat	Mono	Poly	Chol	Na
110	5	4.2	14	1.0	1.3	1.7	0	334

Exchanges: ¼ cup = 1 meat, ½ bread
Recommended for: The Living Heart; Low Calorie; Diabetic; Types IIa, IIb, III, IV, and V Diets

Tuna Spread

1 can (6½ ounces) tuna, drained
1 cup "Help Your Heart" Sour Cream (see recipe, page 89)
3 tablespoons finely chopped celery
2 tablespoons chopped pimento
1 teaspoon Worcestershire sauce
2–3 drops Tabasco
1 tablespoon finely chopped fresh parsley

1. Combine all ingredients except parsley and chill well.
2. Before serving sprinkle top with parsley.
3. Serve as a dip or spread for vegetables or allowed crackers.

Yield: approximately 1½ cups

1 tablespoon contains:

Cal	Prot	Fat	Carb	Sat	Mono	Poly	Chol	Na
20	3	0.6	0	0.2	0.2	0.2	5	96

Exchanges: 1 tablespoon = free; 2 tablespoons = ½ meat
Recommended for: The Living Heart; Low Calorie; Diabetic; Types IIa, IIb, III, IV, and V Diets

Soybean Spread

1 cup dried soybeans
¾ teaspoon salt
½ teaspoon garlic powder
¼ teaspoon dried thyme
¼ teaspoon dried summer savory
⅓ teaspoon paprika
1 tablespoon chopped chives
1 tablespoon chopped parsley

1. Soak soybeans overnight in water.
2. Drain soybeans and combine with remaining ingredients in blender until smooth.
3. Chill in refrigerator overnight to blend flavors.
4. Serve as dip or spread for vegetables or allowed crackers.

Yield: 1½ cups

¼ cup contains:

Cal	Prot	Fat	Carb	Sat	Mono	Poly	Chol	Na
98	8	4.3	8	0.6	0.9	2.2	0	277

Exchanges: ¼ cup = 1½ meats
Recommended for: The Living Heart; Low Calorie; Diabetic; Types IIa, IIb, III, IV, and V Diets

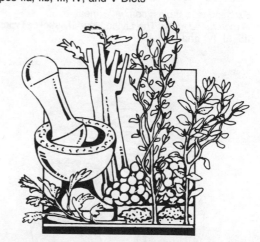

Abbreviations: **Cal,** calories; **Prot,** protein; **Carb,** carbohydrate; **Sat,** saturated fat; **Mono,** monounsaturated fat; **Poly,** polyunsaturated fat; **Chol,** cholesterol; **Na,** sodium. Protein, fat, carbohydrate, saturated fat, monounsaturated fat, and polyunsaturated fat are expressed in *grams*. Cholesterol and sodium are expressed in *milligrams*.

Salmon Ball

2 cans (6½ ounces each) salmon, drained (skin and bones removed)
1 tablespoon lemon juice
2 teaspoons finely chopped onion
2 teaspoons horseradish
¼ teaspoon liquid smoke
⅛ teaspoon salt
⅛ teaspoon pepper
1 cup Mock Cream Cheese (see recipe, page 90)
¼ cup chopped walnuts
2 tablespoons chopped fresh parsley

1. Combine all ingredients except walnuts and parsley.
2. Shape into a ball on waxed paper, wrap, and chill 3–4 hours.
3. Sprinkle with walnuts and parsley before serving.

Yield: 2½ cups

1 tablespoon contains:

Cal	Prot	Fat	Carb	Sat	Mono	Poly	Chol	Na
38	3	2.4	0	0.4	0.6	1.2	4	91

Exchanges: 1 tablespoon = ½ meat
Recommended for: The Living Heart; Diabetic; Types IIa, IIb, III, IV, and V Diets

MEAT, SEAFOOD, CHEESE, EGG APPETIZERS

Oriental Beef Cubes

3½ tablespoons soy sauce
2 tablespoons sherry
1 teaspoon ground ginger
2 cloves garlic, sliced
2 green onions, chopped, including tops
3 small hot red chilies, seeded and finely chopped
1 pound lean beef, well-trimmed, cut into ¾-inch cubes
2 tablespoons oil
1 tablespoon sesame seeds

1. Combine 2 tablespoons soy sauce, sherry, ginger, garlic, onion, and red chilies.
2. Stir beef cubes into mixture and let stand 1 hour at room temperature or overnight in refrigerator.
3. Drain beef cubes and brown on all sides in oil.
4. Place on warm plate or chafing dish and sprinkle with remaining soy sauce and sesame seeds.
5. Serve with frilled toothpick in each beef cube.

Yield: about 24 cubes

2 beef cubes contain:

Cal	Prot	Fat	Carb	Sat	Mono	Poly	Chol	Na
86	8	5.6	0	1.5	1.8	1.6	26	184

Exchanges: 2 cubes = 1 meat, ½ fat
Recommended for: The Living Heart; Low Calorie; Diabetic; Types IIa, IIb, III, IV, and V Diets

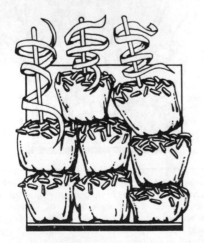

Stuffed Meat Rolls

1½ **cups low-fat cottage cheese**
1 **tablespoon taco seasoning mix**
1 **teaspoon mayonnaise**
¼ **cup chopped walnuts**
1 **package (3 ounces) wafer-thin, sliced luncheon meat**

1. Mix cottage cheese, taco seasoning, mayonnaise, and walnuts together.
2. Put filling into slice of meat folded in half, roll, and secure with a toothpick.
3. Serve on a tray garnished with radish roses and pickles, if desired.

Yield: 10–12 meat rolls

1 roll contains:

Cal	Prot	Fat	Carb	Sat	Mono	Poly	Chol	Na
55	6	3.1	2	0.8	0.8	1.3	5	376

Exchanges: 1 roll = 1 meat
Recommended for: The Living Heart; Low Calorie; Diabetic; Types IIa, IIb, III, IV, and V Diets

Mexican Meatballs

1 **pound very lean ground beef**
1 **package (1¾ ounces) taco seasoning mix**

1. Combine beef and taco seasoning thoroughly.
2. Shape into ¾-inch meatballs and brown in skillet. Drain off fat.
3. Serve with cocktail picks or fondue forks.
4. Serve with Guacamole Dip (see recipe, page 87) or Hearty Cheese Fondue (see recipe, page 88), if desired.

Yield: about 30 meatballs

1 meatball contains:

Cal	Prot	Fat	Carb	Sat	Mono	Poly	Chol	Na
24	3	1.2	0	0.5	0.4	0.1	10	138

Exchanges: 1 meatball = ½ meat
Recommended for: The Living Heart; Low Calorie; Diabetic; Types IIa, IIb, III, IV, and V Diets

Sharon's Sherried Meatballs

2 **pounds very lean ground beef**
1 **cup catsup**
1 **cup sherry**
2 **tablespoons brown sugar, firmly packed**

1. Shape ground beef into 1-inch meatballs.
2. Brown in skillet or chafing dish and drain off fat.
3. Add remaining ingredients and cook until sauce is thick (about 1–2 hours).

Yield: 50 meatballs

1 meatball contains:

Cal	Prot	Fat	Carb	Sat	Mono	Poly	Chol	Na
38	4	1.4	2	0.5	0.5	0.1	12	66

Exchanges: 1 meatball = ½ meat
Recommended for: The Living Heart; Low Calorie; Diabetic; Types IIa, IIb, III, IV, and V Diets

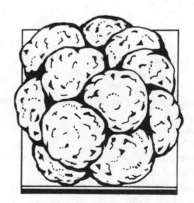

Abbreviations: **Cal,** calories; **Prot,** protein; **Carb,** carbohydrate; **Sat,** saturated fat; **Mono,** monounsaturated fat; **Poly,** polyunsaturated fat; **Chol,** cholesterol; **Na,** sodium. Protein, fat, carbohydrate, saturated fat, monounsaturated fat, and polyunsaturated fat are expressed in *grams.* Cholesterol and sodium are expressed in *milligrams.*

Chicken Curry Sandwiches

  2 **cups cooked chicken, chopped**
 ¾ **teaspoon curry powder**
 ⅓ **cup finely chopped celery**
 ¼ **cup chopped walnuts**
 ¼ **cup raisins**
 ¼ **cup skim milk yogurt**
 ¼ **cup mayonnaise**
  8 **slices bread, crusts removed**

1. Combine all ingredients except bread.
2. Spread on four slices bread and top with remaining bread slices.
3. Cut each sandwich into fourths, cover with plastic wrap, and chill until ready to serve.

Yield: 16 servings

1 serving contains:

Cal	Prot	Fat	Carb	Sat	Mono	Poly	Chol	Na
110	6	5.4	9	1.0	1.3	2.5	18	105

Exchanges: ¼ sandwich = ½ bread, 1 meat, ½ fat
Recommended for: The Living Heart; Diabetic; Types IIa, IIb, III, and IV Diets

Chicken in Fondue Broth

 1½ **pounds chicken breasts, boned, skin and fat removed**
  3 **cups chicken bouillon**
  1 **bay leaf**
  3 **whole cloves**
  1 **teaspoon salt**
 ¼ **teaspoon dried sweet basil**
 ¾ **cup white wine**
  1 **pound fresh mushrooms, sliced**

1. Cut chicken into ¾-inch cubes.
2. Simmer bouillon, bay leaf, cloves, salt, basil, and wine in a saucepan 15 minutes.
3. Pour half of mixture into a fondue pot. Keep remainder hot.
4. Spear chicken cube and mushroom on fork and cook in bouillon 2–3 minutes.
5. Replace broth in fondue pot as needed.

Yield: 16 servings

1 serving contains:

Cal	Prot	Fat	Carb	Sat	Mono	Poly	Chol	Na
55	10	1.0	1	0.3	0.3	0.3	22	23

Exchanges: 1 serving = 1 meat
Recommended for: The Living Heart; Low Calorie; Diabetic; Types I, IIa, IIb, III, IV, and V Diets

Barbecued Chicken Drummettes

 16 **chicken wings, skin and fat removed**
 ¼ **teaspoon salt**
 ⅛ **teaspoon pepper**
  2 **tablespoons tub margarine**
  2 **tablespoons brown sugar, firmly packed**
 ¼ **cup catsup**
  1 **tablespoon prepared mustard**
  1 **tablespoon Worcestershire sauce**

1. Preheat oven to 400°F.
2. Cut off wing tips and straighten remaining sections to resemble a small drumstick.
3. Place in a baking dish and season with salt and pepper.
4. Combine remaining ingredients and spoon half of mixture over chicken.
5. Bake 15 minutes.
6. Turn drummettes and spoon on remaining sauce. Bake an additional 15 minutes until chicken is tender.

Yield: 16 servings

1 drummette contains:

Cal	Prot	Fat	Carb	Sat	Mono	Poly	Chol	Na
48	5	2.0	3	0.4	0.6	0.8	11	134

Exchanges: 1 drummette = 1 meat
Recommended for: The Living Heart; Low Calorie; Diabetic; Types IIa, IIb, III, IV, and V Diets

Tuna Party Mold

1 tablespoon (1 envelope) unflavored gelatin
¼ cup cold water
1 cup mayonnaise
⅓ cup lemon juice
¾ cup chopped celery
⅓ cup chopped green pepper
   salt
   pepper
3 cans (6½ ounces each) water-packed tuna, drained

1. Sprinkle gelatin over water in saucepan.
2. Stir over low heat until gelatin dissolves. Remove from heat.
3. Blend into mayonnaise and add remaining ingredients.
4. Pour into ring mold coated with mayonnaise and chill until firm.
5. Unmold on plate and garnish with endive and radish flowers, if desired.

Yield: 6 cups

1 tablespoon contains:

Cal	Prot	Fat	Carb	Sat	Mono	Poly	Chol	Na
28	2	2.2	0	0.5	0.5	1.0	5	66

Exchanges: 1 tablespoon = free; 2 tablespoons = ½ meat, ½ fat
Recommended for: The Living Heart; Diabetic; Types IIa, IIb, III, and IV Diets

Tasty Tuna Snacks

1 can (6½ ounces) water-packed tuna, drained
⅓ cup Mock Cream Cheese (see recipe, page 90)
2 tablespoons finely chopped celery
2 tablespoons diced pimento
2 teaspoons lemon juice
1½ teaspoons Worcestershire sauce
¼ teaspoon Tabasco
¼ teaspoon garlic salt
⅛ teaspoon salt
⅛ teaspoon pepper
⅓ cup finely chopped fresh parsley

1. Blend tuna and Mock Cream Cheese.
2. Mix in celery, pimento, and all seasoning except parsley.
3. Form mixture into small balls and roll in parsley.
4. Chill. Serve with toothpicks.

Yield: 30 balls

1 snack contains:

Cal	Prot	Fat	Carb	Sat	Mono	Poly	Chol	Na
19	2	1.0	0	0.3	0.3	0.3	4	99

Exchanges: 1 snack = free; 2 snacks = ½ meat
Recommended for: The Living Heart; Low Calorie; Diabetic; Types IIa, IIb, III, IV, and V Diets

Seafood Cocktail

½ cup chili sauce
⅓ cup catsup
2 tablespoons horseradish
1½ teaspoons Worcestershire sauce
2–3 drops Tabasco
   lettuce leaf, lemon slices, or avocado wedges
1 can (6½ ounces) flaked crabmeat, drained and chilled

1. Combine chili sauce, catsup, horseradish, Worcestershire sauce, and Tabasco.
2. Arrange lettuce leaf, lemon slices, or avocado wedges in 4 small cups or salad plates.
3. Add ¼ of crabmeat to each cup.
4. Top with sauce mixture.

Yield: 4 servings

1 serving contains:

Cal	Prot	Fat	Carb	Sat	Mono	Poly	Chol	Na
110	9	0.9	17	0.1	0.2	0.4	46	1188

Exchanges: 1 serving = ½ bread, 1 meat, 1 vegetable
Recommended for: The Living Heart; Diabetic; Types IIa, IIb, III, IV, and V Diets

---

Abbreviations: **Cal,** calories; **Prot,** protein; **Carb,** carbohydrate; **Sat,** saturated fat; **Mono,** monounsaturated fat; **Poly,** polyunsaturated fat; **Chol,** cholesterol; **Na,** sodium. Protein, fat, carbohydrate, saturated fat, monounsaturated fat, and polyunsaturated fat are expressed in *grams.* Cholesterol and sodium are expressed in *milligrams.*

Crunchy Cheese Balls

1 cup low-fat cheese, cubed
1 cup dry curd cottage cheese
½ teaspoon Worcestershire sauce
1 tablespoon finely chopped onion
¼ teaspoon onion salt
¼ teaspoon paprika
¼ cup finely chopped walnuts or sesame seeds

1. Mix cheeses and seasonings in blender until smooth. Depending on the size of your blender you may need to blend one-half at a time.
2. Shape into small balls and roll in walnuts or sesame seeds.

Yield: 32 balls

1 cheese ball contains:

Cal	Prot	Fat	Carb	Sat	Mono	Poly	Chol	Na
18	2	0.8	1	0.3	0.3	0.2	2	82

Exchanges: 1 ball = free; 2 balls = ½ meat
Recommended for: The Living Heart; Diabetic; Types IIa, IIb, III, IV, and V Diets

Cheese Balls

1 cup low-fat cheese, cubed
1 cup dry curd cottage cheese
½ teaspoon Worcestershire sauce
1 tablespoon finely chopped onion
¼ teaspoon onion salt
¼ teaspoon paprika
¼ cup finely chopped fresh parsley

1. Mix cheeses and seasonings in blender until smooth. Depending on the size of your blender you may need to blend one-half at a time.
2. Shape into small balls and roll in parsley.

Yield: 32 balls

1 cheese ball contains:

Cal	Prot	Fat	Carb	Sat	Mono	Poly	Chol	Na
12	2	0.3	1	0.2	0.1	0	2	82

Exchanges: 1–2 balls = free; 3 balls = ½ meat
Recommended for: The Living Heart; Low Calorie; Diabetic; Types IIa, IIb, III, IV, and V Diets

Master Mix Sausage Cheese Balls

1 pound Homemade Sausage (hot variation, see recipe, page 118), uncooked
3½ cups Master Mix (see recipe, page 189)
10 ounces low-fat cheese, melted

1. Preheat oven to 375°F.
2. Combine sausage and Master Mix.
3. Add cheese, stirring until well mixed.
4. Roll into 1-inch balls and place on an ungreased baking sheet.
5. Bake 15–20 minutes.

Yield: 90 cheese balls

Note: Unbaked sausage cheese balls may be frozen. When needed, thaw and bake according to directions.

1 cheese ball contains:

Cal	Prot	Fat	Carb	Sat	Mono	Poly	Chol	Na
36	2	1.5	3	0.4	0.4	0.6	5	122

Exchanges: 2 cheese balls = ½ dairy, ½ fat
Recommended for: The Living Heart; Diabetic; Types IIa, IIb, III, and IV Diets

Okay Deviled Eggs

egg substitute equivalent to 3 eggs
2 tablespoons mayonnaise
2 teaspoons prepared mustard
⅛ teaspoon salt
⅛ teaspoon pepper
1 teaspoon vinegar
6 eggs, hard-boiled and cooled
paprika

1. Cook egg substitute according to package directions for scrambled eggs.
2. Mix egg substitute with mayonnaise, mustard, salt, pepper, and vinegar in blender. Cover and refrigerate until chilled.
3. Halve hard-cooked eggs lengthwise and discard yolk.
4. Fill each egg white half with chilled egg substitute mixture and sprinkle with paprika.

Yield: 12 servings

1 egg half contains:

Cal	Prot	Fat	Carb	Sat	Mono	Poly	Chol	Na
42	3	2.8	1	0.5	0.6	1.5	2	98

Exchanges: 1 egg half = ½ meat, ½ fat
Recommended for: The Living Heart; Diabetic; Types IIa, IIb, III, and IV Diets

BEVERAGES

Herbed Tomato Starter

¾ **cup water**
1 **can (10¾ ounces) condensed beef broth, undiluted**
1 **cup tomato juice**
¼ **teaspoon dried marjoram**
¼ **teaspoon dried thyme**
¼ **teaspoon Tabasco**
¼ **teaspoon Worcestershire sauce**
1 **tablespoon chopped fresh parsley**

1. Combine all ingredients except parsley and simmer for 2 minutes.
2. Serve in mugs garnished with parsley.

Yield: 6 servings

1 serving contains:

Cal	Prot	Fat	Carb	Sat	Mono	Poly	Chol	Na
21	2	0	3	0	0	0	0	409

Exchanges: 1 serving = free
Recommended for: The Living Heart; Low Calorie; Diabetic; Types I, IIa, IIb, III, IV, and V Diets

Fruit Whirl

½ **cup nonfat dry milk powder**
1 **cup apple juice**
2 **cups fresh or unsweetened canned fruit (such as peaches or pineapple)**
1 **teaspoon lemon juice**
⅛ **teaspoon salt**

1. Mix all ingredients in blender until smooth.
2. Add ice cubes or crushed ice if thicker consistency is desired.

Yield: 4 servings

Note: Mixture may be frozen to make sherbet.

1 serving contains:

Cal	Prot	Fat	Carb	Sat	Mono	Poly	Chol	Na
98	4	0.2	22	0	0	0.1	2	116

Exchanges: 1 serving = 1½ fruits, ½ dairy
Recommended for: The Living Heart; Diabetic; Types I, IIa, IIb, III, IV, and V Diets

"Help Your Heart" Nonalcoholic Cocktail

1 **cup tomato juice**
1½ **teaspoons vinegar**
¼ **teaspoon salt**
⅛ **teaspoon dried sweet basil**
⅛ **teaspoon paprika**
½ **medium cucumber, peeled, cut into chunks**
¼ **cup cracked ice**

1. Combine all ingredients except ice in blender until well mixed.
2. Add ice and blend briefly.

Yield: 2 servings

Note: Cucumber may be grated and all ingredients mixed in a shaker.

1 serving contains:

Cal	Prot	Fat	Carb	Sat	Mono	Poly	Chol	Na
35	2	0.2	8	0	0	0.2	0	522

Exchanges: 1 serving = 1 fruit
Recommended for: The Living Heart; Low Calorie; Diabetic; Types I, IIa, IIb, III, IV, and V Diets

---

Abbreviations: **Cal,** calories; **Prot,** protein; **Carb,** carbohydrate; **Sat,** saturated fat; **Mono,** monounsaturated fat; **Poly,** polyunsaturated fat; **Chol,** cholesterol; **Na,** sodium. Protein, fat, carbohydrate, saturated fat, monounsaturated fat, and polyunsaturated fat are expressed in *grams.* Cholesterol and sodium are expressed in *milligrams.*

Fruit Slush

1 cup pineapple juice
½ cup crushed pineapple, packed in own juice
1 tablespoon lemon or lime juice

1. Mix all ingredients in blender until smooth.
2. Pour over finely crushed ice.

Yield: 2 servings

1 serving contains:

Cal	Prot	Fat	Carb	Sat	Mono	Poly	Chol	Na
95	1	0.2	24	0	0	0.2	0	5

Exchanges: 1 serving = 2 fruits
Recommended for: The Living Heart; Diabetic; Types I, IIa, IIb, III, IV, and V Diets

Tropical Smoothee

1½ cups pineapple juice
½ cup nonfat dry milk powder
1 banana, sliced
½ cup pineapple sherbet

1. Combine all ingredients except sherbet in blender 10 seconds.
2. Add sherbet and blend 5 seconds more.

Yield: 2 servings

1 serving contains:

Cal	Prot	Fat	Carb	Sat	Mono	Poly	Chol	Na
283	8	1.4	62	0.7	0.3	0.4	7	118

Exchanges: Not applicable for this recipe
Recommended for: The Living Heart; Type IIa Diets

Wassail

2 quarts apple cider
2 cups orange juice
1 cup lemon juice
5 cups pineapple juice
  sugar or honey to taste
1 cinnamon stick
1½ teaspoons whole cloves

1. Combine juices and sweetener in a large pan. Combine spices in a tea ball.
2. Simmer together for 60 minutes. (If a tea ball is not used, strain liquid after simmering.)
3. Serve in a punch bowl with diced oranges, diced lemons, and whole apples floating for garnish, if desired.

Yield: about 2 quarts

½ cup contains:

Cal	Prot	Fat	Carb	Sat	Mono	Poly	Chol	Na
145	1	0.1	37	0	0	0.1	0	3

Exchanges: Not applicable for this recipe
Recommended for: The Living Heart; Types I and IIa Diets

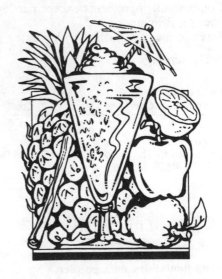

Entrées

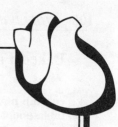

SEAFOOD ENTRÉES

Oven-Fried Fillets

- **1 pound fish fillets**
- **½ teaspoon salt**
- **¼ teaspoon pepper**
- **½ cup fine, dry bread crumbs**
- **3 tablespoons tub margarine**

1. Preheat oven to 500°F.
2. Lightly season fillets with salt and pepper.
3. Roll in bread crumbs.
4. Place in lightly oiled baking dish. Dot each fillet with margarine.
5. Bake 10 minutes or until fish flakes easily with fork.

Yield: 4 servings

1 serving contains:

Cal	Prot	Fat	Carb	Sat	Mono	Poly	Chol	Na
236	23	11.3	9	2.3	4.1	4.7	68	544

Exchanges: 1 serving = 2½ meats, ½ bread, 1 fat
Recommended for: The Living Heart; Diabetic; Types IIa, IIb, III, and IV Diets

Fancy Parisian Fillets

- **1 tablespoon oil**
- **1 onion, chopped**
- **1 tablespoon chopped, fresh parsley**
- **2 pounds fish fillets**
- **1 clove garlic, minced**
- **1 cup white wine**
- **1 can (16 ounces) tomatoes, undrained**
- **2 tablespoons lemon juice**

1. Preheat oven to 350°F.
2. Place oil, half of onion, and the parsley in baking dish. Place fillets on top.
3. Combine remaining ingredients and pour over fish.
4. Bake 35–40 minutes or until fish flakes easily with a fork.

Yield: 8 servings

1 serving contains:

Cal	Prot	Fat	Carb	Sat	Mono	Poly	Chol	Na
147	22	3.9	5	0.8	1.2	1.9	68	152

Exchanges: 1 serving = 2½ meats
Recommended for: The Living Heart; Low Calorie; Diabetic; Types IIa, IIb, III, IV, and V Diets

Abbreviations: **Cal,** calories; **Prot,** protein; **Carb,** carbohydrate; **Sat,** saturated fat; **Mono,** monounsaturated fat; **Poly,** polyunsaturated fat; **Chol,** cholesterol; **Na,** sodium. Protein, fat, carbohydrate, saturated fat, monounsaturated fat, and polyunsaturated fat are expressed in *grams*. Cholesterol and sodium are expressed in *milligrams*.

Baked Fish in Lemon Sauce

¼ cup tub margarine, melted
2 tablespoons lemon juice
2 teaspoons salt
⅛ teaspoon pepper
1 teaspoon paprika
1 fresh fish (2–3 pounds) or 1½ pounds fish fillets
1 green pepper, sliced into rings
1 onion, sliced into rings

1. Preheat oven to 350°F.
2. Combine margarine, lemon juice, salt, pepper, and paprika, and brush over fish.
3. Place green pepper, onion, and fish in a plastic cooking bag.
4. Close bag and puncture according to package directions.
5. Bake 45–50 minutes. (Shorten the cooking time if thin fillets are used.) Fish is done when it flakes with a fork.

Yield: 6 servings

1 serving contains:

Cal	Prot	Fat	Carb	Sat	Mono	Poly	Chol	Na
191	22	9.9	3	2.0	3.5	4.2	68	902

Exchanges: 1 serving = 2½ meats, 1 fat
Recommended for: The Living Heart; Diabetic; Types IIa, IIb, III, and IV Diets

Easy-to-Bake Fish Fillets

¾ cup chopped celery
6 tablespoons chopped onion
¼ cup chopped fresh parsley
4 teaspoons tub margarine, melted
1 pound fish fillets
¼ teaspoon salt
⅛ teaspoon pepper
⅛ teaspoon paprika

1. Preheat oven to 450°F.
2. Mix celery, onion, parsley, and margarine together.
3. Place mixture on top of fillets in a shallow baking dish.

4. Season with salt, pepper, and paprika.
5. Cover and bake 30 minutes or until fish flakes easily with a fork.

Yield: 4 servings

1 serving contains:

Cal	Prot	Fat	Carb	Sat	Mono	Poly	Chol	Na
154	22	6.0	2	1.3	2.1	2.5	68	283

Exchanges: 1 serving = 2½ meats
Recommended for: The Living Heart; Low Calorie; Diabetic; Types IIa, IIb, III, IV, and V Diets

Marinated Fish Fillets

⅔ cup oil
⅓ cup tarragon vinegar
1 teaspoon salt
1 teaspoon Worcestershire sauce
1 onion, sliced
4 peppercorns
1 bay leaf
2 tablespoons chopped parsley
1 pound fish fillets or fish steaks

1. Combine all ingredients, except fish, in baking dish.
2. Add fish, cover, and refrigerate at least 3 hours.
3. Drain fish and reserve marinade.
4. Place fish in baking dish and pour ¼ cup marinade over fish.
5. Bake in a preheated 350°F oven 25–30 minutes or until fish flakes easily with a fork.

Yield: 4 servings

Note: Fish may be broiled if desired. After removing from marinade, place on a preheated broiler rack 3 inches from heat. Broil 5–10 minutes, depending on thickness, turning and basting once.

1 serving contains:

Cal	Prot	Fat	Carb	Sat	Mono	Poly	Chol	Na
196	22	11.2	2	1.7	3.0	6.1	68	360

Exchanges: 1 serving = 3 meats, ½ fat
Recommended for: The Living Heart; Low Calorie; Diabetic; Types IIa, IIb, III, and IV Diets

Fish with Stuffing

1½ **pounds dressed fish or 1 pound fillets**
¼ **cup chopped celery**
2 **tablespoons chopped onion**
1 **tablespoon chopped green pepper**
1 **clove garlic, minced**
¼ **cup tub margarine**
2 **cups soft bread crumbs**
½ **teaspoon salt**
¼ **teaspoon dried thyme**
⅛ **teaspoon ground sage**
⅛ **teaspoon pepper**
2 **tablespoons lemon juice**

1. Preheat oven to 350°F.
2. Sauté celery, onion, green pepper, and garlic in margarine.
3. Mix remaining ingredients together except lemon juice and fish. Combine with the sautéed vegetables.
4. Place whole fish in lightly oiled baking dish and lightly stuff cavity with bread mixture or place half of fillets in lightly oiled baking dish, top with bread mixture, then remaining fillets.
5. Sprinkle lemon juice over fish.
6. Bake whole fish 45 minutes or fillets 30 minutes or until fish flakes easily with fork.

Yield: 4 servings

1 serving contains:

Cal	Prot	Fat	Carb	Sat	Mono	Poly	Chol	Na
279	24	14.3	13	2.8	5.2	6.0	68	610

Exchanges: 1 serving = 3 meats, 1 bread, 1 fat
Recommended for: The Living Heart; Diabetic; Types IIa, IIb, III, and IV Diets

Stuffed Fish Rolls

1 **pound fish fillets**
1 **teaspoon salt**
¼ **cup finely chopped celery**
¼ **cup finely chopped onion**
1 **tablespoon tub margarine**
¼ **pound mushrooms, sliced**
4 **tablespoons chopped, fresh parsley**
2 **tablespoons lemon juice**

1. Preheat oven to 400°F.
2. Season fillets with salt.
3. Sauté celery and onion in margarine until tender.
4. Stir in mushrooms, parsley, and lemon juice.
5. Spread mixture over fillets.
6. Roll up fillets and secure with toothpicks.
7. Place in lightly oiled baking dish and bake 20–25 minutes or until fish flakes easily with fork.

Yield: 4 servings

Note: May also be baked in a microwave oven, 1 minute per roll.

1 serving contains:

Cal	Prot	Fat	Carb	Sat	Mono	Poly	Chol	Na
146	22	5.0	2	1.1	1.8	2.1	68	732

Exchanges: 1 serving = 2½ meats
Recommended for: The Living Heart; Low Calorie; Diabetic; Types IIa, IIb, III, IV, and V Diets

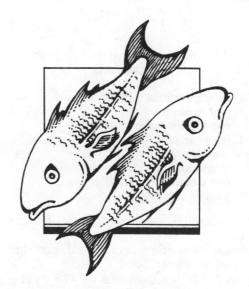

Abbreviations: **Cal,** calories; **Prot,** protein; **Carb,** carbohydrate; **Sat,** saturated fat; **Mono,** monounsaturated fat; **Poly,** polyunsaturated fat; **Chol,** cholesterol; **Na,** sodium. Protein, fat, carbohydrate, saturated fat, monounsaturated fat, and polyunsaturated fat are expressed in *grams.* Cholesterol and sodium are expressed in *milligrams.*

Texas Style Fillets

2 **pounds fish fillets**
⅓ **cup hickory flavored barbecue sauce**
3 **tablespoons oil**
¼ **teaspoon salt**
2 **tablespoons pineapple juice**
1 **tablespoon lemon juice**
3 **tablespoons finely chopped onion**

1. Place the fillets in a shallow baking dish.
2. Combine the remaining ingredients and brush liberally on fillets.
3. Broil 4–6 inches from heat for 5–10 minutes.

Yield: 8 servings

1 serving contains:

Cal	Prot	Fat	Carb	Sat	Mono	Poly	Chol	Na
169	22	7.9	2	1.3	2.2	4.1	68	226

Exchanges: 1 serving = 2½ meats, ½ fat
Recommended for: The Living Heart; Low Calorie; Diabetic; Types IIa, IIb, III, and IV Diets

Herb Flavored Broiled Fish

1 **tablespoon finely chopped onion**
¼ **cup lemon juice**
¼ **cup tub margarine, melted**
1 **teaspoon salt**
¼ **teaspoon pepper**
½ **teaspoon dried marjoram**
¼ **cup chopped fresh parsley**
1½ **pounds fish fillets**

1. Combine all ingredients together except fish fillets.
2. Place fillets on broiler rack and spoon half of herb mixture over fish.
3. Broil 4 inches from heat for 4–6 minutes.
4. Turn fish over and spoon remaining mixture over top.
5. Broil 4–6 minutes more or until fish flakes easily.

Yield: 6 servings

1 serving contains:

Cal	Prot	Fat	Carb	Sat	Mono	Poly	Chol	Na
182	21	9.7	1	2.0	3.5	4.1	68	533

Exchanges: 1 serving = 3 meats
Recommended for: The Living Heart; Low Calorie; Diabetic; Types IIa, IIb, III, and IV Diets

Variation:

Top with ½ cup slivered, toasted almonds.

1 serving contains:

Cal	Prot	Fat	Carb	Sat	Mono	Poly	Chol	Na
239	23	14.9	3	2.4	7.0	5.1	68	533

Exchanges: 1 serving = 3 meats, 1½ fats
Recommended for: The Living Heart; Diabetic; Types IIa, IIb, III, and IV Diets

Zippy Broiled Fillets

1 **pound fish fillets**
1 **tablespoon oil**
1½ **teaspoons soy sauce**
1 **tablespoon Worcestershire sauce**
¼ **teaspoon chili powder**
⅛ **teaspoon garlic powder**
 dash Tabasco

1. Place fillets in single layer in shallow baking dish that has been lightly oiled.
2. Combine remaining ingredients and pour over fillets.
3. Broil about 4 inches from heat for 5–10 minutes or until fish flakes easily with a fork.

Yield: 4 servings

1 serving contains:

Cal	Prot	Fat	Carb	Sat	Mono	Poly	Chol	Na
144	21	5.5	1	1.0	1.6	2.8	68	305

Exchanges: 1 serving = 2½ meats
Recommended for: The Living Heart; Low Calorie; Diabetic; Types IIa, IIb, III, IV, and V Diets

Fish Fillets in Tomato Sauce

1 **onion, sliced into rings**
1 **green pepper, cut into strips**
1 **clove garlic, minced**
1 **tablespoon oil**
1 **can (14 ounces) stewed tomatoes, undrained**
1 **can (8 ounces) tomato sauce**
2 **tablespoons dry red wine**
1 **teaspoon dried sweet basil**
½ **teaspoon salt**
1 **pound fish fillets**

1. In skillet, sauté onion, green pepper, and garlic in oil until tender.
2. Stir in tomatoes, tomato sauce, wine, basil, and salt. Heat to boiling, then reduce heat and cook uncovered about 15 minutes, stirring occasionally.
3. Place fish in tomato mixture.
4. Cover and simmer about 15 minutes or until fish flakes easily with a fork.

Yield: 4 servings

1 serving contains:

Cal	Prot	Fat	Carb	Sat	Mono	Poly	Chol	Na
197	24	5.8	12	1.0	1.6	3.1	68	710

Exchanges: 1 serving = 2½ meats, ½ bread, 1 vegetable
Recommended for: The Living Heart; Low Calorie; Diabetic; Types IIa, IIb, III, IV, and V Diets

Fancy Fillets Poached with Wine

¼ **cup chopped onion**
½ **cup sliced fresh mushrooms**
1 **pound fish fillets**
½ **teaspoon salt**
⅛ **teaspoon pepper**
¼ **cup white wine**
¼ **cup water**
¼ **cup chopped fresh parsley**

1. Preheat oven to 350°F.
2. Sprinkle onion and mushrooms over bottom of lightly oiled baking dish.
3. Place fillets on top of onion-mushroom mixture.

4. Sprinkle with salt and pepper.
5. Combine wine and water and pour over fish.
6. Sprinkle with parsley.
7. Bake 20 minutes or until fish flakes easily.

Yield: 4 servings

1 serving contains:

Cal	Prot	Fat	Carb	Sat	Mono	Poly	Chol	Na
119	22	2.1	2	0.6	0.7	0.8	68	350

Exchanges: 1 serving = 2½ meats
Recommended for: The Living Heart; Low Calorie; Diabetic; Types I, IIa, IIb, III, IV, and V Diets

So-Good Poached Fillets

¾ **cup water**
1 **tablespoon lemon juice**
½ **onion, sliced**
1 **tablespoon vinegar**
3 **peppercorns**
1 **teaspoon salt**
1 **pound fish fillets or fish steaks**

1. Place all ingredients except fish in saucepan and heat 5 minutes.
2. Cut fish in serving size pieces and place in water.
3. Simmer 5–10 minutes or until fish flakes easily.

Yield: 4 servings

1 serving contains:

Cal	Prot	Fat	Carb	Sat	Mono	Poly	Chol	Na
116	21	2.1	1	0.6	0.8	0.8	68	623

Exchanges: 1 serving = 2½ meats
Recommended for: The Living Heart; Low Calorie; Diabetic; Types I, IIa, IIb, III, IV, and V Diets

Abbreviations: **Cal,** calories; **Prot,** protein; **Carb,** carbohydrate; **Sat,** saturated fat; **Mono,** monounsaturated fat; **Poly,** polyunsaturated fat; **Chol,** cholesterol; **Na,** sodium. Protein, fat, carbohydrate, saturated fat, monounsaturated fat, and polyunsaturated fat are expressed in *grams*. Cholesterol and sodium are expressed in *milligrams*.

Tuna Macaroni Casserole

2 tablespoons chopped celery
¼ cup chopped onion
2 tablespoons chopped green pepper
1 tablespoon oil
1 tablespoon flour
½ teaspoon salt
¼ teaspoon pepper
1 cup skim milk
½ cup cubed low-fat cheese
1 cup cooked elbow macaroni
2 fresh tomatoes, chopped
1 can (6½ ounces) water-packed tuna, drained
2 tablespoons chopped fresh parsley
1 tablespoon lemon juice
  paprika

1. Preheat oven to 375°F.
2. Sauté celery, onion, and green pepper in oil until tender.
3. Stir in flour, salt, and pepper until smooth. Gradually stir in milk. Cook, stirring constantly, until thickened.
4. Add cheese and stir until melted.
5. Add macaroni, tomatoes, tuna, parsley, and lemon juice.
6. Pour into casserole and sprinkle paprika over top.
7. Bake 30–35 minutes.

Yield: 4 servings

1 serving contains:

Cal	Prot	Fat	Carb	Sat	Mono	Poly	Chol	Na
238	21	8.0	20	2.3	2.1	3.0	37	946

Exchanges: 1 serving = 2½ meats, 1 bread, ½ fat
Recommended for: The Living Heart; Diabetic; Types IIa, IIb, III, and IV Diets

Salmon-Broccoli Casserole

2 tablespoons tub margarine
1 tablespoon flour
¾ teaspoon salt
¼ teaspoon pepper
¼ teaspoon garlic powder
1 cup skim milk
3 fresh tomatoes, chopped
1 teaspoon lemon juice
1 package (10 ounces) frozen broccoli, thawed
1 can (6¾ ounces) salmon, drained and flaked
2 tablespoons fine, dry bread crumbs

1. Preheat oven to 375°F.
2. Melt 1 tablespoon margarine in saucepan. Blend in flour, salt, pepper, and garlic powder. Add milk and bring to a boil, stirring constantly.
3. Add tomatoes and lemon juice and cook over low heat for 5 minutes.
4. Arrange broccoli on bottom of casserole. Cover with salmon and top with sauce.
5. Sprinkle with bread crumbs and dot with remaining margarine.
6. Bake 30 minutes.

Yield: 4 servings

1 serving contains:

Cal	Prot	Fat	Carb	Sat	Mono	Poly	Chol	Na
194	14	10.0	13	2.0	4.1	3.8	26	574

Exchanges: 1 serving = 1½ meats, 1 bread, ½ fat
Recommended for: The Living Heart; Diabetic; Types IIa, IIb, III, and IV Diets

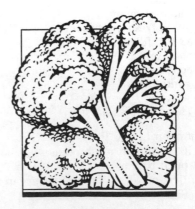

Seafood Croquettes

2 tablespoons finely chopped onion
3 tablespoons tub margarine
2 tablespoons flour
⅓ cup skim milk
1 can (6½ ounces) salmon or water-packed tuna, drained
⅛ teaspoon pepper
4 tablespoons fine dry bread or cracker crumbs

1. Sauté onion in 1 tablespoon margarine until tender.
2. Stir in flour and cook 1 minute, stirring constantly.
3. Blend in milk and cook over medium heat until thick. Cool slightly.
4. Stir in salmon or tuna, pepper, and 2 tablespoons of the bread crumbs.
5. Shape into six patties and roll in remaining bread crumbs.
6. Sauté in remaining margarine until browned.

Yield: 3 servings

1 serving contains:

Cal	Prot	Fat	Carb	Sat	Mono	Poly	Chol	Na
259	14	17.0	12	3.4	7.0	6.3	35	251

Exchanges: 1 serving = 1½ meats, 1 bread, 2 fats
Recommended for: The Living Heart; Diabetic; Types IIa, IIb, III, and IV Diets

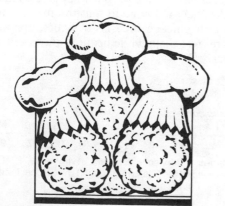

POULTRY ENTRÉES

Quick and Easy Chicken in Wine

3 whole chicken breasts, cut in half, skin and fat removed
1 tablespoon oil
3 onions, quartered
1 can (8 ounces) sliced mushrooms, undrained
½ cup dry white wine
2 tablespoons chopped fresh parsley
½ bay leaf
¾ teaspoon garlic powder
1 teaspoon salt
½ teaspoon pepper
½ cup water
2 cups sliced carrots

1. Brown chicken in oil. Drain off fat.
2. Add remaining ingredients to skillet.
3. Cover and simmer over low heat for 30 minutes or until chicken is tender, adding more water if needed.
4. Remove cover and continue cooking until most of the liquid has evaporated and mixture is thick.

Yield: 6 servings

1 serving contains:

Cal	Prot	Fat	Carb	Sat	Mono	Poly	Chol	Na
153	19	4.4	9	0.9	1.1	1.9	45	426

Exchanges: 1 serving = 2 meats, 1 vegetable
Recommended for: The Living Heart; Low Calorie; Diabetic; Types IIa, IIb, III, IV, and V Diets

Abbreviations: **Cal,** calories; **Prot,** protein; **Carb,** carbohydrate; **Sat,** saturated fat; **Mono,** monounsaturated fat; **Poly,** polyunsaturated fat; **Chol,** cholesterol; **Na,** sodium. Protein, fat, carbohydrate, saturated fat, monounsaturated fat, and polyunsaturated fat are expressed in *grams*. Cholesterol and sodium are expressed in *milligrams*.

Fat-Free Fried Chicken

4 deboned split chicken breasts, skin removed
1 teaspoon seasoned salt
½ teaspoon pepper

1. Sprinkle salt and pepper on both sides of chicken.
2. Place in non-stick surface frying pan and cover.
3. Cook on medium heat 10 to 15 minutes.
4. Turn chicken and continue cooking on medium heat for about 10 minutes.
5. Remove lid and allow moisture to evaporate and chicken to brown.

Yield: 4 servings

1 serving contains:

Cal	Prot	Fat	Carb	Sat	Mono	Poly	Chol	Na
141	27	2.9	0	.9	.8	.6	67	604

Exchanges: 1 serving = 3 meats
Recommended for: The Living Heart; Low Calorie; Diabetic; Type I, IIa, IIb, III, IV, and V Diets

Chinese Chicken

2 tablespoons soy sauce
2 tablespoons dry sherry
1 teaspoon ground ginger or 2 slices ginger root, minced
1 clove garlic, minced
2 whole chicken breasts, skin and fat removed, boned, cut into bite-sized pieces
1 teaspoon oil
2 cups sliced fresh mushrooms
1 cup thinly sliced celery
½ cup chopped green onion
1 package (7 ounces) frozen snow peas
1 can (8 ounces) water chestnuts, drained and sliced
1 tablespoon cornstarch
2 tablespoons water

1. Blend soy sauce, sherry, ginger, and garlic.
2. Marinate chicken in mixture for 30 minutes at room temperature. Drain.

3. Heat oil in wok or heavy skillet. Add chicken, mushrooms, celery, green onion, and snow peas. Sauté 10–15 minutes, stirring constantly, until chicken is tender and vegetables are still crisp.
4. Stir in water chestnuts.
5. Combine cornstarch and water and add to chicken, stirring until thickened.

Yield: 4 servings

1 serving contains:

Cal	Prot	Fat	Carb	Sat	Mono	Poly	Chol	Na
159	20	3.5	11	0.7	0.8	1.5	45	739

Exchanges: 1 serving = 2 meats, 1½ vegetables
Recommended for: The Living Heart; Low Calorie; Diabetic; Types IIa, IIb, III, IV, and V Diets

Lemon Chicken Breasts with Mushrooms

2 whole chicken breasts, cut in half, skin and fat removed
1 tablespoon tub margarine
¼ pound fresh mushrooms, sliced
1 tablespoon chopped green onion
1 lemon
2 tablespoons sherry or white wine

1. Sauté chicken breasts in margarine until brown. Remove from skillet.
2. Sauté mushrooms and onion in skillet.
3. Cut half of the lemon into slices and add to mushroom mixture.
4. Squeeze juice from the other half of the lemon.
5. Add juice and wine to mushroom mixture.
6. Return chicken breasts to skillet, spooning mixture over them while heating. Be careful not to overcook.

Yield: 4 servings

1 serving contains:

Cal	Prot	Fat	Carb	Sat	Mono	Poly	Chol	Na
187	28	5.9	3	1.4	1.8	2.0	67	94

Exchanges: 1 serving = 2 meats, 1 vegetable, 1 fat
Recommended for: The Living Heart; Low Calorie; Diabetic; Types IIa, IIb, III, and IV Diets

Chicken Divan

2 tablespoons tub margarine
2 tablespoons flour
1½ cups chicken bouillon
1 can (4 ounces) mushroom stems and pieces, undrained
½ teaspoon salt
¼ teaspoon pepper
1 package (10 ounces) frozen asparagus spears, cooked according to package directions and drained
2 whole deboned chicken breasts, skin and fat removed, cooked and halved
1½ tablespoons chopped fresh parsley
2 tablespoons fine dry bread crumbs

1. Preheat oven to 375°F.
2. Melt margarine in a small saucepan. Stir in flour and cook for 1 minute.
3. Stir in chicken bouillon until thickened.
4. Add mushrooms, salt, and pepper.
5. Place asparagus spears in a shallow baking dish or four individual casserole dishes.
6. Put chicken over asparagus and top with sauce.
7. Sprinkle with parsley and bread crumbs. Bake for 20 minutes.

Yield: 4 servings

1 serving contains:

Cal	Prot	Fat	Carb	Sat	Mono	Poly	Chol	Na
192	22	8.1	8	1.7	2.6	3.1	45	899

Exchanges: 1 serving = 2½ meats, ½ bread
Recommended for: The Living Heart; Low Calorie; Diabetic; Types IIa, IIb, III, IV, and V Diets

Barbecued Chicken

1 fryer (2–3 pounds), quartered, skin and fat removed
½ teaspoon salt
¼ teaspoon pepper
1 cup Zippy Barbecue Sauce (see recipe, page 176)

1. Season chicken with salt and pepper.
2. Place on broiler rack and brush with sauce.
3. Broil 5–7 inches from heat for 20 minutes on each side, brushing with sauce occasionally.

Yield: 4 servings

1 serving contains:

Cal	Prot	Fat	Carb	Sat	Mono	Poly	Chol	Na
218	25	9.3	8	2.0	2.5	3.5	78	831

Exchanges: 1 serving = 3 meats, ½ bread
Recommended for: The Living Heart; Low Calorie; Diabetic; Types IIa, IIb, III, IV, and V Diets

Variations:

Creole Chicken: Substitute Creole Sauce (see recipe, page 175) for Zippy Barbecue Sauce.

1 serving contains:

Cal	Prot	Fat	Carb	Sat	Mono	Poly	Chol	Na
190	25	8.4	3	2.1	2.6	2.6	78	557

Exchanges: 1 serving = 3 meats, 1 vegetable
Recommended for: The Living Heart; Low Calorie; Diabetic; Types IIa, IIb, III, IV, and V Diets

Abbreviations: **Cal,** calories; **Prot,** protein; **Carb,** carbohydrate; **Sat,** saturated fat; **Mono,** monounsaturated fat; **Poly,** polyunsaturated fat; **Chol,** cholesterol; **Na,** sodium. Protein, fat, carbohydrate, saturated fat, monounsaturated fat, and polyunsaturated fat are expressed in *grams.* Cholesterol and sodium are expressed in *milligrams.*

Crispy Corny Baked Chicken

1 chicken fryer (2–3 pounds), cut up, skin and
fat removed
½ teaspoon salt
⅛ teaspoon pepper
1 cup skim milk
1 cup cornflake crumbs

1. Preheat oven to 400°F.
2. Season chicken with salt and pepper.
3. Dip into milk and roll in crumbs.
4. Place in lightly oiled baking dish being careful that pieces do not touch.
5. Bake 45 minutes or until tender.

Yield: 4 servings

1 serving contains:

Cal	Prot	Fat	Carb	Sat	Mono	Poly	Chol	Na
254	28	5.6	21	1.6	1.6	1.3	79	593

Exchanges: 1 serving = 3 meats, 1 bread
Recommended for: The Living Heart; Low Calorie; Diabetic; Types I, IIa, IIb, III, IV, and V Diets

Citrus Chicken with Gravy

½ cup flour
2 teaspoons grated orange peel
1 teaspoon paprika
¼ teaspoon pepper
1 chicken fryer (2–3 pounds), cut up, skin and
fat removed
1 tablespoon tub margarine
¾ cup water
1½ cups orange juice
1 tablespoon brown sugar, firmly packed
1½ teaspoons salt
⅛ teaspoon ground ginger

1. Combine flour, orange peel, paprika, and pepper. Reserve ½ tablespoon of mixture for gravy.
2. Coat chicken with remaining flour mixture.
3. Brown chicken in margarine over low heat.
4. Add water, cover, and simmer 30 minutes. Add more water if needed.
5. Remove chicken and keep warm.

6. Remove fat from pan. Stir reserved flour into pan.
7. Add remaining ingredients and cook, stirring constantly, until gravy boils.

Yield: 4 servings

1 serving contains:

Cal	Prot	Fat	Carb	Sat	Mono	Poly	Chol	Na
293	26	8.6	26	2.1	2.6	2.7	78	934

Exchanges: 1 serving = 3 meats, 1 bread, 1 fruit
Recommended for: The Living Heart; Diabetic; Types IIa, IIb, III, IV, and V Diets

Acapulco Chicken

2 onions, finely chopped
1 clove garlic, minced
¼ cup oil
1 chicken fryer (2–3 pounds), cut up, skin and
fat removed
½ teaspoon salt
¼ teaspoon pepper
4 tomatoes, chopped
1 jalapeño pepper, seeded and finely chopped
½ teaspoon ground cumin (optional)
2 cups chicken bouillon
1 cup rice, uncooked
pimento (optional)

1. Sauté onion and garlic in oil. Remove onion and garlic from pan.
2. Season chicken with salt and pepper and brown lightly in the seasoned oil.
3. Return onion and garlic to pan and add tomatoes, jalapeño, cumin, and bouillon. Heat to boiling, cover, and simmer 20 minutes.
4. Add rice and cover. Cook until rice and chicken are tender and liquid has been absorbed.
5. Garnish with thin strips of pimento, if desired.

Yield: 4 servings

1 serving contains:

Cal	Prot	Fat	Carb	Sat	Mono	Poly	Chol	Na
475	29	19.4	45	3.3	5.1	9.3	78	854

Exchanges: 1 serving = 3 meats, 3 breads, 2 fats
Recommended for: The Living Heart; Diabetic; Types IIa, IIb, III, and IV Diets

Chicken with Herb Sauce

¼ cup flour
1 teaspoon salt
1 teaspoon pepper
¼ teaspoon dried oregano
¼ teaspoon dried thyme
½ teaspoon dried parsley flakes
1 chicken fryer (2–3 pounds), cut up, skin and fat removed
⅓ cup tub margarine
1½ cups water

1. Combine flour and seasonings. Set aside 2 tablespoons for gravy.
2. Coat chicken pieces with remaining seasoned flour.
3. Brown chicken on all sides in margarine.
4. Cover, reduce heat, and cook 20 minutes.
5. Uncover and cook 10 more minutes.
6. Remove chicken, keeping it warm.
7. Drain fat from pan.
8. Make a paste using the 2 tablespoons of seasoned flour and ½ cup water.
9. Add paste and remaining water to pan.
10. Cook, stirring until thickened, about 2 minutes.
11. Add chicken to sauce and heat thoroughly. This dish may be prepared ahead and frozen.

Yield: 4 servings

1 serving contains:

Cal	Prot	Fat	Carb	Sat	Mono	Poly	Chol	Na
315	25	20.7	7	4.3	7.0	7.9	78	809

Exchanges: 1 serving = 3 meats, ½ bread, 2 fats
Recommended for: The Living Heart; Diabetic; Types IIa, IIb, III, and IV Diets

Chicken Italiano

1 chicken fryer (2–3 pounds), cut up, skin and fat removed
1 teaspoon salt
¼ teaspoon pepper
¼ cup flour
¼ cup oil
1 onion, chopped
½ cup dry white wine (optional)
1 can (16 ounces) tomatoes, undrained
1 clove garlic, minced
1 teaspoon dried sweet basil
1 tablespoon chopped fresh parsley
1 teaspoon dried oregano
¼ pound fresh mushrooms, sliced
¼ cup water

1. Season chicken pieces with salt and pepper and coat with flour.
2. Brown on all sides in oil.
3. Add remaining ingredients to pan except mushrooms. Cover and cook 30 minutes.
4. Add mushrooms and cook 5 more minutes until chicken and mushrooms are tender.

Yield: 4 servings

1 serving contains:

Cal	Prot	Fat	Carb	Sat	Mono	Poly	Chol	Na
342	27	19.5	15	3.3	4.9	9.5	78	915

Exchanges: 1 serving = 3 meats, 1 bread, 2 fats
Recommended for: The Living Heart; Diabetic; Types IIa, IIb, III, and IV Diets
For Low Calorie Diets, omit flour and decrease oil to 2 tablespoons. Count as 3 meats, ½ bread, 1 fat (254 calories).

Abbreviations: **Cal,** calories; **Prot,** protein; **Carb,** carbohydrate; **Sat,** saturated fat; **Mono,** monounsaturated fat; **Poly,** polyunsaturated fat; **Chol,** cholesterol; **Na,** sodium. Protein, fat, carbohydrate, saturated fat, monounsaturated fat, and polyunsaturated fat are expressed in *grams.* Cholesterol and sodium are expressed in *milligrams.*

Lemon Baked Chicken

1   **chicken fryer (2–3 pounds), cut up, skin and fat removed**
2   **tablespoons lemon juice**
3   **tablespoons oil**
1   **clove garlic, minced**
½   **teaspoon salt**
¼   **teaspoon pepper**
¼   **teaspoon paprika**
¼   **teaspoon dried thyme**
2   **tablespoons chopped fresh parsley**

1. Preheat oven to 350°F.
2. Arrange chicken in a shallow baking dish.
3. Combine remaining ingredients and pour over chicken.
4. Cover and bake 40 minutes.
5. Uncover and cook an additional 20 minutes or until brown.
This dish may be prepared ahead and frozen.

Yield: 4 servings

1 serving contains:

Cal	Prot	Fat	Carb	Sat	Mono	Poly	Chol	Na
242	24	15.6	1	2.8	4.1	7.2	78	348

Exchanges: 1 serving = 3 meats, 1½ fats
Recommended for: The Living Heart; Diabetic; Types IIa, IIb, III, and IV Diets

Brunswick Stew

1   **chicken (2–3 pounds), cut up, skin and fat removed**
1   **onion, sliced**
3   **cups water**
1½   **teaspoons salt**
⅛   **teaspoon cayenne pepper**
1   **can (16 ounces) tomatoes, undrained**
1   **can (16 ounces) lima beans, undrained**
1   **can (16 ounces) whole kernel corn, undrained**
1   **tablespoon Worcestershire sauce**

1. Place chicken, onion, water, salt, and pepper into large pan. Cover and cook until chicken is tender, about 2 hours.

2. Remove from heat and chill.
3. Remove chicken from pan and bone. Remove fat and strain liquid through cheesecloth.
4. Combine chicken meat and liquid.
5. Add remaining ingredients to pan and heat thoroughly.

Yield: 8 servings

1 serving contains:

Cal	Prot	Fat	Carb	Sat	Mono	Poly	Chol	Na
167	16	3.3	19	0.9	0.8	1.0	39	758

Exchanges: 1 serving = 1½ meats, 1 bread
Recommended for: The Living Heart; Low Calorie; Diabetic; Types I, IIa, IIb, III, IV, and V Diets

Chicken Gumbo

2   **cups diced cooked chicken**
2   **tablespoons oil**
1   **can (16 ounces) tomatoes, undrained**
1   **can (16 ounces) okra, undrained**
½   **cup chicken bouillon**
1   **cup sliced onion**
1   **jalapeño pepper, seeded (optional)**
⅓   **cup chopped fresh parsley**
1   **teaspoon salt**
¼   **teaspoon pepper**
1   **bay leaf**
1   **clove garlic, minced**
¼   **teaspoon dried thyme**
1   **cup water**
½   **cup rice, uncooked**

1. Brown chicken lightly in oil in large saucepan.
2. Add all ingredients except rice. Cover and simmer 10 minutes.
3. Add rice and cover. Simmer for 25 minutes or until rice is tender, stirring occasionally.

Yield: 6 servings

1 serving contains:

Cal	Prot	Fat	Carb	Sat	Mono	Poly	Chol	Na
240	17	8.0	26	1.5	2.0	3.7	43	851

Exchanges: 1 serving = 1½ meats, 1½ breads, 1 fat
Recommended for: The Living Heart; Diabetic; Types IIa, IIb, III, and IV Diets

Chicken Vegetable Pot Pie

3 carrots, cut into 1-inch pieces
2 onions, chopped
3 tablespoons tub margarine
¼ cup flour
¼ teaspoon dried thyme
½ teaspoon salt
¼ teaspoon pepper
2 cups chicken bouillon
2 cups chopped cooked chicken or turkey
1 unbaked 9-inch pie shell (see recipe, page 215)

1. Cook carrots and onions in a small amount of water until nearly done. Drain.
2. Preheat oven to 400°F.
3. Melt margarine in a saucepan. Blend in flour, thyme, salt, and pepper. Stir in bouillon until thickened.
4. Place vegetables and chicken in a 2-quart casserole and add the sauce.
5. Top with pastry, sealing the edges. Cut small slits on the top to allow steam to escape.
6. Bake 30 minutes or until pastry is browned.

Yield: 6 servings

Variation:

Add 1 can (8 ounces) drained peas, cut-up celery, or other vegetables.

1 serving contains:

Cal	Prot	Fat	Carb	Sat	Mono	Poly	Chol	Na
328	15	18.7	25	3.7	6.4	7.7	35	929

Exchanges: 1 serving = 1½ meats, 1½ breads, 1 vegetable, 2½ fats
Recommended for: The Living Heart; Diabetic; Types IIa, IIb, III, and IV Diets

Mary Dell's Enchiladas

1 can (4 ounces) green chilies, seeded and finely chopped
1 clove garlic, minced
1 tablespoon oil
1 can (28 ounces) tomatoes, drained, chopped reserve liquid
tomato juice
2 cups chopped onion
1 teaspoon salt
½ teaspoon dried oregano
3 cups chopped cooked chicken or turkey
2 cups plain skim milk yogurt
2 cups cubed low-fat cheese
1 teaspoon salt
25 corn tortillas

1. Preheat oven to 350°F.
2. Sauté chilies and garlic in oil.
3. Stir in tomatoes, onion, salt, and oregano. Add enough tomato juice to tomato liquid to make 1 cup and add to mixture. Simmer, uncovered, until thick, about 30 minutes.
4. Meanwhile, combine chicken or turkey, yogurt, cheese cubes, and salt.
5. Dip tortillas into tomato mixture until they become limp.
6. Fill tortillas with chicken or turkey mixture, roll up, and place side by side, seam side down, in a 9 × 13-inch baking dish.
7. Pour chili sauce over top and bake until heated through, about 15–20 minutes.

Yield: 25 enchiladas

Note: May also be baked in an electric skillet at 250°F.

1 enchilada contains:

Cal	Prot	Fat	Carb	Sat	Mono	Poly	Chol	Na
144	9	2.8	19	0.8	0.6	0.6	17	474

Exchanges: 1 serving = 1 dairy, 1 bread
Recommended for: The Living Heart; Low Calorie; Diabetic; Types IIa, IIb, III, IV, and V Diets

Abbreviations: **Cal,** calories; **Prot,** protein; **Carb,** carbohydrate; **Sat,** saturated fat; **Mono,** monounsaturated fat; **Poly,** polyunsaturated fat; **Chol,** cholesterol; **Na,** sodium. Protein, fat, carbohydrate, saturated fat, monounsaturated fat, and polyunsaturated fat are expressed in *grams.* Cholesterol and sodium are expressed in *milligrams.*

Chicken Crêpes

½ cup chopped onion
¼ pound fresh mushrooms, sliced
2 tablespoons oil
6 tablespoons flour
1 chicken bouillon cube
1 teaspoon salt
¼ teaspoon pepper
¼ cup chopped fresh parsley
3 cups skim milk
⅓ cup white wine
3½ cups chopped cooked chicken
9 crêpes (see recipe, page 275)

1. Preheat oven to 350°F.
2. Sauté onion and mushrooms in oil.
3. Sprinkle with flour, add bouillon cube, salt, pepper, and parsley.
4. Gradually stir in milk and cook, stirring constantly, until mixture thickens.
5. Pour in wine and cook 5 minutes longer.
6. Add half of sauce mixture to the chicken.
7. Place ¼ cup chicken mixture on each crêpe.
8. Roll crêpes up and place seam side down in a 9 × 13-inch baking dish.
9. Top with remaining sauce, cover, and bake 20–30 minutes.

Yield: 9 servings

1 serving contains:

Cal	Prot	Fat	Carb	Sat	Mono	Poly	Chol	Na
251	23	9.4	18	2.0	2.6	3.9	52	682

Exchanges: 1 serving = 3 meats, 1 bread
Recommended for: The Living Heart; Low Calorie; Diabetic; Types IIa, IIb, III, IV, and V Diets

Stuffed Cornish Hens

¼ cup chopped celery
¼ cup chopped green pepper
¼ cup chopped onion
¼ cup plus 3 tablespoons tub margarine
¼ teaspoon ground sage
1 clove garlic, minced
⅛ teaspoon salt
⅛ teaspoon pepper
1 tablespoon chopped fresh parsley
1 cup fine, dry bread crumbs
¼ cup chopped walnuts
¼ cup cubed low-fat cheese
4 Rock Cornish hens

1. Preheat oven to 350°F.
2. Sauté celery, green pepper, and onion in 3 tablespoons margarine until celery is tender.
3. Stir in sage, garlic, salt, pepper, parsley and bread crumbs. Remove from heat.
4. Add walnuts and cheese.
5. Spoon mixture into cavities of Cornish hens.
6. Melt remaining margarine and brush hens.
7. Bake breast side up in a shallow pan for 60 minutes. Baste occasionally with the melted margarine.
8. Remove skin and fat before eating.

Yield: 4 servings

1 serving contains:

Cal	Prot	Fat	Carb	Sat	Mono	Poly	Chol	Na
580	60	26.6	22	5.4	8.1	11	138	753

Exchanges: 1 serving = 6½ meats, 1½ breads, 2 fats
Recommended for: The Living Heart; Diabetic; Types IIa, IIb, III, and IV Diets

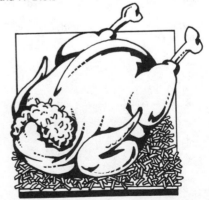

VEAL ENTRÉES

Veal Scallopini

2 tablespoons flour
1 teaspoon salt
¼ teaspoon pepper
¼ teaspoon dried sweet basil
¼ teaspoon dried oregano
1 pound veal cutlets, well trimmed
2 tablespoons oil
1 onion, chopped
1 clove garlic, minced
½ cup white wine
½ pound fresh mushrooms
2 tablespoons chopped fresh parsley
   paprika (optional)

1. Combine flour, salt, pepper, basil, and oregano.
2. Coat veal with flour mixture and brown in oil.
3. Add onion, garlic, and wine. Cover and cook about 20 minutes. Add more wine if necessary.
4. Add mushrooms and parsley.
5. Cover and cook 5–10 minutes longer, until meat and mushrooms are tender.
6. Garnish with paprika, if desired.

Yield: 4 servings

1 serving contains:

Cal	Prot	Fat	Carb	Sat	Mono	Poly	Chol	Na
266	28	13.1	8	3.0	3.6	4.4	78	618

Exchanges: 1 serving = 3 meats, ½ bread, 1 fat
Recommended for: The Living Heart; Diabetic; Types IIa, IIb, III, and IV Diets
For Low Calorie Diets, omit flour and decrease oil to 1 tablespoon. Count as 3 meats, 1½ vegetables (221 calories).

Veal Birds

⅓ cup finely chopped celery
¼ cup finely chopped walnuts
¼ cup chopped stuffed green olives
1½ pounds thinly sliced veal cutlets, well trimmed
¼ cup flour
¼ teaspoon salt
¼ teaspoon pepper
½ teaspoon garlic powder
½ teaspoon paprika
1 tablespoon tub margarine
1 cup beef bouillon
¼ pound mushrooms, sliced

1. Mix celery, walnuts, and olives. Place 2 tablespoons on each veal cutlet.
2. Roll each cutlet up like a jelly roll and secure with toothpicks.
3. Mix together flour and seasonings. Coat veal with seasoned flour and brown lightly on all sides in margarine.
4. Add bouillon. Cover and simmer until tender, about 45 minutes. Turn meat occasionally and add water if needed.
5. Add mushrooms and heat through.

Yield: 6 servings

1 serving contains:

Cal	Prot	Fat	Carb	Sat	Mono	Poly	Chol	Na
248	29	11.9	6	3.6	4.6	3.4	78	627

Exchanges: 1 serving = 3 meats, ½ bread, 1 fat
Recommended for: The Living Heart; Diabetic; Types IIa, IIb, III, and IV Diets

Abbreviations: **Cal,** calories; **Prot,** protein; **Carb,** carbohydrate; **Sat,** saturated fat; **Mono,** monounsaturated fat; **Poly,** polyunsaturated fat; **Chol,** cholesterol; **Na,** sodium. Protein, fat, carbohydrate, saturated fat, monounsaturated fat, and polyunsaturated fat are expressed in *grams.* Cholesterol and sodium are expressed in *milligrams.*

Braised Veal

¼ **cup flour**
1½ **teaspoons salt**
¼ **teaspoon pepper**
2 **pounds veal cutlets, well trimmed**
2 **tablespoons oil**
2 **onions, cut into rings**
1 **clove garlic, minced**
½ **cup water**
2 **tablespoons lemon juice**
1 **teaspoon dried oregano**
2 **tablespoons chopped fresh parsley**

1. Combine flour, ½ of the salt, and pepper and coat veal with flour mixture.
2. Brown veal on both sides in oil. Remove from pan.
3. Sauté onions and garlic until tender.
4. Return veal to pan and add remaining ingredients. Cover pan.
5. Simmer over low heat for 30 minutes. Add more water if needed.

Yield: 8 servings

1 serving contains:

Cal	Prot	Fat	Carb	Sat	Mono	Poly	Chol	Na
217	26	9.6	5	2.6	2.7	2.2	78	474

Exchanges: 1 serving = 3 meats, ½ bread
Recommended for: The Living Heart; Diabetic; Types IIa, IIb, III, IV, and V Diets

Buttermilk Breaded Veal Cutlet

1 **pound veal cutlets, well trimmed**
½ **cup buttermilk**
½ **cup fine, dry bread crumbs**
½ **teaspoon salt**
⅛ **teaspoon pepper**
3 **tablespoons tub margarine**

1. Dip cutlets in buttermilk, then in bread crumbs which have been seasoned with salt and pepper.
2. Melt margarine in skillet. Brown cutlets on low heat for about 5 minutes on each side.

Yield: 4 servings

1 serving contains:

Cal	Prot	Fat	Carb	Sat	Mono	Poly	Chol	Na
301	28	15.3	11	3.9	5.2	4.1	78	568

Exchanges: 1 serving = 3 meats, 1 bread, 1 fat
Recommended for: The Living Heart; Diabetic; Types IIa, IIb, III, and IV Diets

Roast Veal

3 **pound veal leg or shoulder roast, well trimmed**
1 **large onion, cut into rings**
2 **cloves garlic, sliced**
   ground ginger
   salt
   pepper
2 **cups water**
¼ **cup lemon juice**
¼ **teaspoon dried marjoram**

1. Preheat oven to 325°F.
2. Make small deep cuts in veal to insert onion and garlic.
3. Rub roast with ginger, salt, and pepper, and place in baking dish.
4. Pour remaining ingredients over roast.
5. Roast 35 minutes per pound.

Yield: 8 servings

1 serving contains:

Cal	Prot	Fat	Carb	Sat	Mono	Poly	Chol	Na
188	24	8.8	2	3.4	3.3	0.5	78	333

Exchanges: 1 serving = 3 meats
Recommended for: The Living Heart; Low Calorie; Diabetic; Types I, IIa, IIb, III, IV, and V Diets

Veal Curry

1 **cup sliced onion**
½ **cup chopped celery**
1 **apple, cored and sliced**
3 **tablespoons tub margarine**
2 **cups chopped cooked veal, well trimmed**
4 **teaspoons flour**
1 **teaspoon curry powder**
1 **cup beef bouillon**
1 **tablespoon lemon juice**
½ **teaspoon salt**
¼ **teaspoon pepper**

1. Sauté onion, celery, and apple in margarine until tender. Remove from pan.
2. Lightly brown veal in the same pan and remove.
3. Stir in flour, curry powder, and bouillon until smooth. Add lemon juice, salt, and pepper.
4. Return vegetables and veal to pan and heat through.
5. Serve over rice, if desired.

Yield: 4 servings

1 serving contains:

Cal	Prot	Fat	Carb	Sat	Mono	Poly	Chol	Na
230	19	12.4	11	3.4	4.6	4.2	52	676

Exchanges: 1 serving = 2 meats, ½ bread, 1½ fats
Recommended for: The Living Heart; Diabetic; Types IIa, IIb, III, and IV Diets

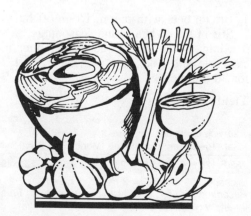

GROUND BEEF ENTRÉES

Main Dish Meatballs

1 **pound very lean ground beef**
¼ **teaspoon garlic salt**
1 **onion, finely chopped**
¼ **cup skim milk**
½ **teaspoon salt**
¼ **teaspoon pepper**
¼ **cup wheat germ**
1 **teaspoon dry mustard**
1 **egg white**
2 **beef bouillon cubes**
1½ **cups plus 1 tablespoon water**
2 **teaspoons chopped fresh parsley**
1 **tablespoon cornstarch**

1. Mix beef, garlic salt, onion, milk, salt, pepper, wheat germ, dry mustard, and egg white together. Form into 12 meatballs. Brown meatballs on all sides. Drain off fat.
2. Add bouillon cubes, 1½ cups water, and parsley. Cover and cook 20 minutes.
3. Stir cornstarch into 1 tablespoon cold water. Stir into meatballs to make a gravy.

Yield: 4 servings

1 serving contains:

Cal	Prot	Fat	Carb	Sat	Mono	Poly	Chol	Na
232	28	9.5	7	3.6	3.4	0.9	78	955

Exchanges: 1 serving = 3½ meats, ½ bread
Recommended for: The Living Heart; Diabetic; Types IIa, IIb, III, IV, and V Diets

Abbreviations: **Cal,** calories; **Prot,** protein; **Carb,** carbohydrate; **Sat,** saturated fat; **Mono,** monounsaturated fat; **Poly,** polyunsaturated fat; **Chol,** cholesterol; **Na,** sodium. Protein, fat, carbohydrate, saturated fat, monounsaturated fat, and polyunsaturated fat are expressed in *grams.* Cholesterol and sodium are expressed in *milligrams.*

Quick Spaghetti and Meatballs

1 clove garlic, minced
1 onion, chopped
½ green pepper, chopped
1 tablespoon oil
1 can (16 ounces) tomatoes, undrained
1 can (8 ounces) tomato sauce
½ teaspoon salt
¼ teaspoon pepper
½ teaspoon dried oregano
1 package (8 ounces) spaghetti
½ cup soft bread crumbs
2 tablespoons skim milk
1 pound very lean ground beef
½ teaspoon salt

1. Sauté garlic, onion, and green pepper in oil until tender.
2. Add tomatoes, tomato sauce, salt, pepper, and oregano. Simmer 15 minutes.
3. Cook spaghetti according to package directions.
4. While spaghetti is cooking, combine bread crumbs, milk, meat, and salt. Shape into 24 small meatballs. Brown in skillet. Drain off fat.
5. Add sauce to meatballs and simmer 5–10 minutes.
6. Serve over hot, drained spaghetti.

Yield: 6 servings

1 serving contains:

Cal	Prot	Fat	Carb	Sat	Mono	Poly	Chol	Na
295	21	8.9	32	2.6	2.8	2.3	52	682

Exchanges: 1 serving = 2½ meats, 2 breads, ½ fat
Recommended for: The Living Heart; Diabetic; Types IIa, IIb, III, and IV Diets

Spaghetti Sauce

1 pound very lean ground beef
1 onion, chopped
1 green pepper, finely chopped
1 clove garlic, minced
¼ cup chopped fresh parsley
½ teaspoon dried oregano

1 teaspoon dried sweet basil
¼ teaspoon fennel seeds
1 can (16 ounces) tomatoes, undrained
1 can (6 ounces) tomato paste
1½ cups water
1 bay leaf
2 tablespoons sugar
1 teaspoon salt
¼ teaspoon pepper

1. Brown meat, onion, and green pepper. Drain off fat.
2. Add remaining ingredients. Cover and simmer 2 hours, stirring occasionally.

Yield: 6 servings

1 serving contains:

Cal	Prot	Fat	Carb	Sat	Mono	Poly	Chol	Na
191	18	6.2	16	2.3	2.2	0.6	52	525

Exchanges: 1 serving = 2 meats, 1 bread
Recommended for: The Living Heart; Low Calorie; Diabetic; Types I, IIa, IIb, III, IV, and V Diets

Main Dish Texas Barbecued Beans

1 pound very lean ground beef
½ cup chopped onion
1 can (28–32 ounces) vegetarian baked beans
½ teaspoon salt
¼ teaspoon pepper
½ cup catsup
3 tablespoons vinegar
¼ teaspoon red pepper sauce

1. Brown beef with onion. Drain off fat.
2. Stir in baked beans and seasonings.
3. Simmer, stirring frequently, or pour into a casserole and bake in a preheated 350°F oven for 30 minutes.

Yield: 6 servings

1 serving contains:

Cal	Prot	Fat	Carb	Sat	Mono	Poly	Chol	Na
330	26	6.7	42	2.5	2.3	0.9	52	962

Exchanges: 1 serving = 2 meats, 3 breads
Recommended for: The Living Heart; Diabetic; Types IIa, IIb, III, IV, and V Diets

Lemon Meat Loaf

1½ **pounds very lean ground beef**
 1 **cup fine, dry bread crumbs**
 ¼ **cup lemon juice**
 ¼ **cup finely chopped onion**
   egg substitute equivalent to 1 egg
 2 **teaspoons salt**
 ½ **cup catsup**
 ⅓ **cup brown sugar, firmly packed**
 1 **teaspoon dry mustard**
 ¼ **teaspoon ground allspice**
 ¼ **teaspoon ground cloves**

1. Preheat oven to 350°F.
2. Combine all ingredients and place in a 9 × 5-inch loaf pan.
3. Bake 60 minutes.

Yield: 8 servings

1 serving contains:

Cal	Prot	Fat	Carb	Sat	Mono	Poly	Chol	Na
250	21	7.7	24	2.8	2.9	0.8	58	879

Exchanges: 1 serving = 2½ meats, 1 bread, 1 vegetable
Recommended for: The Living Heart; Diabetic; Types IIa, IIb, III, IV, and V Diets

Stuffed Meat Loaf

Meatloaf
 2 **pounds very lean ground beef**
 1 **can (8 ounces) tomato sauce with onion**
1½ **teaspoons garlic salt**
 1 **teaspoon dried oregano**
 ½ **teaspoon dried sweet basil**

Filling
1½ **cups dry curd cottage cheese**
   egg substitute equivalent to 1 egg
 ½ **teaspoon salt**
 ½ **teaspoon pepper**

1. Preheat oven to 350°F.
2. Mix meatloaf ingredients together.
3. Place half of the mixture in a loaf pan and form a well in the center.
4. Combine filling ingredients and place in well. Cover with remaining meat, sealing edges.

5. Bake 60 minutes.

Yield: 8 servings

1 serving contains:

Cal	Prot	Fat	Carb	Sat	Mono	Poly	Chol	Na
224	30	9.4	3	3.6	3.4	0.7	79	687

Exchanges: 1 serving = 3½ meats, 1 vegetable
Recommended for: The Living Heart; Low Calorie; Diabetic; Types IIa, IIb, III, IV, and V Diets

Variation:
Heat 2 cups tomato sauce with onion to serve over meat loaf (245 calories per serving).

Applesauce Meat Loaf

1½ **pounds very lean ground beef**
 ¾ **cup fine, dry bread crumbs**
 ½ **cup catsup**
 ½ **cup applesauce**
 ¾ **teaspoon salt**
 ½ **teaspoon pepper**

1. Preheat oven to 350°F.
2. Combine all ingredients and place in a 9 × 5-inch loaf pan.
3. Bake 90 minutes.

Yield: 8 servings

1 serving contains:

Cal	Prot	Fat	Carb	Sat	Mono	Poly	Chol	Na
206	20	7.1	15	2.7	2.7	0.5	58	496

Exchanges: 1 serving = 2½ meats, 1 bread
Recommended for: The Living Heart; Low Calorie; Types IIa, IIb, III, IV, and V Diets

Abbreviations: **Cal,** calories; **Prot,** protein; **Carb,** carbohydrate; **Sat,** saturated fat; **Mono,** monounsaturated fat; **Poly,** polyunsaturated fat; **Chol,** cholesterol; **Na,** sodium. Protein, fat, carbohydrate, saturated fat, monounsaturated fat, and polyunsaturated fat are expressed in *grams.* Cholesterol and sodium are expressed in *milligrams.*

Pizza

Dough
1 package active dry yeast
1⅔ cups lukewarm water (95–105°F)
3 tablespoons oil
4 cups flour
1 teaspoon salt

Tomato Sauce
1 cup finely chopped onion
3 tablespoons oil
1 clove garlic, minced
2 cans (16 ounces each) tomatoes, undrained, chopped
1 can (6 ounces) tomato paste
1 tablespoon dried oregano
1 teaspoon dried sweet basil
1 bay leaf
1 tablespoon salt

Topping
8 ounces low-fat cheese, sliced
1 can (4 ounces) anchovies
¼ pound fresh mushrooms, sliced
1 cup chopped green pepper
1 pound very lean ground beef or Homemade Sausage (see recipe, this page), browned

Dough
1. Dissolve yeast in lukewarm water in a bowl. Add oil and stir in flour and salt.
2. Turn onto a lightly floured board and knead until smooth.
3. Place dough in an oiled bowl, turning once to oil surface. Cover and let rise until double in bulk, 1½–2 hours. At this point dough can be punched down, refrigerated for a day or two, or frozen for future use.
4. Preheat oven to 400°F.
5. Punch down and knead again for a few minutes. Divide in half and pat into two oiled 14-inch pans.
6. Add tomato sauce (see instructions below) and topping ingredients.
7. Bake for 20–25 minutes.

Sauce (prepare while dough is rising)
1. Sauté onions in oil until soft and tender. Add garlic and cook 2 minutes. Add remaining ingredients and simmer, uncovered, for 60 minutes, stirring occasionally.
2. Remove bay leaf. If a smoother sauce is desired, it may be either puréed or put through a sieve.

Yield: 2 pizzas

Note: Half of the dough (after step 4) and half of the sauce may be frozen if only one pizza is desired.

⅛ pizza contains:

Cal	Prot	Fat	Carb	Sat	Mono	Poly	Chol	Na
271	15	9.1	32	2.2	2.5	3.7	34	923

Exchanges: ⅛ pizza = 2 meats, 2 breads, ½ fat
Recommended for: The Living Heart; Diabetic; Types IIa, IIb, III, and IV Diets

Homemade Sausage

1 pound very lean ground beef
½ teaspoon ground sage
¼ teaspoon dried thyme
1 teaspoon salt
1 teaspoon pepper
1 teaspoon liquid smoke

1. Mix all ingredients together thoroughly and shape into patties.
2. Broil or pan fry patties. If pan frying, pour off fat as it collects.
3. Drain patties on paper towels.

Yield: 6 servings

Variation:
Hot Sausage: Add 1 teaspoon crushed red pepper.

1 serving contains:

Cal	Prot	Fat	Carb	Sat	Mono	Poly	Chol	Na
122	16	5.8	0	2.3	2.2	0.3	52	404

Exchanges: 1 serving = 2 meats
Recommended for: The Living Heart; Low Calorie; Diabetic; Types I, IIa, IIb, III, IV, and V Diets

Better Broiled Burgers

To 1 pound very lean ground beef, add one of the following combinations:

¼ **cup Worcestershire sauce**
¼ **cup tomato juice**
¼ **cup finely chopped onion**
¼ **teaspoon red pepper sauce**
or
¼ **cup finely chopped onion**
2½ **tablespoons prepared mustard**
1 **tablespoon Worcestershire sauce**

1. Combine all ingredients and form into 4 patties.
2. Place on broiler rack and broil 3 inches from heat for about 4 minutes on each side.

Yield: 4 servings

1 serving contains:

Cal	Prot	Fat	Carb	Sat	Mono	Poly	Chol	Na
195	25	8.8	3	3.4	3.3	0.5	78	355

Exchanges: 1 serving = 3 meats, 1 vegetable
Recommended for: The Living Heart; Low Calorie; Diabetic; Types IIa, IIb, III, IV, and V Diets

Easy Enchiladas

1 **onion, chopped**
1 **pound very lean ground beef**
3 **tablespoons tub margarine**
3 **tablespoons flour**
3 **cups beef bouillon**
1 **tablespoon chili powder**
½ **teaspoon ground cumin**
8 **soft corn tortillas**
8 **ounces low-fat cheese, cubed or shredded**

1. Preheat oven to 350°F.
2. Brown onion and beef. Drain off fat and remove from pan.
3. Melt margarine in skillet. Add flour and beef bouillon to make gravy. Stir in spices and simmer 5 minutes.
4. Dip each tortilla in the gravy until soggy.
5. Spread meat mixture and half of the cheese

on tortillas, roll, and place seam side down in 9 × 13-inch baking pan.
6. Pour remaining gravy over enchiladas and top with remaining cheese.
7. Bake 15 minutes until cheese is melted and bubbly.

Yield: 8 servings

1 serving contains:

Cal	Prot	Fat	Carb	Sat	Mono	Poly	Chol	Na
269	20	11.3	20	3.6	3.7	2.2	49	880

Exchanges: 1 serving = 2½ meats, 1 bread, 1 fat
Recommended for: The Living Heart; Diabetic; Types IIa, IIb, III, and IV Diets

Barbecue on a Bun

1 **pound very lean ground beef**
1 **onion, chopped**
1 **tablespoon prepared mustard**
½ **cup catsup**
1 **can (8 ounces) tomato sauce**
¼ **teaspoon ground cloves**
1 **tablespoon vinegar**
1 **teaspoon sugar**
2–3 **drops red pepper sauce**
4 **hamburger buns**

1. Brown meat and onion. Drain off fat.
2. Add seasonings and simmer at least 15 minutes.
3. Serve on hamburger buns.

Yield: 4 servings

1 serving contains:

Cal	Prot	Fat	Carb	Sat	Mono	Poly	Chol	Na
373	31	10.6	38	4.4	4.4	1.3	78	884

Exchanges: 1 serving = 3 meats, 2½ breads, 1 vegetable, ½ fat
Recommended for: The Living Heart; Diabetic; Types IIa, IIb, III, and IV Diets

Abbreviations: **Cal,** calories; **Prot,** protein; **Carb,** carbohydrate; **Sat,** saturated fat; **Mono,** monounsaturated fat; **Poly,** polyunsaturated fat; **Chol,** cholesterol; **Na,** sodium. Protein, fat, carbohydrate, saturated fat, monounsaturated fat, and polyunsaturated fat are expressed in *grams.* Cholesterol and sodium are expressed in *milligrams.*

Chili

1 pound very lean ground beef
1½ cups chopped onion
1 cup water
1 can (8 ounces) tomato sauce
1 teaspoon salt
4 teaspoons chili powder
½ green pepper, chopped
1 bay leaf (optional)
⅛ teaspoon dried sweet basil (optional)

1. Brown meat and onion. Drain off fat.
2. Add remaining ingredients.
3. Cover and simmer for 30 minutes, stirring occasionally.

Yield: 4 servings

1 serving contains:

Cal	Prot	Fat	Carb	Sat	Mono	Poly	Chol	Na
236	26	9.3	12	3.4	3.3	0.6	78	859

Exchanges: 1 serving = 3 meats, 1 bread
Recommended for: The Living Heart; Diabetic; Types IIa, IIb, III, IV, and V Diets

Variation:

Chili with Beans: Add 2 cans (16 ounces each) undrained kidney beans.

Yield: 6 servings

1 serving contains:

Cal	Prot	Fat	Carb	Sat	Mono	Poly	Chol	Na
311	27	6.8	36	2.4	2.2	0.7	52	578

Exchanges: 1 serving = 3 meats, 2 breads
Recommended for: The Living Heart; Diabetic; Types IIa, IIb, III, IV, and V Diets

MEAT AND GAME ENTRÉES

Home-Cooked Beef Stew

1½ pounds lean beef, well trimmed, cut into 1-inch cubes
¼ cup flour
¼ cup oil
2½ cups water
2 tablespoons chopped fresh parsley
1 clove garlic, minced
2 bay leaves
2 teaspoons salt
½ teaspoon dried thyme
¼ teaspoon pepper
4 potatoes, peeled and cubed
5 carrots, cut into 1-inch pieces
3 stalks celery, cut into 1-inch pieces
2 onions, cut into eighths

1. Coat beef cubes with flour and brown in oil.
2. Add water and simmer 20 minutes.
3. Remove from heat and chill. Skim off fat that rises to surface.
4. Add parsley, garlic, bay leaves, salt, thyme, and pepper. Simmer 1 hour or until meat is tender. Add more water if needed.
5. Add vegetables.
6. Cook an additional 30 minutes or until vegetables are tender.

Yield: 6 servings

1 serving contains:

Cal	Prot	Fat	Carb	Sat	Mono	Poly	Chol	Na
360	27	18.1	22	4.6	5.5	6.0	78	836

Exchanges: 1 serving = 3 meats, 1 bread, 1 vegetable, 2 fats
Recommended for: The Living Heart; Diabetic; Types IIa, IIb, III, and IV Diets
For Low Calorie Diets, omit flour and decrease oil to 2 tablespoons. Count as 3 meats, 1 bread, 1 vegetable, ½ fat (286 calories).

Teriyaki Strip Steak

¼ **cup soy sauce**
2 **tablespoons sugar**
½ **teaspoon ground ginger**
1 **clove garlic, minced**
1 **tablespoon vinegar**
1½ **pounds lean beef, well trimmed, cut into ½-inch strips**

1. Combine soy sauce, sugar, ginger, garlic, and vinegar. Marinate meat in this mixture at least 1 hour or overnight in refrigerator.
2. Remove meat from marinade. Broil 6 inches from heat 3–5 minutes on each side.
3. Serve with rice, if desired.

Yield: 6 servings

1 serving contains:

Cal	Prot	Fat	Carb	Sat	Mono	Poly	Chol	Na
189	26	6.2	6	2.2	1.9	0.3	78	936

Exchanges: 1 serving = 3 meats
Recommended for: The Living Heart; Low Calorie; Diabetic; Types I, IIa, IIb, III, IV, and V Diets

Garden Kabobs

½ **cup oil**
½ **cup wine vinegar**
½ **cup chopped onion**
1 **teaspoon salt**
½ **teaspoon garlic powder**
½ **teaspoon pepper**
2 **pounds lean beef or lamb, well trimmed, cut into 1-inch cubes**
10–15 **small white onions or 3 yellow onions, quartered**
1 **green pepper, cut into chunks**
¼ **pound whole fresh mushrooms**
10–15 **cherry tomatoes**

1. Combine oil, vinegar, onion, salt, garlic powder, and pepper. Pour over meat cubes and marinate several hours or overnight in refrigerator.
2. Remove meat from marinade. Thread meat with vegetables on skewers. Brush with marinade.

3. Broil 6–8 minutes, turning once, until done.

Yield: 8 servings

1 serving contains:

Cal	Prot	Fat	Carb	Sat	Mono	Poly	Chol	Na
271	26	15.7	6	4.3	5.0	4.6	78	203

Exchanges: 1 serving = 3 meats, 1 vegetable, 1½ fats
Recommended for: The Living Heart; Diabetic; Types IIa, IIb, III, and IV Diets

Beef Sukiyaki

1 **pound lean round steak, well trimmed, cut into 1-inch strips**
2 **tablespoons water**
½ **cup celery, diagonally cut**
1 **green pepper, sliced**
1½ **cups sliced fresh mushrooms or 1 can (8 ounces) mushrooms, drained**
½ **cup green pepper, chopped**
1 **can (10¾ ounces) condensed beef broth, undiluted**
1 **tablespoon soy sauce**
½ **cup sliced water chestnuts**
1 **tablespoon cornstarch**

1. Brown meat in pan with 1 tablespoon water.
2. Add vegetables, beef broth, and soy sauce. Cook over low heat 5 minutes or until vegetables are tender, stirring frequently.
3. Add water chestnuts and stir 30 seconds.
4. Combine remaining water with cornstarch. Add to meat mixture, stirring until thickened.

Yield: 4 servings

1 serving contains:

Cal	Prot	Fat	Carb	Sat	Mono	Poly	Chol	Na
223	31	6.4	10	2.2	1.9	0.5	78	899

Exchanges: 1 serving = 3 meats, 2 vegetables
Recommended for: The Living Heart; Low Calorie; Diabetic; Types IIa, IIb, III, IV, and V Diets

Abbreviations: **Cal,** calories; **Prot,** protein; **Carb,** carbohydrate; **Sat,** saturated fat; **Mono,** monounsaturated fat; **Poly,** polyunsaturated fat; **Chol,** cholesterol; **Na,** sodium. Protein, fat, carbohydrate, saturated fat, monounsaturated fat, and polyunsaturated fat are expressed in *grams*. Cholesterol and sodium are expressed in *milligrams*.

Herb Garden Steak

  1 **pound round steak, well trimmed**
  ¼ **teaspoon salt**
  ⅛ **teaspoon pepper**
  2 **tablespoons tub margarine**
  ¼ **cup chopped onion**
  1 **clove garlic, minced**
  1 **tablespoon flour**
  ½ **teaspoon dried oregano**
  ¼ **teaspoon dried marjoram**
  ¼ **teaspoon dried thyme**
  ¾ **cup water**
  1 **tablespoon lemon juice**

1. Season steak lightly with salt and pepper. Brown in margarine in large skillet. Remove from pan.
2. Add onion and garlic to skillet and cook until tender. Stir in flour.
3. Add herbs, water, lemon juice, and steak. Cover and simmer 30 minutes or until meat is tender.
4. Serve meat topped with the sauce.

Yield: 4 servings

1 serving contains:

Cal	Prot	Fat	Carb	Sat	Mono	Poly	Chol	Na
228	26	11.9	3	3.2	3.9	2.7	78	268

Exchanges: 1 serving = 3 meats, 1 fat
Recommended for: The Living Heart; Low Calorie; Diabetic; Types IIa, IIb, III, and IV Diets

Polynesian Kabobs

  1 **teaspoon dry mustard**
  ¼ **teaspoon ground ginger**
  ¼ **teaspoon pepper**
  1 **clove garlic, minced**
  3 **tablespoons Worcestershire sauce**
  3 **tablespoons lemon juice**
  3 **tablespoons oil**
  1 **can (7 ounces) pineapple chunks, packed in own juice, drained, reserve liquid**
  2 **pounds lean round steak, well trimmed, cut into ½-inch strips**
  1 **green pepper, cut into 1-inch chunks**

1. Combine mustard, ginger, pepper, garlic, Worcestershire sauce, lemon juice, oil, and ¼ cup reserved pineapple liquid. Add steak strips and marinate 4 hours or overnight.
2. Thread strips on skewers accordion style, alternating beef with pineapple and green pepper chunks.
3. Broil about 4 inches from heat 6–8 minutes, turning once and brushing occasionally with marinade.

Yield: 8 servings

1 serving contains:

Cal	Prot	Fat	Carb	Sat	Mono	Poly	Chol	Na
238	26	11.3	7	2.8	3.1	3.3	78	159

Exchanges: 1 serving = 3 meats, 1 fruit, ½ fat
Recommended for: The Living Heart; Diabetic; Types IIa, IIb, III, and IV Diets

Burgundy Flank Steak

  ¾ **cup dry red or rosé wine**
  1 **onion, sliced**
  1 **clove garlic, minced**
  1 **teaspoon salt**
  1 **teaspoon pepper**
  ¼ **teaspoon dried rosemary**
  1 **bay leaf**
  1½ **pounds flank steak**

1. Combine all ingredients and pour over flank steak. Marinate 2–3 hours at room temperature, turning steak frequently. Drain, reserving marinade.
2. Place meat on broiler rack and broil 3 inches from heat for 3–4 minutes on each side, basting frequently with marinade.
3. Slice diagonally into very thin slices before serving.

Yield: 6 servings

1 serving contains:

Cal	Prot	Fat	Carb	Sat	Mono	Poly	Chol	Na
167	26	6.1	1	2.2	1.9	0.2	78	240

Exchanges: 1 serving = 3 meats
Recommended for: The Living Heart; Low Calorie; Diabetic; Types I, IIa, IIb, III, IV, and V Diets

London Broil Our Way

1½ **pounds flank steak**
¾ **cup low-calorie Italian dressing**
2 **tablespoons soy sauce**
⅛ **teaspoon onion powder**
⅛ **teaspoon lemon pepper**
½ **teaspoon dried thyme**
½ **teaspoon salt**

1. Score steak diagonally on both sides.
2. Combine Italian dressing, soy sauce, onion powder, lemon pepper, and thyme. Pour over steak. Cover and let stand at room temperature 2–3 hours, turning steak frequently.
3. Drain marinade from meat. Place meat on broiler rack. Broil 3 inches from heat for 4 minutes on each side.
4. Season lightly with salt. Slice on the diagonal in very thin slices before serving.

Yield: 6 servings

1 serving contains:

Cal	Prot	Fat	Carb	Sat	Mono	Poly	Chol	Na
183	26	7.5	1	2.4	2.2	1.0	78	934

Exchanges: 1 serving = 3 meats
Recommended for: The Living Heart; Low Calorie; Diabetic; Types I, IIa, IIb, III, IV, and V Diets

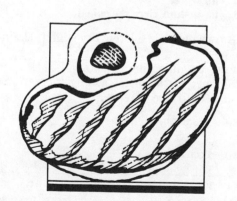

Oven-Dried Beef Jerky

2–2½ **pounds flank steak or lean roast, well trimmed**
1 **cup water**
2 **tablespoons liquid smoke**
2 **teaspoons salt**
1 **teaspoon garlic powder (optional)**
1 **teaspoon onion powder (optional)**
¼ **teaspoon black pepper**

1. Cut meat into strips 4–6 inches long, ½–1 inch wide, and ⅛–¼ inch thick. Meat is easier to work with if partially frozen. For chewy jerky, cut with grain of meat. For more tender jerky, cut across grain.
2. Mix water and seasonings and marinate beef in mixture overnight in refrigerator.
3. Drain beef strips and pat dry with paper towels.
4. Cover bottom rack of oven with baking sheet or aluminum foil.
5. Hang or lay strips on top oven rack so they do not touch or overlap.
6. Dry meat at lowest oven temperature (150–200°F) until it has turned brown, feels hard, and is dry to the touch, about 4–5 hours.
7. Let cool, then remove from racks.
8. Store in a cool dry place in a tightly covered container.

Yield: 24 strips (approximately 1 ounce each)

1 strip contains:

Cal	Prot	Fat	Carb	Sat	Mono	Poly	Chol	Na
62	10	2.3	0	0.8	0.7	0.1	29	204

Exchanges: 1 strip = 1 meat
Recommended for: The Living Heart; Low Calorie; Diabetic; Types I, IIa, IIb, III, IV, and V Diets

Abbreviations: **Cal,** calories; **Prot,** protein; **Carb,** carbohydrate; **Sat,** saturated fat; **Mono,** monounsaturated fat; **Poly,** polyunsaturated fat; **Chol,** cholesterol; **Na,** sodium. Protein, fat, carbohydrate, saturated fat, monounsaturated fat, and polyunsaturated fat are expressed in *grams*. Cholesterol and sodium are expressed in *milligrams*.

Baked Beef Hash

¼ **cup finely chopped onion**
¼ **teaspoon dried marjoram**
¼ **teaspoon dried thyme**
¼ **teaspoon dried savory**
¼ **cup chopped fresh parsley**
¼ **cup tub margarine**
4 **cups chopped cooked lean roast beef, well trimmed**
½ **cup red wine**
4 **cups boiled potatoes, cubed**
½ **cup skim milk**
2 **tablespoons soy sauce**
    paprika

1. Sauté onion, marjoram, thyme, savory, and parsley in margarine until onions are tender.
2. Combine roast beef, wine, potatoes, milk, and soy sauce. Add onion-herb mixture.
3. Refrigerate 3 hours or overnight, stirring occasionally.
4. Pour into a casserole and sprinkle generously with paprika. Bake in a preheated 350°F oven 30 minutes.

Yield: 6 servings

1 serving contains:

Cal	Prot	Fat	Carb	Sat	Mono	Poly	Chol	Na
298	26	13.3	18	3.4	4.4	3.7	69	597

Exchanges: 1 serving = 3 meats, 1 bread, 1 fat
Recommended for: The Living Heart; Diabetic; Types IIa, IIb, III, and IV Diets

Louisiana Creole Roast

3 **pounds lean beef roast, well trimmed**
2 **tablespoons oil**
1 **teaspoon salt**
½ **teaspoon pepper**
1 **onion, cut into rings**
½ **cup chopped celery**
½ **green pepper, cut into rings**
2 **cans (16 ounces each) tomatoes (tomatoes with okra, if desired), undrained**
½ **cup sliced stuffed green olives**
6 **drops red pepper sauce**

1. Brown meat in oil in large pan or Dutch oven. Season with salt and pepper.
2. Add onion rings, celery, and green pepper, stirring until tender.
3. Add remaining ingredients.
4. Cover and simmer 1½–2 hours until tender or bake in a 350°F oven.
5. Remove fat from pan drippings and thicken with cornstarch for gravy, if desired.

Yield: 8 servings

1 serving contains:

Cal	Prot	Fat	Carb	Sat	Mono	Poly	Chol	Na
265	26	14.7	7	4.1	5.9	2.9	78	927

Exchanges: 1 serving = 3 meats, 1½ vegetables, 1 fat
Recommended for: The Living Heart; Diabetic; Types IIa, IIb, III, and IV Diets
For Low Calorie Diets, omit olives. Count as 3 meats, 1½ vegetables, ½ fat (245 calories).

Pork Chops in Spanish Rice

1 **pound lean pork chops, well trimmed**
¼ **cup chopped onion**
¼ **cup chopped green pepper**
1 **can (16 ounces) tomatoes, undrained**
1 **can (8 ounces) tomato sauce**
1 **teaspoon salt**
1 **cup water**
1 **cup instant rice, uncooked**

1. Brown chops in a large, dry skillet. Drain off fat.
2. Add remaining ingredients.
3. Simmer 20 minutes, adding more water if needed, until rice is tender.

Yield: 4 servings

1 serving contains:

Cal	Prot	Fat	Carb	Sat	Mono	Poly	Chol	Na
344	30	8.9	36	2.7	3.5	1.2	75	980

Exchanges: 1 serving = 3 meats, 2 breads, 1 vegetable
Recommended for: The Living Heart; Diabetic; Types I, IIa, IIb, III, IV, and V Diets

Barbecued Pork Chops

1 **pound lean pork chops, well trimmed**
3 **slices lemon or 3 tablespoons lemon juice**
1 **tablespoon brown sugar, firmly packed**
⅓ **cup catsup**
¼ **cup water**

1. Brown chops in dry skillet. Drain off fat.
2. Combine remaining ingredients and pour over meat.
3. Cover and simmer 20 minutes. Remove cover and simmer 10 minutes more, adding more water if needed.

Yield: 4 servings

1 serving contains:

Cal	Prot	Fat	Carb	Sat	Mono	Poly	Chol	Na
222	26	8.5	10	2.6	3.5	0.9	75	288

Exchanges: 1 serving = 3 meats, ½ bread
Recommended for: The Living Heart; Low Calorie; Diabetic; Types I, IIa, IIb, III, IV, and V Diets

Curried Lamb

1 **pound lean lamb, well trimmed, cut into 1-inch cubes**
1 **tablespoon oil**
½ **cup finely chopped onion**
½ **teaspoon salt**
2 **teaspoons curry powder**
¼ **teaspoon pepper**
1 **teaspoon ground allspice**
1 **bay leaf**
2 **teaspoons ground cinnamon**
1½ **cups water**
½ **cup raisins**

1. Brown meat on all sides in oil.
2. Add remaining ingredients. Cook over medium heat for about 1 hour or until meat is tender, stirring occasionally.
3. Serve over cooked rice, if desired.

Yield: 4 servings

1 serving contains:

Cal	Prot	Fat	Carb	Sat	Mono	Poly	Chol	Na
275	25	12.2	17	3.9	4.1	2.5	78	339

Exchanges: 1 serving = 3 meats, 1 vegetable, 1 fruit, ½ fat
Recommended for: The Living Heart; Diabetic; Types IIa, IIb, III, and IV Diets
For Low Calorie Diets, omit raisins. Count as 3 meats, 1 vegetable, ½ fat (223 calories).

Swissed Venison Steak

1½ **pounds venison round steak, cut 1½ inches thick, well trimmed**
1 **teaspoon salt**
¼ **teaspoon pepper**
¼ **cup flour**
3 **tablespoons oil**
3 **onions, sliced**
1 **stalk celery, chopped**
1 **can (8 ounces) tomatoes, undrained**
2 **tablespoons Worcestershire sauce**

1. Season venison with salt and pepper and coat with flour.
2. Brown meat in oil.
3. Remove from pan and place in baking dish. Add other ingredients over meat.
4. Cover and bake at 300°F 90 minutes or until tender.

Yield: 6 servings

1 serving contains:

Cal	Prot	Fat	Carb	Sat	Mono	Poly	Chol	Na
267	27	13.0	9	3.0	3.6	4.3	78	573

Exchanges: 1 serving = 3 meats, ½ bread, 1 fat
Recommended for: The Living Heart; Diabetic; Types IIa, IIb, III, and IV Diets

Abbreviations: **Cal,** calories; **Prot,** protein; **Carb,** carbohydrate; **Sat,** saturated fat; **Mono,** monounsaturated fat; **Poly,** polyunsaturated fat; **Chol,** cholesterol; **Na,** sodium. Protein, fat, carbohydrate, saturated fat, monounsaturated fat, and polyunsaturated fat are expressed in *grams*. Cholesterol and sodium are expressed in *milligrams*.

EGG ENTRÉES

Cheesy Scrambled Eggs

**2 tablespoons tub margarine
egg substitute equivalent to 4 eggs
½ pound low-fat cheese, cubed**

1. Melt margarine in medium skillet.
2. Add egg substitute, stirring over low heat until almost firm.
3. Stir in cheese until melted.

Yield: 4 servings

Variations:
Add one or more of the following with cheese:
6 tablespoons chopped onion
6 tablespoons chopped green pepper
6 tablespoons chopped mushrooms
¼ teaspoon curry powder

1 serving contains:

Cal	Prot	Fat	Carb	Sat	Mono	Poly	Chol	Na
217	18	12.9	7	3.8	4.0	4.6	20	1034

Exchanges: 1 serving = 2 meats, ½ dairy, 1½ fats
Recommended for: The Living Heart; Diabetic; Types IIa, IIb, III, and IV Diets

Easy Cheese Omelet

**egg substitute equivalent to 4 eggs
¼ teaspoon salt
⅛ teaspoon pepper
1 tablespoon tub margarine
½ cup cubed low-fat cheese**

1. Combine egg substitute and seasonings.
2. Melt margarine in omelet pan or 8-inch skillet over medium heat, tilting pan to grease sides.
3. Add egg substitute mixture to pan. Do not stir. As egg substitute sets, lift edges with spatula and allow uncooked portion to run underneath.

4. When omelet is nearly set, sprinkle cheese on one half. When completely set, fold second half over the half with cheese.
5. Slide omelet from pan onto warm plate.

Yield: 2 servings

1 serving contains:

Cal	Prot	Fat	Carb	Sat	Mono	Poly	Chol	Na
232	18	14.9	6	3.3	4.4	6.7	11	989

Exchanges: 1 serving = 2 meats, ½ dairy, 1½ fats
Recommended for: The Living Heart; Diabetic; Types IIa, IIb, III, and IV Diets

Scrambled Whites

**2 egg whites
1 tablespoon skim milk
⅛ teaspoon salt
2–3 drops yellow food coloring
1 teaspoon oil**

1. Beat egg whites until stiff.
2. Fold in milk, salt, and coloring.
3. Heat oil in skillet. Add whites mixture. Cook over low heat, stirring often.

Yield: 1 serving

Variation:
Season mixture before cooking with 1 teaspoon of the following: minced onion, chives, green pepper, imitation bacon bits.

1 serving contains:

Cal	Prot	Fat	Carb	Sat	Mono	Poly	Chol	Na
77	7	4.6	2	0.6	1.1	2.6	0	371

Exchanges: 1 serving = 1 meat
Recommended for: The Living Heart; Low Calorie; Diabetic; Types IIa, IIb, III, and IV Diets
1 serving with bacon bits counts as 1 meat, ½ fat (92 calories).

Meatless Entrées

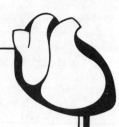

Nutty Cheese Loaf

  1 **cup low-fat cottage cheese**
  ½ **cup peanut butter**
  1 **cup tomato sauce**
  1 **cup cracker crumbs**
  1 **cup skim milk**
  1 **onion, minced**
    egg substitute equivalent to 2 eggs
  1 **tablespoon flour**
  ½ **teaspoon salt**
  ½ **teaspoon sage**
  ¾ **teaspoon garlic powder**

1. Preheat oven to 325°F.
2. Combine all ingredients except ¼ cup cracker crumbs.
3. Coat loaf pan with vegetable oil spray and ¼ cup cracker crumbs. Place cheese mixture in pan.
4. Bake for 70 minutes.

Yield: 8 servings

1 serving contains:

Cal	Prot	Fat	Carb	Sat	Mono	Poly	Chol	Na
203	12	10.8	16.1	2.5	4.7	3.2	3	600

Exchanges: 1 serving = 1 meat, 1 bread, 1½ fats
Recommended for: The Living Heart; Types IIa, IIb, III, and IV Diets

Mary Pat's Wheat Germ Patties

  1 **cup wheat germ**
  ½ **cup plain skim milk yogurt**
  ½ **cup shredded low-fat cheese**
  3 **tablespoons finely chopped green pepper**
  ¼ **cup chopped walnuts**
  ½ **teaspoon dried oregano**
  ⅛ **teaspoon garlic powder**

1. Combine all ingredients.
2. Form into patties and brown in skillet coated with vegetable oil spray.
3. Serve with pita bread, if desired.

Yield: 4 patties

1 serving contains:

Cal	Prot	Fat	Carb	Sat	Mono	Poly	Chol	Na
184	13	8.5	17	1.6	1.4	4.9	5.5	237

Exchanges: 1 serving = 1½ meats, 1 bread, 1 fat
Recommended for: The Living Heart; Low Calorie; Diabetic; Types IIa, IIb, III, and IV Diets

Abbreviations: **Cal,** calories; **Prot,** protein; **Carb,** carbohydrate; **Sat,** saturated fat; **Mono,** monounsaturated fat; **Poly,** polyunsaturated fat; **Chol,** cholesterol; **Na,** sodium. Protein, fat, carbohydrate, saturated fat, monounsaturated fat, and polyunsaturated fat are expressed in *grams.* Cholesterol and sodium are expressed in *milligrams.*

Cottage Cheese–Spinach Casserole

2 cups low-fat cottage cheese, rinsed and drained
   egg substitute equivalent to 3 eggs
3 tablespoons flour
4 ounces low-fat cheese, cubed
½ package (10 ounces) frozen chopped spinach, partially thawed
⅛ teaspoon salt

1. Preheat oven to 350°F.
2. Combine cottage cheese, egg substitute, and flour.
3. Add cheese.
4. Add spinach in chunks along with salt.
5. Place in baking dish and bake uncovered for 60 minutes.

Yield: 4 servings

1 serving contains:

Cal	Prot	Fat	Carb	Sat	Mono	Poly	Chol	Na
197	26	5.0	12	1.7	1.3	1.8	15	618

Exchanges: 1 serving = 3 meats, 1 bread
Recommended for: The Living Heart; Low Calorie; Diabetic; Types IIa, IIb, III, IV, and V Diets

Cottage Cheese Mushroom Rollups

1 cup low-fat cottage cheese, rinsed and drained
   egg substitute equivalent to 2 eggs
3 tablespoons flour
⅛ teaspoon salt
⅛ teaspoon seasoned salt
1 tablespoon finely chopped onion
1 can (6 ounces) sliced mushrooms, drained
1 cup White Sauce (see recipe, page 177)

1. Preheat oven to 350°F.
2. Combine cottage cheese, egg substitute, flour, salt, and seasoned salt. Drop mixture using a large spoon into a skillet coated with vegetable oil spray. Each pattie should be about 4 inches in diameter.
3. Brown lightly on both sides. Drain on paper towels.
4. Place mushrooms on each pattie and roll up.

Place smooth side up in baking dish and pour on White Sauce.
5. Bake for 20 minutes.

Yield: 6 rolls

1 serving contains:

Cal	Prot	Fat	Carb	Sat	Mono	Poly	Chol	Na
121	9	5.4	9	1.0	1.7	2.4	2.4	401

Exchanges: 1 serving = 1 meat, 2 vegetables
Recommended for: The Living Heart; Low Calorie; Diabetic; Types IIa, IIb, III, IV, and V Diets

Cheesy Potato Puff

   egg substitute equivalent to 1 egg
¼ cup skim milk
3 cups mashed potatoes
1 tablespoon finely chopped onion
1 tablespoon chopped fresh parsley
2 cups cubed low-fat cheese
3 egg whites

1. Preheat oven to 375°F.
2. Combine egg substitute and milk. Mix in potatoes, onion, parsley, and cheese.
3. Beat egg whites until stiff and fold into mixture.
4. Place mixture in baking dish that has been greased with margarine.
5. Bake 40–45 minutes or until a knife inserted in center comes out clean.

Yield: 6 servings

1 serving contains:

Cal	Prot	Fat	Carb	Sat	Mono	Poly	Chol	Na
158	14	3.6	17	1.9	1.0	0.5	17	763

Exchanges: 1 serving = 1 dairy, 1 bread
Recommended for: The Living Heart; Low Calorie; Diabetic; Types IIa, IIb, III, and IV Diets

Stuffed Manicotti

12 **manicotti pasta shells, cooked and drained**
1 **package (10 ounces) frozen chopped spinach, thawed**
1 **tablespoon chopped green onions**
¼ **teaspoon ground nutmeg**
1 **cup low-fat cottage cheese, rinsed and drained**
¼ **cup skim milk**
2 **teaspoons chopped fresh parsley**
1 **egg white**
2 **cups tomato sauce**
¼ **cup tomato paste**
½ **teaspoon garlic powder**
¾ **teaspoon dried oregano**
½ **teaspoon dried basil**
2 **tablespoons grated Parmesan cheese**

1. Preheat oven to 350°F.
2. Cook the spinach, onions, and nutmeg in a small amount of water and drain.
3. Mash the cottage cheese with skim milk and parsley and add to spinach.
4. Beat egg white with a fork until frothy and add to spinach mixture.
5. Combine remaining ingredients and cook over low heat 3–5 minutes.
6. Stuff spinach mixture into manicotti shells.
7. Spoon a layer of tomato sauce on the bottom of a baking dish and arrange stuffed shells on top. Pour remaining sauce over manicotti and sprinkle with Parmesan cheese.
8. Bake for 30 minutes.

Yield: 6 servings

1 serving contains:

Cal	Prot	Fat	Carb	Sat	Mono	Poly	Chol	Na
320	17	1.6	60	0.6	0.6	0.6	3.2	370

Exchanges: 1 serving = 4 breads, 1 meat
Recommended for: The Living Heart; Low Calorie; Diabetic; Types IIa, IIb, III, IV, and V Diets

Macaroni and Cheese

1½ **cups elbow macaroni, uncooked**
3 **tablespoons tub margarine**
2 **tablespoons flour**
½ **teaspoon salt**
¼ **teaspoon pepper**
¼ **teaspoon dry mustard (optional)**
2 **cups skim milk**
½ **cup chopped onion**
2 **cups cubed low-fat cheese**
paprika

1. Cook macaroni in boiling water until tender. Drain.
2. Preheat oven to 350°F.
3. Melt margarine in saucepan. Blend in flour, salt, pepper, and mustard.
4. Stir in milk until thick and bubbly.
5. Add onion and cheese, stirring until cheese is melted.
6. Stir in cooked macaroni. Pour into a casserole greased with margarine. Sprinkle with paprika.
7. Bake for 35–40 minutes.

Yield: 6 servings

1 serving contains:

Cal	Prot	Fat	Carb	Sat	Mono	Poly	Chol	Na
239	13	8.5	27	2.6	2.9	2.7	15	868

Exchanges: 1 serving = 1 meat, 2 breads, 1 fat
Recommended for: The Living Heart; Diabetic; Types IIa, IIb, III, and IV Diets

Abbreviations: **Cal,** calories; **Prot,** protein; **Carb,** carbohydrate; **Sat,** saturated fat; **Mono,** monounsaturated fat; **Poly,** polyunsaturated fat; **Chol,** cholesterol; **Na,** sodium. Protein, fat, carbohydrate, saturated fat, monounsaturated fat, and polyunsaturated fat are expressed in *grams*. Cholesterol and sodium are expressed in *milligrams*.

Spinach Lasagna

¾ **pound fresh spinach, washed**
2 **tablespoons Parmesan cheese**
1 **cup low-fat cottage cheese**
¼ **teaspoon nutmeg**
¼ **teaspoon salt**
⅛ **teaspoon pepper**
10 **lasagna noodles, cooked and drained**
2 **cups Tomato and Garlic Sauce (see recipe, page 177)**

1. Preheat oven to 350°F.
2. Steam spinach until limp but not mushy.
3. Chop spinach and combine with Parmesan, cottage cheese, nutmeg, salt, and pepper.
4. In a baking pan, layer noodles, spinach filling, and sauce three times.
5. Bake for 20 minutes.

Yield: 4 servings

1 serving contains:

Cal	Prot	Fat	Carb	Sat	Mono	Poly	Chol	Na
580	27	8	100	2.1	2.3	3.8	6.8	919

Exchanges: 1 serving = 6 breads, 2 meats, 1 vegetable
Recommended for: The Living Heart; Low Calorie; Diabetic; Types IIa, IIb, III, IV, and V Diets

Spinach Quiche

2 **pounds fresh spinach, cooked, drained thoroughly, and chopped**
1 **tablespoon lemon juice**
⅛ **teaspoon ground nutmeg**
1 **teaspoon dried tarragon**
⅛ **teaspoon salt**
⅛ **teaspoon pepper**
2 **tablespoons chopped fresh parsley**
½ **cup shredded low-fat cheese**
 egg substitute equivalent to 4 eggs
¾ **cup evaporated skim milk, undiluted**
½ **cup plain skim milk yogurt**
2 **9-inch partially baked Margarine Pastry shells (see recipe, page 214)**

1. Preheat oven to 350°F.
2. Combine spinach, lemon juice, and seasonings. Place in bottom of pastry shells. Sprinkle cheese on top of spinach mixture.

3. Beat egg substitute 5 minutes. Add milk and yogurt and beat well. Pour over spinach mixture.
4. Bake 30 minutes or until set.

Yield: 12 servings

1 serving contains:

Cal	Prot	Fat	Carb	Sat	Mono	Poly	Chol	Na
369	12	22.9	31	4.3	7.8	10.2	3	555

Exchanges: 1 serving = 1 meat, ½ dairy, 1½ breads, 3½ fats
Recommended for: The Living Heart; Diabetic; Types IIa, IIb, III, and IV Diets

Stuffed Onions

6 **onions, peeled**
4 **tablespoons tub margarine**
¼ **cup chopped celery**
¼ **cup chopped green pepper**
¼ **teaspoon ground sage**
1 **clove garlic, minced**
⅛ **teaspoon salt**
⅛ **teaspoon pepper**
1 **tablespoon chopped fresh parsley**
1 **cup fine, dry bread crumbs**
¼ **cup chopped walnuts**
¼ **cup cubed low-fat cheese**

1. Preheat oven to 350°F.
2. Cut a thin slice of onion from each end. Pierce each onion from top through the center several times with a fork.
3. Place onions upright, side by side (these should fit snugly) in saucepan and cover with salted water. Cover and simmer 30 minutes or until onions are tender but not soft. Drain.
4. When onions are cool, scoop out centers and set aside.
5. Brush cooked onions with 1 tablespoon melted margarine.
6. Sauté celery, green pepper, and chopped onion centers in remaining margarine until celery is tender. Stir in sage, garlic, salt, pepper, parsley, and bread crumbs.
7. Remove from heat and add nuts and cheese.
8. Spoon mixture into onion cups. Bake for 20 minutes.

Yield: 6 servings

1 serving contains:

Cal	Prot	Fat	Carb	Sat	Mono	Poly	Chol	Na
209	5	12.1	21	2.1	3.7	5.8	2	729

Exchanges: 1 serving = ½ meat, 1 bread, 1 vegetable, 2 fats
Recommended for: The Living Heart; Low Calorie; Diabetic; Types IIa, IIb, III, and IV Diets

Stuffed Peppers

- **4** green peppers
- **¼** cup chopped onion
- **2** tablespoons tub margarine
- **1** cup long-cooking rice or brown rice, uncooked
- **2** cups water
- **½** teaspoon garlic powder
- **½** teaspoon salt
- **½** teaspoon paprika
- **1** teaspoon Worcestershire sauce
- **1** can (8 ounces) tomatoes, undrained
- **½** teaspoon dried oregano
- **½** teaspoon dried sweet basil
  egg substitute equivalent to 2 eggs
- **½** package (10 ounces) frozen green peas, thawed
- **½** cup cubed low-fat cheese

1. Preheat oven to 350°F.
2. Cut off top of green peppers. Remove seeds and membrane. Boil peppers in salted water 5 minutes. Drain.
3. Cook onion in margarine until tender.
4. Add rice, water, garlic powder, salt, paprika, Worcestershire sauce, tomatoes, oregano, and basil. Cover and cook until rice soaks the liquid and is tender.
5. Stir egg substitute, peas, and cheese into rice mixture.
6. Stuff green peppers and stand upright in a baking dish.
7. Bake for 20 minutes.

Yield: 4 servings

1 serving contains:

Cal	Prot	Fat	Carb	Sat	Mono	Poly	Chol	Na
368	16	10.0	54	2.4	3.2	4.1	10	979

Exchanges: 1 serving = 1 meat, 3 breads, 1 vegetable, 1½ fats
Recommended for: The Living Heart; Diabetic; Types IIa, IIb, III, and IV Diets

Vegetable Chop Suey

- **¼** teaspoon salt
- **¼** teaspoon pepper
- **½** teaspoon ground ginger
- **¼** teaspoon garlic powder
- **1** cup chicken broth or bouillon
- **2** teaspoons oil
- **4** cups celery, diagonally sliced
- **3** cups fresh mushrooms, sliced
- **¼** cup chopped onion
- **4** green onions, sliced
- **½** cup chopped green pepper
- **1** cup shredded red cabbage
- **1½** cups bean sprouts
- **1** tablespoon cornstarch
- **2** tablespoons cold water
- **1** tablespoon soy sauce
- **¼** cup toasted almonds

1. Stir salt, pepper, ginger, and garlic powder into chicken broth. Set aside.
2. Heat heavy skillet or wok until a drop of water dances on the surface.
3. Add oil and heat.
4. Add celery, mushrooms, onions, green pepper, and cabbage. Stir-fry about 5 minutes.
5. Add bouillon mixture.
6. Cover and simmer until celery is tender but crisp, 3–5 minutes.
7. Add bean sprouts.
8. Combine cornstarch, water, and soy sauce.
9. Stir into vegetables until thickened. Add almonds.
10. Serve over rice or bulgur, if desired.

Yield: 6 servings

1 serving contains:

Cal	Prot	Fat	Carb	Sat	Mono	Poly	Chol	Na
92	4	4.5	11	0.4	2.1	1.8	0	553

Exchanges: 1 serving = 2 vegetables, 1 fat
Recommended for: The Living Heart; Low Calorie; Diabetic; Types IIa, IIb, III, and IV Diets

Abbreviations: **Cal,** calories; **Prot,** protein; **Carb,** carbohydrate; **Sat,** saturated fat; **Mono,** monounsaturated fat; **Poly,** polyunsaturated fat; **Chol,** cholesterol; **Na,** sodium. Protein, fat, carbohydrate, saturated fat, monounsaturated fat, and polyunsaturated fat are expressed in *grams.* Cholesterol and sodium are expressed in *milligrams.*

Preparation of Dried Legumes

1. Sort the dried legumes carefully, removing any rocks, or moldy and discolored beans.

2. Place the dried legumes in a colander and rinse thoroughly with cold water.

METHOD I: Overnight soaking

METHOD II: Boiling and cooking

METHOD III: Pressure cooking

3. Place the legumes in a large container and soak them overnight (preferably in the refrigerator) in three to four times their volume of water.

4. Transfer the soaked legumes and the water used for soaking to a large saucepan.

3. Place the legumes with three to four times their volume of water in a large saucepan and bring to a full boil. Continue boiling for 2 minutes.

4. Remove from heat. Cover tightly and let stand for an hour or more.

3. Cover the washed legumes with three to four times their volume of water in the cooker.

4. Cover and bring the pressure cooker to 15 pounds of pressure.

5. Length of cooking time varies with legume (see Table 1). Cook as directed and cool immediately.

5. Heat the legumes and liquid to boiling. Lower the heat and simmer partially covered (adding water if necessary), until they are tender and well done. See Table 1 for individual legume cooking times.

6. Drain the cooked legumes. They are now ready for use in any recipe.

Helpful Hints: It is important that legumes be covered with liquid at all times—during soaking and cooking. Grease the inside top edge of the pan to prevent liquid from boiling over. Keep the saucepan partially covered during cooking— the legumes will boil over if tightly covered. Do not add salt to the legumes until they are tender; adding salt during cooking may make them tough. Save the drained liquid. This can be used as a base for soups, gravies, main dishes, etc.

TABLE 1. *Cooking times for dried legumes*

Legume (1 cup dry measure)	Cooking time		Yield
	Soaked Stove-top	No soaking Pressure cooker	
Black beans	1 hour	*a*	2 cups
Garbanzos (chick peas)	4 hours	40–45 minutes	2¼ cups
Great Northern beans	2 hours	20–25 minutes	2¼ cups
Kidney beans	1½ hours	15–20 minutes	2¼ cups
Lentils	1 hour	10–15 minutes	2½ cups
Lima beans	1½ hours	*a*	1¼ cups
Baby limas	1½ hours	*a*	1¾ cups
Navy beans	2 hours	30–35 minutes	2¼ cups
Pinto beans	2 hours	25–30 minutes	2¼ cups
Red beans	3 hours	30–35 minutes	2¼ cups
Soybeans	4–5 hours	30 minutes	2¼ cups
Split peas	1 hour	*a*	2¼ cups

*a*Pressure cooking is not recommended with these legumes as they get foamy and may clog the pressure cooker vent.

Vegetable Bean Noodle Bake

1 **cup dried soybeans (2 cups cooked)**
6 **ounces uncooked noodles (3 cups cooked)**
1 **onion, chopped**
½ **bunch celery, chopped**
5 **tablespoons flour**
2 **cups water**
2 **carrots, sliced**
1 **potato, cubed**
½ **package (10 ounces) frozen corn**
4 **tomatoes**
1 **tablespoon salt**
¼ **teaspoon pepper**
½ **teaspoon dried mustard**
½ **teaspoon dried sage**
2 **teaspoons dried sweet basil**
⅓ **cup finely chopped fresh parsley**

1. Place dried beans in water and soak overnight. Simmer for 4 hours and drain (see Preparation of Dried Legumes, page 132).
2. Preheat oven to 350°F.
3. Cook noodles and drain.
4. Sauté onions and celery in small amount of water until tender and transparent. Stir in flour and cook several minutes, stirring over medium heat. Slowly add 2 cups water, stirring constantly over low heat.
5. Add carrots, potato, corn, 1 chopped tomato, and seasonings. Bring to a boil to thicken, stirring constantly. Remove from heat.
6. In a 9 × 13-inch baking dish sprayed with vegetable oil spray, alternate layers of beans and noodles, pouring some of the vegetable gravy over each layer. Liquid should come almost to the top. Slice remaining 3 tomatoes and arrange on top. Sprinkle with parsley.
7. Bake 60 minutes.

Yield: 8 servings

1 serving contains:

Cal	Prot	Fat	Carb	Sat	Mono	Poly	Chol	Na
226	10	1.7	45	0.4	0.5	0.6	20	860

Exchanges: 1 serving = 1½ meats, 2½ breads
Recommended for: The Living Heart; Low Calorie; Diabetic; Types IIa, IIb, III, IV, and V Diets

Abbreviations: **Cal,** calories; **Prot,** protein; **Carb,** carbohydrate; **Sat,** saturated fat; **Mono,** monounsaturated fat; **Poly,** polyunsaturated fat; **Chol,** cholesterol; **Na,** sodium. Protein, fat, carbohydrate, saturated fat, monounsaturated fat, and polyunsaturated fat are expressed in *grams.* Cholesterol and sodium are expressed in *milligrams.*

Black Beans with Tangy Sauce

1¼ cups dried black beans (3 cups cooked)
1 can (16 ounces) tomatoes, chopped, undrained
1¾ cups chopped onion
½ teaspoon garlic powder
1½ teaspoons salt
⅛ teaspoon red pepper sauce
2 whole cloves
1 onion, peeled
1 clove garlic, minced
1 green pepper, cored, seeded, and chopped
2⅔ cups cooked rice

1. Place beans in 4 cups water, cover, and soak overnight in a cool place.
2. Combine tomatoes, ¾ cup chopped onion, garlic powder, ½ teaspoon salt, and red pepper sauce. Cover and refrigerate overnight to blend flavors of sauce.
3. Add 1 teaspoon salt to beans and bring to a boil. Cover pan, reduce heat, and simmer 60 minutes.
4. Stick whole cloves in peeled onion and add to beans along with garlic. Cover and simmer 60 minutes, adding more water if needed.
5. About 15 minutes before beans are done, sauté 1 cup chopped onion and green pepper in small amount of water in a small skillet until onion is tender and transparent.
6. Remove whole onion from beans, add cooked chopped onion and green pepper, and simmer a few minutes to blend flavors.
7. Serve beans over rice and top with refrigerated sauce.

Yield: 6 servings

1 serving contains:

Cal	Prot	Fat	Carb	Sat	Mono	Poly	Chol	Na
162	9	0.8	31	0.1	0	0.5	0	667

Exchanges: 1 serving = 2½ meats
Recommended for: The Living Heart; Low Calorie; Diabetic; Types I, IIa, IIb, III, IV, and V Diets

Chili

2 cups dried kidney beans (5–6 cups cooked)
⅔ cup chopped onion
1 clove garlic, minced
1 bay leaf
1 can (6 ounces) tomato paste
2 tablespoons oil
2½ tablespoons flour
2 tablespoons chili powder
1 tablespoon ground cumin
¼ teaspoon garlic powder
½ teaspoon salt
⅛ teaspoon pepper

1. Place dried beans in water and soak overnight. Simmer for 3 hours and drain (see Preparation of Dried Legumes, pages 132–133).
2. Combine beans, 6 cups water, ⅓ cup chopped onion, minced garlic, bay leaf, and tomato paste, and simmer 2 hours.
3. Heat oil in separate pan, gradually stir in flour, chili powder, cumin, ⅓ cup onion, and garlic powder. Heat 5 minutes.
4. Stir into beans and cook 1 hour until beans are soft and chili is thickened.
5. Add salt and pepper.
6. May be served over rice or with tortillas, if desired.

Yield: 8 servings

1 serving contains:

Cal	Prot	Fat	Carb	Sat	Mono	Poly	Chol	Na
229	12	4.5	37	0.6	0.9	2.4	0	173

Exchanges: 1 serving = 2½ meats, 1 bread
Recommended for: The Living Heart; Low Calorie; Diabetic; Types IIa, IIb, III, IV, and V Diets

Variation:

Chili Pie: Combine 1 cup cornmeal with 4 cups water in saucepan. Simmer 30 minutes or until cornmeal is thick enough to hold shape when dropped from a spoon. Spread in oiled 9-inch pie pan and top with chili. Bake in a preheated 350°F oven 30 minutes.

Yield: 8 servings

1 serving contains:

Cal	Prot	Fat	Carb	Sat	Mono	Poly	Chol	Na
285	13	4.7	49	0.6	0.9	2.5	0	170

Exchanges: 1 serving = 2½ meats, 1½ breads, 1 vegetable
Recommended for: The Living Heart; Low Calorie; Diabetic; Types IIa, IIb, III, IV, and V Diets

Chili Macaroni

1 cup dried kidney beans (2½ cups cooked)
½ cup dried lentils (1½ cups cooked)
1 onion, chopped
1 stalk celery, chopped
1 clove garlic, minced
2 teaspoons chili powder
¼ teaspoon pepper
1 can (16 ounces) tomatoes, undrained
2 tablespoons tomato paste
1 cup macaroni, cooked
6 ounces low-fat cheese, shredded

1. Place dried beans and dried lentils in water and soak overnight.
2. Drain beans and lentils and set aside.
3. Sauté onion, celery, garlic and chili powder in a small amount of water until vegetables are tender.
4. Place beans and lentils in large saucepan and add vegetables, pepper, tomatoes, and tomato paste. Cover and cook until beans are tender, about 60 minutes, adding water if needed.
5. Add the cooked macaroni and shredded cheese. Mix thoroughly.

Yield: 6 servings

1 serving contains:

Cal	Prot	Fat	Carb	Sat	Mono	Poly	Chol	Na
261	18	2.8	43	1.2	0.6	0.6	10	558

Exchanges: 1 serving = 2 meats, 2 breads
Recommended for: The Living Heart; Low Calorie; Diabetic; Types IIa, IIb, III, IV, and V Diets

Chili Stuffed Peppers

1 cup dried kidney beans (2½ cups cooked)
6 large green peppers, cored and seeded
1 onion, chopped
1 cup cooked rice
2 teaspoons chili powder
1 can (8 ounces) corn, drained, reserve liquid
½ cup catsup
1 tablespoon cornstarch
¾ cup water

1. Place dried beans in water and soak overnight. Simmer for 3 hours and drain (see Preparation of Dried Legumes, pages 132–133).
2. Parboil peppers 5 minutes and drain.
3. Mix onion, rice, beans, chili powder, corn, and catsup.
4. Mix cornstarch with 1 tablespoon reserved corn liquid and add to vegetable mixture. Fill pepper with mixture and stand upright in a pan coated with vegetable oil spray.
5. Pour water around peppers and cover. Bake 30 minutes.

Yield: 6 servings

1 serving contains:

Cal	Prot	Fat	Carb	Sat	Mono	Poly	Chol	Na
222	10	1.3	46	0.1	0.1	0.8	0	457

Exchanges: 1 serving = 1½ meats, 2 breads
Recommended for: The Living Heart; Low Calorie; Diabetic; Types I, IIa, IIb, III, IV, and V Diets

Abbreviations: **Cal,** calories; **Prot,** protein; **Carb,** carbohydrate; **Sat,** saturated fat; **Mono,** monounsaturated fat; **Poly,** polyunsaturated fat; **Chol,** cholesterol; **Na,** sodium. Protein, fat, carbohydrate, saturated fat, monounsaturated fat, and polyunsaturated fat are expressed in *grams.* Cholesterol and sodium are expressed in *milligrams.*

Easy One-Dish Dinner

½ cup dried kidney beans (1 cup cooked)
1 can (8 ounces) corn, drained
1 can (8 ounces) whole tomatoes, lightly drained
¾ teaspoon salt
¼ teaspoon dried oregano
¼ teaspoon dried sweet basil
1 teaspoon brown sugar
1 teaspoon finely chopped onion
3 tablespoons fine, dry bread crumbs

1. Place dried beans in water and soak overnight.
2. Drain and simmer 3 hours (see Preparation of Dried Legumes, pages 132–133).
3. Preheat oven to 350°F.
4. Mix all ingredients together except bread crumbs. Place in casserole coated with vegetable oil spray and sprinkle with bread crumbs.
5. Bake 45 minutes.

Yield: 4 servings

1 serving contains:

Cal	Prot	Fat	Carb	Sat	Mono	Poly	Chol	Na
128	6	0.9	26	0.2	0.2	0.5	0	624

Exchanges: 1 serving = ½ meat, 1 bread, 1 vegetable
Recommended for: The Living Heart; Low Calorie; Diabetic; Types I, IIa, IIb, III, IV, and V Diets

Zucchini Garbanzos

2 onions, thinly sliced
½ pound zucchini, sliced
1 can (16 ounces) garbanzos, drained
½ teaspoon dried oregano
¼ teaspoon dried sweet basil
¼ teaspoon sugar
¼ teaspoon garlic powder
½ teaspoon salt
⅛ teaspoon red pepper sauce
3 tomatoes, chopped
1 cup frozen green peas, thawed

1. Sauté onions in small amount of water until tender and transparent.

2. Add zucchini, garbanzos, oregano, basil, sugar, garlic powder, salt, and red pepper sauce. Cover and simmer 5 minutes.
3. Add tomatoes and green peas, cover, and simmer 10 minutes, stirring occasionally. Be careful not to overcook. Serve immediately.

Yield: 6 servings

1 serving contains:

Cal	Prot	Fat	Carb	Sat	Mono	Poly	Chol	Na
131	8	0.7	25	0.04	0.03	0.5	0	222

Exchanges: 1 serving = 1 meat, 1 bread
Recommended for: The Living Heart; Low Calorie; Diabetic; Types I, IIa, IIb, III, IV, and V Diets

Two Bean Casserole

¼ cup dried garbanzo beans (½ cup cooked)
⅓ cup dried soybeans (1 cup cooked)
1 can (8 ounces) corn, drained
1 cup chopped tomatoes
¼ teaspoon paprika
¾ teaspoon salt
½ teaspoon sugar
1 teaspoon finely chopped onion
1 teaspoon chili powder
½ teaspoon ground cumin
¼ cup catsup
2 ounces low-fat cheese, shredded

1. Preheat oven to 350°F.
2. Mix all ingredients together except cheese and place in a casserole dish coated with vegetable oil spray.
3. Top with cheese. Bake 45 minutes.

Yield: 4 servings

1 serving contains:

Cal	Prot	Fat	Carb	Sat	Mono	Poly	Chol	Na
190	12	4.3	29	1	0.8	1.9	5.0	912

Exchanges: 1 serving = 2 meats, 1 bread
Recommended for: The Living Heart; Low Calorie; Diabetic; Types IIa, IIb, III, IV, and V Diets

Pita Bread Tacos

1¼ cups dried garbanzo beans (3 cups cooked)
2 cloves garlic
2 tablespoons lemon juice
2 teaspoons onion salt
½ teaspoon ground cumin
¼ teaspoon cayenne pepper
10 pita breads
1 cup chopped onion
3 cups shredded lettuce
1 cup chopped tomatoes
1 cup chopped cucumber
1½ cups plain skim milk yogurt

1. Place dried beans in water and soak overnight.
2. Simmer for 4 hours and drain (see Preparation of Dried Legumes, pages 132–133).
3. Purée beans, garlic, lemon juice, salt, cumin, and cayenne in blender until smooth. Let stand at room temperature 30 minutes to blend flavors.
4. Fill pita bread with mixture and garnish with onion, lettuce, tomato, cucumber, and yogurt.

Yield: 10 tacos

1 taco contains:

Cal	Prot	Fat	Carb	Sat	Mono	Poly	Chol	Na
233	10	1.4	47	0.3	0.4	0.5	0	123

Exchanges: 1 taco = 1 meat, 1 bread, 2 vegetables, ½ dairy
Recommended for: The Living Heart; Low Calorie; Diabetic; Types I, IIa, IIb, III, IV, and V Diets

Chinese Style Vegetable Dinner

1 cup dried pinto beans (2½ cups cooked)
1 tablespoon cornstarch
¼ cup soy sauce
½ cup water
½ teaspoon ground ginger
½ teaspoon curry powder
⅛ teaspoon pepper
4 stalks celery, thinly sliced on the diagonal
2 onions, sliced
1 green pepper, seeded, cored, and cut in thin strips

1 package (10 ounces) frozen French cut green beans, thawed
¼ cup chopped fresh parsley
3 tomatoes, cut in wedges
5 cups cooked rice

1. Soak beans overnight.
2. Drain and cook in 3 cups water until tender, approximately 2 hours. Drain and set aside (see Preparation of Dried Legumes, pages 132–133).
3. Combine cornstarch, soy sauce, and water. Set aside.
4. Heat a small amount of water in skillet and add ginger, pepper, and curry powder.
5. Add celery and onion and stir-fry until crisp.
6. Add cornstarch mixture and stir well.
7. Add beans, green pepper, green beans, parsley, and tomatoes, cooking only until all vegetables are heated through.
8. Serve over rice.

Yield: 6 servings

1 serving contains:

Cal	Prot	Fat	Carb	Sat	Mono	Poly	Chol	Na
347	13	1.2	73	0.1	0.1	0.8	0	927

Exchanges: 1 serving = 4 breads, 1½ meats
Recommended for: The Living Heart; Low Calorie; Diabetic; Types I, IIa, IIb, III, IV, and V Diets

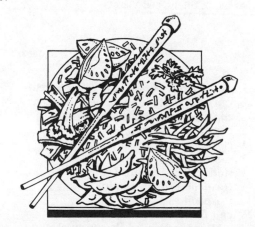

Abbreviations: **Cal,** calories; **Prot,** protein; **Carb,** carbohydrate; **Sat,** saturated fat; **Mono,** monounsaturated fat; **Poly,** polyunsaturated fat; **Chol,** cholesterol; **Na,** sodium. Protein, fat, carbohydrate, saturated fat, monounsaturated fat, and polyunsaturated fat are expressed in *grams.* Cholesterol and sodium are expressed in *milligrams.*

Bean-Filled Pitas

2 cans (16 ounces each) white beans (kidney, Great Northern, or white navy), drained
2 tablespoons lemon juice
½ cup plain skim milk yogurt
1 teaspoon dried oregano
½ teaspoon salt
½ teaspoon ground cumin
¼ teaspoon pepper
¼ cup low-fat cottage cheese, rinsed and drained
2 tomatoes, coarsely chopped
1 cucumber, peeled and chopped
4 pita breads

1. In large bowl, toss beans, lemon juice, yogurt, oregano, salt, cumin, and pepper. Gently stir in cheese, tomatoes, and cucumber.
2. Cover and chill about 2 hours.
3. Fill pita breads.

Yield: 4 servings

1 serving contains:

Cal	Prot	Fat	Carb	Sat	Mono	Poly	Chol	Na
435	25	2.6	82	0.6	0.6	1.0	1.7	454

Exchanges: 1 serving = 4 meats, 3½ breads
Recommended for: The Living Heart; Low Calorie; Diabetic· Types IIa, IIb, III, IV, and V Diets

Soybean Stew

1 cup dried soybeans (2½ cups cooked)
1 can (8 ounces) tomato sauce
⅓ cup chopped onions
1 cup frozen green peas
1 clove garlic, minced
2 carrots, chopped
1 stalk celery, chopped
½ teaspoon ground cumin
½ teaspoon salt
½ cup finely chopped green pepper
4 tablespoons grated Parmesan cheese

Abbreviations: **Cal,** calories; **Prot,** protein; **Carb,** carbohydrate; **Sat,** saturated fat; **Mono,** monounsaturated fat; **Poly,** polyunsaturated fat; **Chol,** cholesterol; **Na,** sodium. Protein, fat, carbohydrate, saturated fat, monounsaturated fat, and polyunsaturated fat are expressed in *grams.* Cholesterol and sodium are expressed in *milligrams.*

1. Place dried beans in water and soak overnight. Simmer for 4 hours and drain (see Preparation of Dried Legumes, pages 132–133).
2. In Dutch oven, combine soybeans with remaining ingredients except green pepper and cheese. Cook 30 minutes over low heat, adding water if needed.
3. Remove from heat and stir in green pepper and cheese.

Yield: 6 servings

1 serving contains:

Cal	Prot	Fat	Carb	Sat	Mono	Poly	Chol	Na
162	12	5.4	18	1.3	1.2	2.4	2.7	447

Exchanges: 1 serving = 2½ meats
Recommended for: The Living Heart; Low Calorie; Diabetic; Types IIa, IIb, III, IV, and V Diets

New England Baked Soybeans

2 cups dried soybeans
2 whole cloves
1 onion
3 tablespoons tub margarine
½ teaspoon salt
½ teaspoon dry mustard
¼ cup molasses
2–3 drops Worcestershire sauce

1. Cover beans with cold water and soak overnight. Simmer until tender, about 2 hours.
2. Stick cloves in onion and place in a casserole.
3. Pour in beans with liquid. (Reserve some of the liquid if beans are soupy.)
4. Add margarine, salt, mustard, molasses, and Worcestershire sauce.
5. Cover and bake in a 275°F oven for 8 hours. Add reserved bean liquid or hot water if needed.
6. Uncover and bake 30–40 minutes longer to brown.

Yield: 10 servings

1 cup contains:

Cal	Prot	Fat	Carb	Sat	Mono	Poly	Chol	Na
343	20	17.2	31	2.8	4.6	8.3	0	316

Exchanges: 1 cup = 2 meats, 2 breads, 2 fats
Recommended for: The Living Heart; Types IIa, IIb, III, and IV Diets

Tofu

Tofu is prepared from soybeans which have been blended or ground, cooked in water, pressed into a cake, and solidified into a curd. Tofu is an excellent source of protein that contains no cholesterol and very little fat. Because of its protein content, tofu is an excellent substitute for meat. Fresh tofu packed in water may be purchased in the produce section of most large grocery stores, health food and natural food stores, and specialty shops that sell Japanese or Chinese foods.

We recommend that you try fresh tofu before trying the canned, dried, or frozen varieties. Fresh tofu has a very mild, subtle flavor and a soft, light texture, slightly denser than gelatin and less dense than soft cheese. The texture varies slightly from brand to brand. Very soft tofu crumbles easily and would not be as satisfactory for cutting into small cubes as would a denser, drier tofu. As soon as you bring it home, rinse it in cold water and repack it in your own container (plastic, glass, or stainless steel, not aluminum), covering it completely with cold water. It should have very little odor; if it smells strong or sour, return it to the store as spoiled. Keep tofu refrigerated at all times; it should remain fresh for at least a week. Rinse the tofu every 2 days and cover it with cold water to preserve its fresh, delicate flavor. As tofu ages, it develops a stronger taste and aroma. Older tofu may be used in more strongly flavored dishes in which the slightly stronger taste will not be noticed. It can also be cut into cubes, placed in enough cold water to cover it, and then boiled and allowed to simmer for a few minutes. This technique restores its freshness. Also, if your tofu is beginning to age and you are not ready to use it, place it in a plastic bag and freeze it. When thawed, this tofu is somewhat drier than fresh tofu and rather meatlike, a characteristic many persons prefer.

Because tofu has such a mild flavor, it is frequently marinated or combined with other foods. It has an exceptional ability to absorb flavors and tastes exactly like the seasoned sauce in which you cook or marinate it. For example, soy sauce and vinegar make an excellent sauce in which to marinate cubes of tofu for about half an hour; you might then combine the marinated tofu with stir-fried vegetables. Tofu may be broiled or sautéed in seasoned liquid for a simple side dish, or it may be combined with almost any vegetable. You may broil an entire curd of tofu whole, or you may prefer to cut it into 1-inch cubes, which allows more absorption of the sauce. Tofu cubes that have been creatively marinated add a nice flavor to fruit or vegetable salads. Plain tofu cubes make an excellent appetizer when served with several dipping sauces.

Before using tofu in any recipe, drain the excess water which has accumulated in the curd by placing it on a paper towel for 15 to 30 minutes.

Crumbled Tofu

Crumbled tofu has much the same texture as crumbly, cooked hamburger and may be used in place of it in your favorite recipes.

1. Combine tofu and 2 cups water in saucepan. Break tofu into very small pieces with a wooden spoon or spatula while bringing water to a boil.
2. Place a colander in the sink and line with a large cloth. Pour heated tofu onto the cloth. Hold the corners of the cloth to form a sack, then twist closed. Press the sack of tofu firmly against the bottom of the colander, expelling as much water as possible. Empty the pressed tofu into a large bowl and cool for several minutes.
3. With fingertips or a spoon, crumble the tofu into very small pieces.

Pressed Tofu

1. Drain tofu and place on top of a dry towel.
2. Cover with another dry towel and place a 2- to 3-pound weight on top.
3. Replace the damp towels with dry ones after 30 minutes. Press tofu for a minimum of 60 minutes.

Pita Vegetable Pot Pie

  1   cup skim milk
  2   tablespoons flour
 ⅛   teaspoon pepper
 ⅛   teaspoon dried sage
  1   tablespoon chopped fresh parsley
 ½   cup chopped green pepper
  1   stalk celery, chopped
 1¼ cups frozen peas, thawed
  1   cup chopped carrots
 ⅜   cup chopped onion
 1¼ cups frozen corn, thawed
  1   can (4 ounces) water chestnuts, drained (optional)
  1   can (4 ounces) sliced mushrooms, drained (optional)
 ½   cup cooked rice
  8   ounces tofu, pressed and crumbled
  3   pita breads

1. Preheat oven to 350°F.
2. Combine milk, flour, pepper, sage, and parsley in large saucepan. Heat, stirring constantly, until sauce thickens.
3. Add vegetables and tofu and heat about 5 minutes.
4. Fill pita breads with mixture. Place in a baking dish and bake for 25 minutes.

Yield: 3 servings

1 serving contains:

Cal	Prot	Fat	Carb	Sat	Mono	Poly	Chol	Na
476	24	5.4	90	1.0	1.1	2.7	1.3	592

Exchanges: 1 serving = 6 breads, 1½ meats
Recommended for: The Living Heart; Low Calorie; Diabetic; Types IIa, IIb, III, IV, and V Diets

Tofu Stir-Fry

 1¼ tablespoons oil
 24   ounces tofu, well pressed and broken into ¾-inch pieces
  8   ounces bean sprouts
  4   green onions, cut in 2-inch lengths
 ¾   cup chopped celery
 ½   green pepper, slivered
  1   package (10 ounces) frozen chopped broccoli, thawed
 ¼   cup soy sauce
 ⅓   cup water
  2   tablespoons cornstarch

1. Heat a wok or skillet and coat with oil.
2. Add tofu and stir-fry until golden brown.
3. Add vegetables and cook 2–3 minutes until heated through.
4. Blend soy sauce, water, and cornstarch in a bowl.
5. Add to vegetables, stirring constantly, until thickened.

Yield: 4 servings

1 serving contains:

Cal	Prot	Fat	Carb	Sat	Mono	Poly	Chol	Na
238	19	12.1	19	1.6	2.5	6.8	0	1375

Exchanges: 1 serving = 2 meats, 1 bread, 1 fat, 1 vegetable
Recommended for: The Living Heart; Low Calorie; Diabetic; Types IIa, IIb, III, and IV Diets

Tofu Stuffed Green Peppers

  5   green onions, chopped
 ½   cup cooked brown rice
 12   ounces tofu, pressed
 ¼   cup sliced water chestnuts
  2   tablespoons catsup
 ½   teaspoon salt
  3   large green peppers, cut horizontally in half and seeded

1. Preheat oven to 350°F.
2. Heat skillet or wok and sauté onion in small amount of water until tender and transparent.
3. Add rice and sauté 1 minute more.

4. Add tofu, mashing it in the pan, and sauté about 2 minutes.
5. Add water chestnuts, catsup, and salt.
6. Stuff each green pepper half with tofu mixture.
7. Place in baking dish coated with vegetable oil spray and bake 20 minutes.

Yield: 3 servings

1 serving contains:

Cal	Prot	Fat	Carb	Sat	Mono	Poly	Chol	Na
178	12	5.5	24	0.8	1.0	3.0	0	601

Exchanges: 1 serving = 1 meat, 1½ breads, ½ fat
Recommended for: The Living Heart; Low Calorie; Diabetic; Types IIa, IIb, III, IV, and V Diets

Tofu Burgers

1 onion, finely chopped
24 ounces tofu, crumbled and cool
2 cups water
½ cup fine, dry bread crumbs
2 tablespoons Worcestershire sauce
¾ teaspoon salt
⅛ teaspoon pepper

1. Sauté onion in small amount of water until tender and transparent. Remove from heat and cool.
2. Mix onion with rest of ingredients and form into 8 patties.
3. Heat a nonstick skillet and coat with vegetable oil spray.
4. Add 4 patties, cover, and cook over low heat about 5 minutes per side.
5. Repeat with remaining 4 patties.

Yield: 8 patties

1 patty contains:

Cal	Prot	Fat	Carb	Sat	Mono	Poly	Chol	Na
91	8	3.9	8	0.6	0.9	2.0	0	326

Exchanges: 1 patty = 1 meat, 1 vegetable
Recommended for: The Living Heart; Low Calorie; Diabetic; Types IIa, IIb, III, IV, and V Diets

Lynn's Tofu Enchiladas

1 package (1½ ounces) enchilada sauce mix
1 can (6 ounces) tomato paste
½ onion, chopped
¼ green pepper, chopped
8 ounces tofu, pressed and crumbled
5 corn tortillas

1. Preheat oven to 350°F.
2. Prepare enchilada sauce mix with tomato paste according to package directions.
3. Sauté onion and green pepper in a small amount of water until tender.
4. Add tofu and heat through.
5. Add ½ cup sauce to tofu mixture.
6. Place on tortillas, roll up, and place in baking dish.
7. Cover with remaining sauce and bake 25 minutes until hot and bubbly.

Yield: 5 enchiladas

1 serving contains:

Cal	Prot	Fat	Carb	Sat	Mono	Poly	Chol	Na
140	7	2.7	23	0.3	0.4	1.1	0	789

Exchanges: 1 serving = 1½ breads, ½ meat
Recommended for: The Living Heart; Low Calorie; Diabetic; Types I, IIa, IIb, III, IV, and V Diets

Variation:

Add 2 cups homemade refried beans to the tofu mixture.

With Refried Beans
1 serving contains:

Cal	Prot	Fat	Carb	Sat	Mono	Poly	Chol	Na
152	8	2.8	25	0.3	0.4	1.1	0	829

Exchanges: 1 serving = ½ meat, 1 bread, 2 vegetables
Recommended for: The Living Heart; Low Calorie; Diabetic; Types IIa, IIb, III, IV, and V Diets

---

Abbreviations: **Cal,** calories; **Prot,** protein; **Carb,** carbohydrate; **Sat,** saturated fat; **Mono,** monounsaturated fat; **Poly,** polyunsaturated fat; **Chol,** cholesterol; **Na,** sodium. Protein, fat, carbohydrate, saturated fat, monounsaturated fat, and polyunsaturated fat are expressed in *grams.* Cholesterol and sodium are expressed in *milligrams.*

Tofu Tacos

12 ounces tofu, drained
⅔ cup cooked brown rice
½ green pepper, chopped
¼ cup catsup
½ teaspoon salt
½ package (1¼ ounces) taco seasoning mix
6 corn tortillas
½ cup chopped tomato
½ cup chopped onion
1½ cups shredded lettuce

1. Combine tofu, rice, green pepper, catsup, salt, and taco seasoning, mixing thoroughly.
2. Heat skillet and warm tortillas until soft and pliable.
3. Fill each tortilla with tofu mixture and garnish with tomato, onion, and lettuce.
4. Season with hot sauce, if desired.

Yield: 6 tacos

1 serving contains:

Cal	Prot	Fat	Carb	Sat	Mono	Poly	Chol	Na
166	8	3	27	0.4	0.5	1.5	0	647

Exchanges: 1 serving = 1 meat, 1 bread, 1 vegetable
Recommended for: The Living Heart; Low Calorie; Diabetic; Types IIa, IIb, III, IV, and V Diets

Tofu Tortilla Casserole

1 can (16 ounces) pinto beans
½ package (1½ ounces) enchilada sauce mix
½ can (6 ounces) tomato paste
10 corn tortillas, torn in pieces
12 ounces tofu, pressed

1. Preheat oven to 350°F.
2. Drain pinto beans. Place in saucepan and heat, stirring constantly and mashing with spoon until thickened.
3. Prepare enchilada sauce with tomato paste according to package directions.
4. In a baking dish, layer tortillas, beans, sauce, and tofu, repeating three times.

5. Bake 30 minutes until hot and bubbly.

Yield: 4 servings

1 serving contains:

Cal	Prot	Fat	Carb	Sat	Mono	Poly	Chol	Na
364	19	5.7	60	0.6	0.8	2.2	0	428

Exchanges: 1 serving = 2½ meats, 3 breads
Recommended for: The Living Heart; Low Calorie; Diabetic; Types IIa, IIb, III, IV, and V Diets

Tofu Pizza

3 pita breads, split into 6 rounds
1½ cups Tomato and Garlic Sauce, drained (see recipe, page 177)
1 pound tofu, pressed
½ pound fresh mushrooms, sliced
½ cup chopped green pepper
1½ tablespoons Parmesan cheese

1. Preheat oven to 375°F.
2. Place pita bread rounds on cookie sheet and spread with Tomato and Garlic Sauce. Crumble tofu over each pizza crust. Top with green pepper and mushrooms. Sprinkle with cheese.
3. Bake 15 minutes.

Yield: six 6-inch pizzas

1 serving contains:

Cal	Prot	Fat	Carb	Sat	Mono	Poly	Chol	Na
190	11	6.6	24	1.2	1.5	3.3	1.0	320

Exchanges: 1 serving = 1½ breads, 1 meat, 1 fat
Recommended for: The Living Heart; Low Calorie; Diabetic; Types IIa, IIb, III, and IV Diets

Tofu Sandwich Spread

8 ounces tofu, squeezed
   egg substitute equivalent to 3 eggs, cooked and diced
2 tablespoons lemon juice
¹⁄₁₆ teaspoon garlic powder
2 teaspoons prepared mustard
¾ tablespoon chopped green onion
¹⁄₁₆ teaspoon pepper
1½ tablespoons chopped fresh parsley

1. Combine all ingredients except parsley in blender. Blend until smooth.
2. Stir in parsley and spread mixture over bread.

Yield: filling for 4 sandwiches

1 serving contains:

Cal	Prot	Fat	Carb	Sat	Mono	Poly	Chol	Na
95	9	5.3	4	0.8	1.2	2.9	0.3	151

Exchanges: 1 serving = 1 meat, 1 vegetable
Recommended for: The Living Heart; Low Calorie; Diabetic; Types IIa, IIb, III, IV, and V Diets

Grilled Tofu Sandwiches

4 slices bread
2 teaspoons mustard
¼ cup Tofu Mayonnaise (see recipe, page 171)
4 slices tomato
12 ounces tofu, pressed and cut into 8 slices
2 teaspoons soy sauce
2 ounces low-fat cheese, sliced

1. Spread bread with mustard and Tofu Mayonnaise.
2. Top with slices of tomato and tofu. Sprinkle with soy sauce and top with cheese.
3. Place under broiler until cheese melts.

Yield: 4 sandwiches

1 sandwich contains:

Cal	Prot	Fat	Carb	Sat	Mono	Poly	Chol	Na
174	13	5.9	18	1.4	1.5	2.5	5	655

Exchanges: 1 sandwich = 1½ meats, 1 bread
Recommended for: The Living Heart; Low Calorie; Diabetic; Types IIa, IIb, III, IV, and V Diets

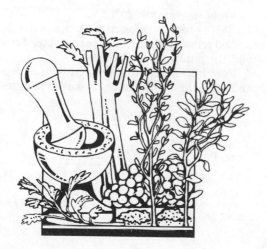

Abbreviations: **Cal,** calories; **Prot,** protein; **Carb,** carbohydrate; **Sat,** saturated fat; **Mono,** monounsaturated fat; **Poly,** polyunsaturated fat; **Chol,** cholesterol; **Na,** sodium. Protein, fat, carbohydrate, saturated fat, monounsaturated fat, and polyunsaturated fat are expressed in *grams*. Cholesterol and sodium are expressed in *milligrams*.

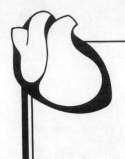

Vegetables

Cheesy Asparagus

2 tablespoons tub margarine
2 tablespoons flour
6 tablespoons chicken bouillon
6 tablespoons skim milk
⅓ cup cubed low-fat cheese
¼ teaspoon salt
⅛ teaspoon pepper
1 package (10 ounces) frozen asparagus spears, cooked and drained

1. Melt margarine in saucepan. Blend in flour.
2. Add chicken bouillon and milk, stirring constantly until thickened.
3. Stir in cheese, salt, and pepper until cheese is melted.
4. Place cooked asparagus in a shallow baking dish and pour sauce over spears. Broil until bubbly.

Yield: 4 servings

1 serving contains:

Cal	Prot	Fat	Carb	Sat	Mono	Poly	Chol	Na
113	6	6.7	8	1.5	2.3	2.7	4	460

Exchanges: 1 serving = ½ dairy, 1 vegetable, 1 fat
Recommended for: The Living Heart; Diabetic; Types IIa, IIb, III, and IV Diets

Green Bean Casserole

1 onion, chopped
½ green pepper, chopped
1 tablespoon oil
1 package (10 ounces) frozen green beans, cooked until almost tender
1 can (8 ounces) tomatoes, drained
¼ teaspoon salt
⅛ teaspoon crushed red pepper
⅛ teaspoon garlic powder
1 tablespoon mayonnaise
¼ cup bread crumbs

1. Preheat oven to 375°F.
2. Sauté onion and green pepper in oil.
3. Add remaining ingredients except bread crumbs and stir until heated through.
4. Pour into a casserole greased with margarine and sprinkle with crumbs. Bake 30 minutes.

Yield: 8 servings

1 serving contains:

Cal	Prot	Fat	Carb	Sat	Mono	Poly	Chol	Na
52	1	3.2	5	0.5	0.7	1.8	1	128

Exchanges: 1 serving = 1 vegetable, ½ fat
Recommended for: The Living Heart; Diabetic; Types IIa, IIb, III, and IV Diets

Oriental Green Beans

½ cup bouillon
2 tablespoons chopped green onion, including tops
¼ teaspoon garlic salt
1 tablespoon soy sauce
⅛ teaspoon ground ginger
4 teaspoons cold water
2 teaspoons cornstarch
1 package (10 ounces) frozen green beans, partially cooked and drained

1. Simmer bouillon, onion, garlic salt, soy sauce, and ginger together until onion is soft, about 10 minutes.
2. Combine cold water and cornstarch. Add to soy sauce mixture, cooking until thickened.
3. Stir in green beans and heat thoroughly.

Yield: 4 servings

1 serving contains:

Cal	Prot	Fat	Carb	Sat	Mono	Poly	Chol	Na
27	1	0.1	6	0	0	0.1	0	572

Exchanges: 1 serving = 1 vegetable
Recommended for: The Living Heart; Low Calorie; Diabetic; Types I, IIa, IIb, III, IV, and V Diets

Savory Green Beans

⅓ cup chopped onion
1 clove garlic, minced
1 teaspoon oil
1 tomato, chopped
2 tablespoons finely chopped green pepper
2 tablespoons finely chopped celery
2 tablespoons dry white wine
1 tablespoon chopped fresh parsley
½–1 teaspoon dried savory
1 teaspoon salt
¼ teaspoon pepper
1 package (10 ounces) frozen French style green beans, cooked and drained

1. Sauté onion and garlic in oil.
2. Add remaining ingredients except green beans. Simmer 10 minutes.
3. Stir sauce into green beans.

Yield: 4 servings

1 serving contains:

Cal	Prot	Fat	Carb	Sat	Mono	Poly	Chol	Na
41	2	1.3	7	0.1	0.3	0.8	0	556

Exchanges: 1 serving = 1 vegetable
Recommended for: The Living Heart; Low Calorie; Diabetic; Types IIa, IIb, III, and IV Diets

Oriental Bean Sprouts

1 can (16 ounces) bean sprouts, drained
2 green onions, chopped
1 tablespoon soy sauce
1 tablespoon sesame seeds
1 tablespoon water
⅛ teaspoon paprika
⅛ teaspoon salt

1. Place all ingredients in saucepan.
2. Stir until heated thoroughly.

Yield: 4 servings

1 serving contains:

Cal	Prot	Fat	Carb	Sat	Mono	Poly	Chol	Na
36	3	1.3	5	0.2	0.4	0.7	0	399

Exchanges: 1 serving = 1 vegetable
Recommended for: The Living Heart; Low Calorie; Diabetic; Types IIa, IIb, III, and IV Diets

Abbreviations: **Cal,** calories; **Prot,** protein; **Carb,** carbohydrate; **Sat,** saturated fat; **Mono,** monounsaturated fat; **Poly,** polyunsaturated fat; **Chol,** cholesterol; **Na,** sodium. Protein, fat, carbohydrate, saturated fat, monounsaturated fat, and polyunsaturated fat are expressed in *grams.* Cholesterol and sodium are expressed in *milligrams.*

Spicy Beets

2 teaspoons cornstarch
¾ cup orange juice
1 teaspoon grated orange peel
¼ teaspoon ground allspice
¼ teaspoon salt
1 can (16 ounces) sliced beets, drained

1. Stir cornstarch into orange juice over medium heat until juice is thickened.
2. Stir in remaining ingredients and heat through.

Yield: 4 servings

1 serving contains:

Cal	Prot	Fat	Carb	Sat	Mono	Poly	Chol	Na
55	1	0.1	13	0	0	0.1	0	313

Exchanges: 1 serving = 1 vegetable, ½ fruit
Recommended for: The Living Heart; Low Calorie; Diabetic; Types I, IIa, IIb, III, IV, and V Diets

Florida Beets

1 can (16 ounces) sliced beets, drained
1 teaspoon grated orange peel
½ cup orange juice concentrate, undiluted
1 tablespoon sugar
½ teaspoon salt
1 tablespoon tub margarine

1. Preheat oven to 350°F.
2. Place beets in a shallow baking dish. Combine remaining ingredients and pour over beets.
3. Cover and bake 45 minutes.

Yield: 4 servings

1 serving contains:

Cal	Prot	Fat	Carb	Sat	Mono	Poly	Chol	Na
129	2	3.0	25	0.5	1.0	1.4	0	511

Exchanges: 1 serving = 1 vegetable, 1½ fruits, 1 fat
Recommended for: The Living Heart; Diabetic; Types IIa, IIb, III, and IV Diets

Broccoli Soufflé

2 tablespoons tub margarine
2 tablespoons flour
½ teaspoon salt
¼ teaspoon pepper
½ cup skim milk
⅔ cup puréed broccoli (½ of 10-ounce package frozen broccoli cooked according to package directions, drained and puréed)
1 tablespoon finely chopped onion
egg substitute equivalent to 3 eggs

1. Preheat oven to 350°F.
2. Melt margarine in saucepan and blend in flour, salt, and pepper, stirring until bubbly.
3. Remove from heat and stir in milk.
4. Stir mixture over low heat until it begins to simmer. Cook 1 minute and remove from heat.
5. Stir in broccoli and onion.
6. Beat egg substitute at high speed 5 minutes.
7. Fold broccoli mixture into beaten egg substitute.
8. Place in a greased 6-inch casserole. Place casserole in a pan of hot water and bake for 40 minutes.

Yield: 4 servings

1 serving contains:

Cal	Prot	Fat	Carb	Sat	Mono	Poly	Chol	Na
135	7	8.8	8	1.6	2.8	4.2	1	447

Exchanges: 1 serving = 1 meat, 1 vegetable, 1 fat
Recommended for: The Living Heart; Diabetic; Types IIa, IIb, III, and IV Diets

Sesame Broccoli

1 tablespoon sesame seeds
1 tablespoon lemon juice
1 tablespoon soy sauce
¼ teaspoon salt
1 package (10 ounces) frozen broccoli or 1 pound fresh broccoli, cooked and drained

1. Spread sesame seeds on cookie sheet and heat in a 350°F oven for 5–10 minutes or until brown.

2. Combine lemon juice, soy sauce, salt, and sesame seeds in a small saucepan. Heat to boiling.

3. Pour over broccoli, coating all spears.

Yield: 4 servings

1 serving contains:

Cal	Prot	Fat	Carb	Sat	Mono	Poly	Chol	Na
33	3	1.4	4	0.2	0.4	0.7	0	478

Exchanges: 1 serving = 1 vegetable
Recommended for: The Living Heart; Low Calorie; Diabetic; Types IIa, IIb, III, and IV Diets

Stir-Fried Cabbage

¼ **cup chopped onion**
1 **tablespoon oil**
1 **pound cabbage, shredded**
1 **teaspoon sugar**
⅛ **teaspoon dried tarragon**
⅛ **teaspoon dried savory**
½ **teaspoon salt**
¼ **teaspoon pepper**

1. Sauté onion in oil.
2. Add cabbage and stir until lightly browned.
3. Add remaining ingredients and cover.
4. Cook until cabbage is tender but crisp.

Yield: 4 servings

1 serving contains:

Cal	Prot	Fat	Carb	Sat	Mono	Poly	Chol	Na
53	1	3.6	5	0.4	0.8	2.1	0	286

Exchanges: 1 serving = 1 vegetable, ½ fat
Recommended for: The Living Heart; Diabetic; Types IIa, IIb, III, and IV Diets

Glazed Carrots

2 **packages (10 ounces each) frozen carrots or 1 pound fresh carrots, sliced or julienne cut**
1 **cup orange juice**
2 **teaspoons lemon juice**
⅛ **teaspoon grated lemon peel**
½ **teaspoon salt**
⅛ **teaspoon pepper**

1. Combine ingredients in a saucepan. Cover and simmer 15 minutes, stirring occasionally.

2. Uncover and continue to simmer, stirring frequently, until most of the liquid is evaporated and carrots are tender and glazed. If a thicker glaze is desired, add 2 teaspoons cornstarch to ¼ cup water (stir until thoroughly combined) and add to carrots.

3. Continue cooking until sauce is desired thickness.

Yield: 4 servings

1 serving contains:

Cal	Prot	Fat	Carb	Sat	Mono	Poly	Chol	Na
67	1	0.3	16	0	0	0.3	0	313

Exchanges: 1 serving = 1 vegetable, 1 fruit
Recommended for: The Living Heart; Low Calorie; Diabetic; Types I, IIa, IIb, III, IV, and V Diets

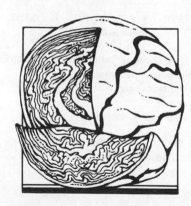

Abbreviations: **Cal,** calories; **Prot,** protein; **Carb,** carbohydrate; **Sat,** saturated fat; **Mono,** monounsaturated fat; **Poly,** polyunsaturated fat; **Chol,** cholesterol; **Na,** sodium. Protein, fat, carbohydrate, saturated fat, monounsaturated fat, and polyunsaturated fat are expressed in *grams*. Cholesterol and sodium are expressed in *milligrams*.

Creamed Carrots and Celery

2 cups sliced carrots
1 cup celery, thinly sliced
¼ cup finely chopped onion
1 cup skim milk
1 tablespoon cornstarch
1 teaspoon chopped fresh parsley
¼ teaspoon salt
⅛ teaspoon pepper

1. Place vegetables in saucepan and cover with water.
2. Cover and simmer 10 minutes or until tender but not soft. Drain.
3. Mix cold milk and cornstarch together. Stir into vegetables and cook, stirring constantly, until sauce is thick.
4. Add remaining ingredients.

Yield: 4 servings

1 serving contains:

Cal	Prot	Fat	Carb	Sat	Mono	Poly	Chol	Na
62	3	0.3	12	0.1	0	0.2	1	228

Exchanges: 1 serving = ½ dairy, 1 vegetable
Recommended for: The Living Heart; Low Calorie; Diabetic; Types I, IIa, IIb, III, IV, and V Diets

Glazed Carrots and Raisins

6 carrots, sliced or julienne cut, partially cooked
2 tablespoons tub margarine
2 tablespoons sugar
½ cup raisins
2 tablespoons lemon juice

1. Drain carrots when nearly cooked.
2. Add remaining ingredients.
3. Cook slowly, stirring constantly, until glazed.

Yield: 6 servings

1 serving contains:

Cal	Prot	Fat	Carb	Sat	Mono	Poly	Chol	Na
110	1	4.0	19	0.7	1.4	1.8	0	76

Exchanges: 1 serving = 1 vegetable, 1 fruit, 1 fat
Recommended for: The Living Heart; Diabetic; Types IIa, IIb, III, and IV Diets

Southern Corn

¼ cup imitation bacon bits
½ green pepper, chopped
¼ cup chopped onion
1 tablespoon oil
1 can (16 ounces) cream-style corn
¼ teaspoon salt
⅛ teaspoon pepper

1. Sauté bacon bits, green pepper, and onion in oil until onions are tender.
2. Stir in remaining ingredients and heat through.

Yield: 4 servings

1 serving contains:

Cal	Prot	Fat	Carb	Sat	Mono	Poly	Chol	Na
186	7	5.9	30	0.8	1.5	3.0	0	788

Exchanges: 1 serving = 2 breads, 1 fat
Recommended for: The Living Heart; Diabetic; Types IIa, IIb, III, and IV Diets

Tangy Buttered Corn

1 can (16 ounces) whole kernel corn, undrained
1 tablespoon prepared mustard
1 tablespoon tub margarine
¼ teaspoon salt

1. Heat corn. Drain most of liquid from the corn.
2. Stir in remaining ingredients and heat through.

Yield: 4 servings

1 serving contains:

Cal	Prot	Fat	Carb	Sat	Mono	Poly	Chol	Na
98	2	3.7	17	0.7	1.1	1.7	0	414

Exchanges: 1 serving = 1 bread, ½ fat
Recommended for: The Living Heart; Diabetic; Types IIa, IIb, III, and IV Diets

Eggplant Vegetable Medley

1 **eggplant, peeled and chopped**
2 **cloves garlic, minced**
1 **tablespoon oil**
1 **green pepper, chopped**
3 **tomatoes, chopped**
1 **onion, chopped**
½ **pound fresh mushrooms, sliced**
1 **teaspoon salt**
1 **teaspoon dried sweet basil**
2 **tablespoons chopped fresh parsley**

1. Sauté eggplant and garlic in oil until lightly browned.
2. Add remaining ingredients. Simmer 8 minutes or until tender.

Yield: 6 servings

Variation:
Top with 2 ounces grated low-fat cheese and broil until cheese melts.

1 serving contains:

Cal	Prot	Fat	Carb	Sat	Mono	Poly	Chol	Na
60	2	2.6	8	0.3	0.6	1.7	0	472

Exchanges: 1 serving = 1½ vegetables, ½ fat
1 serving with cheese = 1 vegetable, 1 fat (76 calories)
Recommended for: The Living Heart; Low Calorie; Diabetic; Types IIa, IIb, III, and IV Diets

Scalloped Eggplant

1 **green pepper, chopped**
1 **onion, chopped**
¼ **cup tub margarine**
1 **eggplant, peeled, cooked, and mashed**
1 **egg white**
1 **cup skim milk**
2 **tablespoons chopped pimento**
½ **teaspoon salt**
⅛ **teaspoon pepper**
1 **cup cracker crumbs**
  paprika

1. Preheat oven to 350°F.
2. Sauté green pepper and onion in margarine until tender.
3. Combine with eggplant, egg white, milk, pimento, salt, and pepper.
4. Pour into a casserole greased with margarine and top with crumbs and paprika.
5. Bake 30–40 minutes or until lightly browned.

Yield: 6 servings

1 serving contains:

Cal	Prot	Fat	Carb	Sat	Mono	Poly	Chol	Na
165	5	9.4	17	1.8	3.4	3.9	1	458

Exchanges: 1 serving = 1 bread, 2 fats
Recommended for: The Living Heart; Diabetic; Types IIa, IIb, III, and IV Diets

Eggplant with Tomatoes

1 **eggplant, peeled, cut into ½-inch slices**
1½ **teaspoons salt**
¼ **teaspoon garlic powder**
2 **tablespoons oil**
1 **can (16 ounces) tomatoes, undrained**
1½ **tablespoons chopped fresh parsley**
½ **teaspoon pepper**
½ **teaspoon dried sweet basil**
½ **teaspoon dried oregano**

1. Sprinkle both sides of eggplant slices with garlic powder and 1 teaspoon salt. Brown in oil.
2. Add tomatoes and seasonings.
3. Heat thoroughly.

Yield: 6 servings

1 serving contains:

Cal	Prot	Fat	Carb	Sat	Mono	Poly	Chol	Na
73	2	4.9	7	0.6	1.1	3.0	0	654

Exchanges: 1 serving = 1 vegetable, 1 fat
Recommended for: The Living Heart; Diabetic; Types IIa, IIb, III, and IV Diets

Abbreviations: **Cal,** calories; **Prot,** protein; **Carb,** carbohydrate; **Sat,** saturated fat; **Mono,** monounsaturated fat; **Poly,** polyunsaturated fat; **Chol,** cholesterol; **Na,** sodium. Protein, fat, carbohydrate, saturated fat, monounsaturated fat, and polyunsaturated fat are expressed in *grams.* Cholesterol and sodium are expressed in *milligrams.*

Baked Okra and Tomatoes

1 **pound whole okra, fresh or frozen**
1 **tablespoon oil**
1 **onion, chopped**
3 **tomatoes, chopped**
1 **teaspoon salt**
¼ **teaspoon pepper**
¼ **teaspoon garlic powder**

1. Preheat oven to 400°F.
2. Wash okra and cut off tip ends.
3. Heat oil in saucepan and add okra and remaining ingredients. Cover and simmer until okra is tender, about 15 minutes.
4. Turn into lightly oiled casserole and bake 30 minutes.

Yield: 6 servings

Variation:
Top with ¼ cup fine, dry bread crumbs before baking.

1 serving contains:

Cal	Prot	Fat	Carb	Sat	Mono	Poly	Chol	Na
66	2	2.5	10	0.3	0.6	1.5	0	371

Exchanges: 1 serving = 2 vegetables, ½ fat
1 serving with bread crumbs = 1 vegetable, ½ bread, ½ fat (82 calories)
Recommended for: The Living Heart; Low Calorie; Diabetic; Types IIa, IIb, III, and IV Diets

Broiled Onions

2 **sweet Spanish onions, peeled and halved**
¾ **cup chicken bouillon**
¾ **cup dry white wine**
2 **teaspoons tub margarine**
¼ **cup fine, dry bread crumbs**
½ **teaspoon celery salt**
½ **teaspoon dried summer savory**

1. Simmer onion halves in bouillon and wine for 30–40 minutes or until tender. Drain.

2. Remove center from each onion and chop. Place halves on a baking sheet.
3. Combine chopped onion centers and remaining ingredients. Stuff ¼ of mixture into each onion half.
4. Brown lightly under broiler.

Yield: 4 servings

1 serving contains:

Cal	Prot	Fat	Carb	Sat	Mono	Poly	Chol	Na
69	2	2.3	11	0.4	0.8	1.0	0	359

Exchanges: 1 serving = 2 vegetables, ½ fat
Recommended for: The Living Heart; Low Calorie; Diabetic; Types IIa, IIb, III, and IV Diets

Honey Glazed Onions

16 **white onions, about 1½ inches in diameter**
¼ **cup tub margarine**
2 **tablespoons honey**
2 **teaspoons chopped fresh parsley**

1. Preheat oven to 400°F.
2. Blanch onions about 1 minute.
3. Drain and remove skins and tops. Place in a single layer in a small baking dish.
4. Melt margarine in a saucepan, stir in honey and parsley, and heat through. Pour over onions.
5. Bake for 45 minutes, basting occasionally.

Yield: 6 servings

Note: These may be baked in a microwave oven 15 minutes.

1 serving contains:

Cal	Prot	Fat	Carb	Sat	Mono	Poly	Chol	Na
135	2	7.8	16	1.4	2.7	3.5	0	105

Exchanges: 1 serving = 1 bread, 1½ fats
Recommended for: The Living Heart; Diabetic; Types IIa, IIb, III, and IV Diets

Spiced Peas

1   package (10 ounces) frozen peas
½   cup water
¼   cup chopped celery
3   tablespoons chopped onion
2   tablespoons chopped pimento
¼   teaspoon dried marjoram
⅛   teaspoon salt
⅛   teaspoon pepper

1. Cook peas in water until tender.
2. Add remaining ingredients. Simmer for a few more minutes.

Yield: 4 servings

1 serving contains:

Cal	Prot	Fat	Carb	Sat	Mono	Poly	Chol	Na
47	3	0.2	8	0	0	0.2	0	172

Exchanges: 1 serving = ½ bread
Recommended for: The Living Heart; Low Calorie; Diabetic; Types I, IIa, IIb, III, IV, and V Diets

German Potatoes

¼   cup flour
4   potatoes, peeled and grated
1   onion, grated
    egg substitute equivalent to 1 egg
1   teaspoon salt
¼   teaspoon pepper
3   tablespoons oil

1. Combine all ingredients except oil.
2. Heat oil in skillet.
3. Drop batter from a tablespoon into the hot oil. Fry until golden brown on both sides.

Yield: 12 servings

1 serving contains:

Cal	Prot	Fat	Carb	Sat	Mono	Poly	Chol	Na
96	2	3.8	14	0.5	0.9	2.2	0	195

Exchanges: 1 serving = 1 bread, ½ fat
Recommended for: The Living Heart; Diabetic; Types IIa, IIb, III, and IV Diets

Fluffy Stuffed Baked Potatoes

2   potatoes, baked
1   egg white
½   teaspoon salt
⅛   teaspoon pepper
½   teaspoon instant minced onion
½   teaspoon chives
4–6   tablespoons skim milk
2   tablespoons shredded low-fat cheese
      paprika

1. Preheat oven to 425°F.
2. Whip egg white and salt until stiff peaks form. Set aside.
3. Cut potatoes in half lengthwise and scoop out insides.
4. Whip potato insides, pepper, onion, and chives with an electric mixer, adding the milk a little at a time, until fluffy.
5. Fold in egg white. Put mixture back into potato skins.
6. Sprinkle with shredded cheese and paprika.
7. Bake until cheese is melted and potatoes are hot.

Yield: 4 servings

1 serving contains:

Cal	Prot	Fat	Carb	Sat	Mono	Poly	Chol	Na
90	4	0.4	18	0.2	0.1	0.1	2	362

Exchanges: 1 serving = 1½ breads
Recommended for: The Living Heart; Low Calorie; Diabetic; Types I, IIa, IIb, III, IV, and V Diets

Abbreviations: **Cal,** calories; **Prot,** protein; **Carb,** carbohydrate; **Sat,** saturated fat; **Mono,** monounsaturated fat; **Poly,** polyunsaturated fat; **Chol,** cholesterol; **Na,** sodium. Protein, fat, carbohydrate, saturated fat, monounsaturated fat, and polyunsaturated fat are expressed in *grams*. Cholesterol and sodium are expressed in *milligrams*.

Cottage Cheese Stuffed Baked Potatoes

2 potatoes, baked
1 cup low-fat cottage cheese
2 teaspoons chives
1 teaspoon onion powder
  paprika

1. Preheat oven to 425°F.
2. Cut potatoes in half lengthwise and scoop out insides.
3. Return shell to oven and bake until crisp.
4. Whip potato insides with remaining ingredients except paprika with an electric mixer.
5. Put mixture back into potato skins. Sprinkle with paprika.
6. Bake until heated through.

Yield: 4 servings

1 serving contains:

Cal	Prot	Fat	Carb	Sat	Mono	Poly	Chol	Na
124	10	1.2	19	0.7	0.3	0.2	5	233

Exchanges: 1 serving = 1 bread, 1 meat
Recommended for: The Living Heart; Diabetic; Types IIa, IIb, III, IV, and V Diets

Spicy New Potatoes

1 teaspoon concentrated instant liquid crab and shrimp boil
8 small new potatoes

1. Pour crab and shrimp boil into water and bring to a boil.
2. Add potatoes and simmer until potato skins barely pop and potatoes are tender.

Yield: 4 servings

1 serving contains:

Cal	Prot	Fat	Carb	Sat	Mono	Poly	Chol	Na
104	3	0.1	23	0	0	0.1	0	158

Exchanges: 1 serving = 1½ breads
Recommended for: The Living Heart; Low Calorie; Diabetic; Types I, IIa, IIb, III, IV, and V Diets

Creamed Potatoes

4 potatoes
1 cup cold skim milk
1 tablespoon cornstarch
2 tablespoons tub margarine
¼ cup grated onion
½ teaspoon salt
⅛ teaspoon pepper
¼ cup chopped fresh parsley
  paprika

1. Pare, slice, boil, and drain potatoes.
2. Heat cold milk and cornstarch in a saucepan until thickened.
3. Add remaining ingredients except paprika and heat through.
4. Garnish with paprika.

Yield: 4 servings

1 serving contains:

Cal	Prot	Fat	Carb	Sat	Mono	Poly	Chol	Na
114	3	3.0	19	0.6	1.0	1.4	1	329

Exchanges: 1 serving = 1 bread, 1 fat
Recommended for: The Living Heart; Diabetic; Types IIa, IIb, III, and IV Diets

Glorified Sauerkraut

2 onions, chopped
1 green pepper, chopped
1 can (4 ounces) mushrooms, drained
1 tablespoon tub margarine
1 can (16 ounces) sauerkraut, drained
1 can (16 ounces) peeled tomatoes, undrained, chopped

1. Preheat oven to 350°F.
2. Sauté onion, green pepper, and mushrooms in margarine.
3. Add sauerkraut and tomatoes and pour into a casserole.
4. Cover and bake 60 minutes. Uncover and continue baking 30 minutes more.

Yield: 6 servings

1 serving contains:

Cal	Prot	Fat	Carb	Sat	Mono	Poly	Chol	Na
61	2	2.3	9	0.4	0.7	1.2	0	586

Exchanges: 1 serving = 2 vegetables, ½ fat
Recommended for: The Living Heart; Diabetic; Types IIa, IIb, III, and IV Diets

Chinese Spinach

1 package (10 ounces) frozen chopped spinach, cooked, undrained
1 cup bean sprouts
⅓ cup sliced water chestnuts
1 cup sliced fresh mushrooms or 1 can (2 ounces) mushrooms, drained
4 teaspoons soy sauce

1. To cooked spinach, add remaining vegetables and heat.
2. Drain and toss with soy sauce.

Yield: 4 servings

1 serving contains:

Cal	Prot	Fat	Carb	Sat	Mono	Poly	Chol	Na
42	4	0.4	8	0	0	0.4	0	484

Exchanges: 1 serving = 1½ vegetables
Recommended for: The Living Heart; Low Calorie; Diabetic; Types I, IIa, IIb, III, IV, and V Diets

Spinach Soufflé

1 package (10 ounces) frozen chopped spinach, cooked, drained
3 tablespoons chopped onion
½ cup low-fat cottage cheese
1 teaspoon lemon juice
¼ teaspoon salt
⅛ teaspoon pepper
1 egg white, whipped

1. Preheat oven to 350°F.
2. Combine all ingredients except egg white and purée in blender.

3. Fold in whipped egg white. Place in ungreased small casserole or muffin tins.
4. Bake 25 minutes. Serve immediately.

Yield: 3 servings

1 serving contains:

Cal	Prot	Fat	Carb	Sat	Mono	Poly	Chol	Na
67	10	1.0	6	0.5	0.2	0.3	3	407

Exchanges: 1 serving = ½ dairy, 1 vegetable
Recommended for: The Living Heart; Low Calorie; Diabetic; Types IIa, IIb, III, and IV Diets

Orange Acorn Squash

2 acorn squash, cut in half, seeds removed
1 tablespoon butter flavoring
1 cup orange juice
½ teaspoon salt
¾ teaspoon ground allspice

1. Preheat oven to 350°F.
2. Place squash halves in a casserole dish.
3. Combine remaining ingredients and pour into squash cavities.
4. Cover and bake 60 minutes or until squash is tender.

Yield: 4 servings

1 serving contains:

Cal	Prot	Fat	Carb	Sat	Mono	Poly	Chol	Na
127	3	0.7	31	0	0	0.7	0	277

Exchanges: 1 serving = 2 breads
Recommended for: The Living Heart; Diabetic; Types I, IIa, IIb, III, IV, and V Diets

Abbreviations: **Cal,** calories; **Prot,** protein; **Carb,** carbohydrate; **Sat,** saturated fat; **Mono,** monounsaturated fat; **Poly,** polyunsaturated fat; **Chol,** cholesterol; **Na,** sodium. Protein, fat, carbohydrate, saturated fat, monounsaturated fat, and polyunsaturated fat are expressed in *grams.* Cholesterol and sodium are expressed in *milligrams.*

Seasoned Squash

1 clove garlic, minced
1 tablespoon tub margarine
1¼ pounds yellow crookneck or zucchini squash, peeled, sliced ¼ inch thick
½ teaspoon seasoned salt
¼ cup chopped green onion
¼ cup water
1 can (8 ounces) tomatoes, undrained
2 tablespoons chopped fresh parsley

1. Sauté garlic in margarine for 3 minutes.
2. Add squash, salt, onion, and water.
3. Cover and simmer, stirring occasionally, until squash is tender.
4. Add tomatoes and parsley.
5. Heat through.

Yield: 6 servings

1 serving contains:

Cal	Prot	Fat	Carb	Sat	Mono	Poly	Chol	Na
35	1	2.1	4	0.4	0.7	1.0	0	179

Exchanges: 1 serving = 1 vegetable
Recommended for: The Living Heart; Low Calorie; Diabetic; Types IIa, IIb, III, and IV Diets

Herbed Tomatoes

4 tomatoes, cut in half
4 teaspoons tub margarine
½ teaspoon salt
¼ teaspoon pepper
¼ teaspoon dried oregano
¼ teaspoon dried thyme
¼ teaspoon dried rosemary

1. Preheat oven to 325°F.
2. Place tomatoes in a shallow baking dish, cut side up, and dot with margarine.
3. Combine seasonings and sprinkle over tomatoes.
4. Bake 20 minutes.

Yield: 4 servings

1 serving contains:

Cal	Prot	Fat	Carb	Sat	Mono	Poly	Chol	Na
55	1	4.0	5	0.7	1.4	1.8	0	326

Exchanges: 1 serving = 1 vegetable, 1 fat
Recommended for: The Living Heart; Diabetic; Types IIa, IIb, III, and IV Diets

Spinach Tomatoes

3 tomatoes, cut in half
2 tablespoons grated onion
¼ cup chopped fresh parsley
2 tablespoons tub margarine
1 can (8 ounces) or half of a 10-ounce package frozen spinach, cooked, drained, and chopped
2 tablespoons fine, dry bread crumbs

1. Preheat oven to 350°F.
2. Place tomatoes in a shallow baking pan, cut side up.
3. Mix onion, parsley, margarine, and spinach. Spread on tomatoes and sprinkle with crumbs.
4. Bake 20 minutes.

Yield: 6 servings

1 serving contains:

Cal	Prot	Fat	Carb	Sat	Mono	Poly	Chol	Na
55	2	4.0	4	0.7	1.4	1.8	0	67

Exchanges: 1 serving = 1 vegetable, 1 fat
Recommended for: The Living Heart; Diabetic; Types IIa, IIb, III, and IV Diets

Baked Zucchini

1 pound zucchini squash, unpeeled, sliced
¼ cup sliced green onion
1 tablespoon oil
3 tomatoes, chopped
½ teaspoon salt
⅛ teaspoon pepper
1 clove garlic, minced
½ green pepper, chopped

1. Preheat oven to 350°F.
2. Sauté zucchini and green onion in oil.

3. Place in casserole dish and top with remaining ingredients.
4. Cover and bake 30 minutes.

Yield: 6 servings

1 serving contains:

Cal	Prot	Fat	Carb	Sat	Mono	Poly	Chol	Na
43	1	2.4	5	0.3	0.6	1.5	0	187

Exchanges: 1 serving = 1 vegetable, ½ fat
Recommended for: The Living Heart; Low Calorie; Diabetic; Types IIa, IIb, III, and IV Diets

Lemon Zucchini

4–5 **zucchini squash, unpeeled, sliced**
1½ **teaspoons salt**
¾ **cup water**
2 **tablespoons finely chopped onion**
⅓ **cup chopped fresh parsley**
1 **tablespoon tub margarine**
¼ **teaspoon grated lemon peel**
1 **tablespoon lemon juice**

1. Cook zucchini in salted water 8–10 minutes or until tender. Drain.
2. While zucchini is cooking, briefly sauté onion and parsley in margarine. Add lemon peel and lemon juice. Heat through and pour over zucchini.

Yield: 4 servings

1 serving contains:

Cal	Prot	Fat	Carb	Sat	Mono	Poly	Chol	Na
36	1	2.9	2	0.5	1.0	1.3	0	173

Exchanges: 1 serving = 1 vegetable, ½ fat
Recommended for: The Living Heart; Low Calorie; Diabetic; Types IIa, IIb, III, and IV Diets

Stir-Fried Vegetable Medley

1 **tablespoon oil**
1 **onion, sliced into rings**
1 **clove garlic, minced**
2 **large carrots, peeled and sliced on diagonal**
1 **zucchini squash, unpeeled and sliced**
2 **yellow crookneck squash, unpeeled and sliced**
1 **green pepper, cut into strips**
8 **fresh mushrooms, sliced**
½ **cup bamboo shoots**
4 **water chestnuts, sliced**
2 **tablespoons soy sauce**

1. Heat large skillet or wok until a drop of water dances on the surface.
2. Add oil and heat.
3. Cook onion rings and garlic until just tender.
4. Add carrots, stirring with wooden spoon until lightly coated with oil.
5. Cover and cook 3–4 minutes.
6. Add zucchini and yellow squash, stirring lightly.
7. Cover and allow vegetables to steam in their own juices 2–3 minutes.
8. Add remaining vegetables and stir another 1–2 minutes until tender but crisp.
9. Add soy sauce, cover, and steam 1 additional minute. Serve immediately.

Yield: 8 servings

1 serving contains:

Cal	Prot	Fat	Carb	Sat	Mono	Poly	Chol	Na
43	1	1.9	6	0.2	0.4	1.2	0	377

Exchanges: 1 serving = 1 vegetable, ½ fat
Recommended for: The Living Heart; Low Calorie; Diabetic; Types IIa, IIb, III, and IV Diets

Abbreviations: **Cal,** calories; **Prot,** protein; **Carb,** carbohydrate; **Sat,** saturated fat; **Mono,** monounsaturated fat; **Poly,** polyunsaturated fat; **Chol,** cholesterol; **Na,** sodium. Protein, fat, carbohydrate, saturated fat, monounsaturated fat, and polyunsaturated fat are expressed in *grams.* Cholesterol and sodium are expressed in *milligrams.*

Herbed Rice

1½ cups water
 1 chicken bouillon cube
 ¾ cup long-cooking rice, uncooked
 1 stalk celery, chopped
 ¼ teaspoon dried oregano
 1 bay leaf
 ½ teaspoon salt
 1 tablespoon chopped fresh parsley
 1 teaspoon tub margarine

1. Heat water and bouillon cube until dissolved.
2. Add remaining ingredients and cover.
3. Cook until water is absorbed and rice is tender.

Yield: 6 servings

1 serving contains:

Cal	Prot	Fat	Carb	Sat	Mono	Poly	Chol	Na
92	2	0.8	19	0.1	0.3	0.3	0	359

Exchanges: 1 serving = 1½ breads
Recommended for: The Living Heart; Low Calorie; Diabetic; Types IIa, IIb, III, IV, and V Diets

Almond Rice with Curry

 2 tablespoons chopped onion
 ¼ cup thinly sliced celery
 1 tablespoon tub margarine
 2 tablespoons slivered almonds
 1 cup long-cooking rice, uncooked
 ½ teaspoon curry powder
 2 cups hot water

1. In saucepan, sauté onion and celery in margarine until tender.
2. Add almonds, rice, and curry powder.
3. Cook until slightly browned.
4. Add water, mix well, and heat to boiling.
5. Cover and simmer 15 minutes or until liquid is absorbed and rice is tender.
6. Remove from heat and toss lightly.

Yield: 8 servings

1 serving contains:

Cal	Prot	Fat	Carb	Sat	Mono	Poly	Chol	Na
121	2	2.6	22	0.4	1.2	0.9	0	357

Exchanges: 1 serving = 1½ breads, ½ fat
Recommended for: The Living Heart; Diabetic; Types IIa, IIb, III, and IV Diets

Tasty Rice Casserole

 7 cups water
 2 beef bouillon cubes
 ½ cup brown rice, uncooked
 ½ cup long-cooking white rice, uncooked
 1 onion, finely chopped
 2 stalks celery, finely chopped
 ½ pound mushrooms, sliced
 1 can (8 ounces) water chestnuts, drained and sliced
 2 tablespoons soy sauce

1. Preheat oven to 350°F.
2. In a large kettle, bring the water and bouillon cubes to a boil.
3. Add brown rice and cook 25 minutes.
4. Add white rice and continue to cook an additional 15–20 minutes, or until tender. Drain.
5. In skillet, steam onions in a small amount of water until they are limp and transparent.
6. Add celery and mushrooms. Cook an additional 5 minutes.
7. Add vegetables and water chestnuts to rice. Season with soy sauce and mix thoroughly.
8. Place in a lightly oiled casserole.
9. Bake uncovered for 30 minutes.

Yield: 6 servings

1 serving contains:

Cal	Prot	Fat	Carb	Sat	Mono	Poly	Chol	Na
188	5.2	1.0	40	0.2	0.2	0.5	0	975

Exchanges: 1 serving = 2 breads, 2 vegetables
Recommended for: The Living Heart; Low Calorie; Diabetic; Types I, IIa, IIb, III, IV, and V Diets

Spanish Rice

½ **onion, finely chopped**
¼ **green pepper, chopped**
1 **cup long-cooking rice, uncooked**
1 **tablespoon tub margarine**
2 **cups tomato juice**
½ **teaspoon dried sweet basil**
¼ **teaspoon pepper**
¼ **teaspoon garlic powder**

1. Sauté onion, green pepper, and rice in margarine until lightly browned.
2. Stir in remaining ingredients and cover.
3. Cook over low heat until juice is absorbed and rice is tender.

Yield: 8 servings

1 serving contains:

Cal	Prot	Fat	Carb	Sat	Mono	Poly	Chol	Na
124	2	1.7	25	0.3	0.6	0.8	0	476

Exchanges: 1 serving = 1½ breads, ½ fat
Recommended for: The Living Heart; Diabetic; Types IIa, IIb, III, and IV Diets

Macaroni Fiesta

¾ **cup macaroni, uncooked**
¼ **cup chopped onion**
1 **tablespoon oil**
2 **tablespoons chopped pimento**
1 **can (8 ounces) peas, drained**
¼ **teaspoon salt**
⅛ **teaspoon pepper**

1. Cook macaroni according to package directions. Drain.
2. Sauté onion in oil until tender.
3. Add macaroni and remaining ingredients. Stir until heated through.

Yield: 4 servings

Variation:

Macaroni Fiesta Salad: Chill 2 hours or overnight and serve cold.

1 serving contains:

Cal	Prot	Fat	Carb	Sat	Mono	Poly	Chol	Na
131	4	3.9	21	0.4	1.0	2.3	0	267

Exchanges: 1 serving = 1 vegetable, 1 bread, 1 fat
Recommended for: The Living Heart; Diabetic; Types IIa, IIb, III, and IV Diets

Herb Bread Stuffing

1 **onion, finely chopped**
1 **stalk celery, finely chopped**
⅓ **cup tub margarine**
2 **chicken bouillon cubes**
1 **cup boiling water**
8 **cups bread cubes**
¾ **teaspoon dried sage**
¾ **teaspoon dried thyme**
¼ **teaspoon garlic powder**
1 **teaspoon salt**
½ **teaspoon chopped fresh parsley**
¼ **teaspoon pepper**
1 **can (4 ounces) mushroom pieces, drained**

1. Sauté onion and celery in margarine.
2. Dissolve bouillon cubes in water and add to bread cubes.
3. Add remaining ingredients and toss together.
4. Stuff lightly into bird.

Yield: enough for 10-pound bird or 12 servings

1 serving contains:

Cal	Prot	Fat	Carb	Sat	Mono	Poly	Chol	Na
142	3	6.2	18	1.2	2.3	2.5	0	623

Exchanges: 1 serving = 1 bread, 1½ fats
Recommended for: The Living Heart; Diabetic; Types IIa, IIb, III, and IV Diets

Abbreviations: **Cal,** calories; **Prot,** protein; **Carb,** carbohydrate; **Sat,** saturated fat; **Mono,** monounsaturated fat; **Poly,** polyunsaturated fat; **Chol,** cholesterol; **Na,** sodium. Protein, fat, carbohydrate, saturated fat, monounsaturated fat, and polyunsaturated fat are expressed in *grams.* Cholesterol and sodium are expressed in *milligrams.*

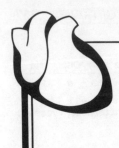

Salads and Dressings

VEGETABLE SALADS

Guacamole

2 avocados, peeled and mashed
½ tomato, finely chopped, discard juice and seeds
¼ onion, finely chopped
1½ teaspoons lemon juice
½ teaspoon garlic salt
½ teaspoon mayonnaise
5–6 drops red pepper sauce
½ cup finely shredded lettuce

1. Combine all ingredients except lettuce.
2. Store in covered container with avocado seed in center.
3. Remove seed and serve on shredded lettuce.

Yield: 4 servings

1 serving contains:

Cal	Prot	Fat	Carb	Sat	Mono	Poly	Chol	Na
197	3	18.9	8	3.7	8.3	2.7	0	251

Exchanges: 1 serving = 1½ vegetables, 3½ fats
Recommended for: The Living Heart; Diabetic; Types IIa, IIb, III, and IV Diets

Sugarless Three Bean Salad

1 can (16 ounces) green beans, drained
1 can (16 ounces) wax beans, drained
1 can (16 ounces) kidney beans, drained
1 can (16 ounces) Italian beans, drained (optional)
½ green pepper, chopped
¾ cup chopped onion
¾ cup chopped celery
¼ cup chopped pimento
½ cup vinegar
⅓ cup oil
¾ teaspoon pepper
¾ teaspoon salt
¾ teaspoon Worcestershire sauce
¾ teaspoon celery seed
¼ teaspoon garlic salt

1. Combine the beans, green pepper, onion, celery, and pimento.
2. Combine remaining ingredients.
3. Pour dressing over bean mixture and stir.
4. Refrigerate in covered container for 12 hours before serving, stirring occasionally.
5. This salad will keep for several days in the refrigerator.

Yield: 16 servings

1 serving contains:

Cal	Prot	Fat	Carb	Sat	Mono	Poly	Chol	Na
82	2	4.7	9	0.6	1.1	2.8	0	263

Exchanges: 1 serving = ½ bread, 1 fat
Recommended for: The Living Heart; Low Calorie; Diabetic; Types IIa, IIb, III, and IV Diets

Cabbage Slaw

⅓ **cup mayonnaise**
¼ **cup vinegar**
¼ **cup sugar**
1 **teaspoon salt**
¼ **cup finely chopped green pepper**
2 **tablespoons chopped fresh parsley**
2 **tablespoons finely chopped onion**
3 **cups shredded cabbage**
½ **cup grated carrots**
¼ **cup thinly sliced radishes**

1. Combine mayonnaise, vinegar, sugar, salt, green pepper, parsley, and onion.
2. Toss with cabbage, carrots, and radishes.
3. Chill before serving.

Yield: 6 servings

1 serving contains:

Cal	Prot	Fat	Carb	Sat	Mono	Poly	Chol	Na
143	1	9.9	14	1.7	2.1	5.1	8	455

Exchanges: 1 serving = 2 vegetables, 2 fats
Recommended for: The Living Heart; Types IIa, IIb, III, and IV Diets

Caraway Slaw

2 **teaspoons vinegar**
½ **teaspoon caraway seed**
1 **teaspoon prepared mustard**
½ **teaspoon salt**
½ **teaspoon garlic salt**
1 **cup plain skim milk yogurt**
2 **carrots, grated**
4 **cups shredded cabbage**
½ **cup chopped green pepper**

1. Combine vinegar, caraway seed, mustard, salt and garlic salt.
2. Fold in yogurt.
3. Cover and chill.
4. Toss carrots, cabbage, and green pepper with chilled dressing.

Yield: 8 servings

1 serving contains:

Cal	Prot	Fat	Carb	Sat	Mono	Poly	Chol	Na
37	3	0.2	7	0	0	0.2	1	306

Exchanges: 1 serving = 1½ vegetables
Recommended for: The Living Heart; Low Calorie; Diabetic; Types I, IIa, IIb, III, IV, and V Diets

Mexican Slaw Salad

1 **tablespoon (1 envelope) unflavored gelatin**
½ **teaspoon salt**
1½ **cups boiling water**
¼ **cup vinegar**
¼ **cup chopped celery**
½ **cup shredded cabbage**
¼ **cup chopped green pepper**
¼ **cup grated carrot**
2 **tablespoons chopped sweet red pepper or pimento**

1. Dissolve gelatin and salt in boiling water. Stir in vinegar.
2. Chill until partially thickened.
3. Fold in vegetables.
4. Pour into mold and chill until firm.

Yield: 4 servings

1 serving contains:

Cal	Prot	Fat	Carb	Sat	Mono	Poly	Chol	Na
19	2	0.1	3	0	0	0.1	0	319

Exchanges: 1 serving = 1 vegetable
Recommended for: The Living Heart; Low Calorie; Diabetic; Types I, IIa, IIb, III, IV, and V Diets

Abbreviations: **Cal,** calories; **Prot,** protein; **Carb,** carbohydrate; **Sat,** saturated fat; **Mono,** monounsaturated fat; **Poly,** polyunsaturated fat; **Chol,** cholesterol; **Na,** sodium. Protein, fat, carbohydrate, saturated fat, monounsaturated fat, and polyunsaturated fat are expressed in *grams.* Cholesterol and sodium are expressed in *milligrams.*

Cole Slaw

6 cups shredded cabbage
3 carrots, shredded
½ cup chopped green pepper
¼ cup finely chopped onion
¼ teaspoon salt
⅛ teaspoon pepper
1 cup Cole Slaw Dressing (see recipe, page 169)

1. Combine all ingredients.
2. Chill until flavors are blended.

Yield: 8 servings

1 serving contains:

Cal	Prot	Fat	Carb	Sat	Mono	Poly	Chol	Na
43	2	0.2	9	0	0	0.2	0	491

Exchanges: 1 serving = 2 vegetables
Recommended for: The Living Heart; Low Calorie; Diabetic; Types IIa, IIb, III, IV, and V Diets

Carrot Raisin Salad

3 cups grated carrots
¾ cup raisins
⅓ cup mayonnaise
1 teaspoon sugar
¼ teaspoon salt
2 tablespoons evaporated skim milk, undiluted
1 tablespoon lemon juice

1. Combine carrots and raisins in large bowl.
2. Mix together the mayonnaise, sugar, salt, milk, and lemon juice.
3. Toss with carrots and raisins.
4. Chill well before serving.

Yield: 6 servings

1 serving contains:

Cal	Prot	Fat	Carb	Sat	Mono	Poly	Chol	Na
170	2	9.8	21	1.7	2.1	5.0	9	201

Exchanges: 1 serving = 2 fruits, 2 fats
Recommended for: The Living Heart; Diabetic; Types IIa, IIb, III, and IV Diets

Mexican Marinated Salad

1 head cauliflower (about 1½ pounds), thinly sliced
½ cup thinly sliced green pepper
¼ cup thinly sliced red pepper
¾ cup Basic Oil and Vinegar Dressing (see recipe, page 167)
romaine lettuce
4 tomatoes, sliced
1 cucumber, sliced

1. Combine cauliflower and peppers in a bowl.
2. Add Basic Oil and Vinegar Dressing.
3. Refrigerate several hours.
4. Line a large plate with romaine leaves. Mound cauliflower and peppers in the center.
5. Garnish around the edge with tomato and cucumber slices.

Yield: 8 servings

1 serving contains:

Cal	Prot	Fat	Carb	Sat	Mono	Poly	Chol	Na
156	2	13.5	9	2.3	2.8	7.2	0	471

Exchanges: 1 serving = 1 vegetable, 3 fats
Recommended for: The Living Heart; Diabetic; Types IIa, IIb, III, and IV Diets

Cauliflower Salad

1 package (10 ounces) frozen cauliflower
1 stalk celery, chopped
¼ cup chopped green pepper
2 tablespoons pickle relish
2 teaspoons prepared mustard
2 tablespoons finely chopped onion
3 teaspoons chopped fresh parsley
½ teaspoon salt
2 teaspoons sugar
½ teaspoon Worcestershire sauce
½ teaspoon lemon juice

1. Cook cauliflower according to package directions. Drain well. Chop into small pieces.
2. Toss with other ingredients.
3. Chill salad well before serving.

Yield: 4 servings

1 serving contains:

Cal	Prot	Fat	Carb	Sat	Mono	Poly	Chol	Na
43	2	0.4	9	0	0	0.4	0	394

Exchanges: 1 serving = 2 vegetables
Recommended for: The Living Heart; Low Calorie; Diabetic; Types I, IIa, IIb, III, IV, and V Diets

1 serving contains:

Cal	Prot	Fat	Carb	Sat	Mono	Poly	Chol	Na
21	2	0.1	4	0	0	0.1	0	561

Exchanges: 1 serving = 1 vegetable
Recommended for: The Living Heart; Low Calorie; Diabetic; Types I, IIa, IIb, III, IV, and V Diets

Cool Cuke Salad

1 large cucumber, cut in diagonal slices
2 green onions, chopped
¼ cup buttermilk
1 tablespoon tarragon vinegar
⅛ teaspoon paprika
½ teaspoon salt
⅛ teaspoon pepper

1. Combine all ingredients.
2. Chill well.

Yield: 4 servings

1 serving contains:

Cal	Prot	Fat	Carb	Sat	Mono	Poly	Chol	Na
21	1	0.1	4	0	0	0.1	0	300

Exchanges: 1 serving = 1 vegetable
Recommended for: The Living Heart; Low Calorie; Diabetic; Types IIa, IIb, III, IV, and V Diets

Marinated Okra Salad

1 package (10 ounces) frozen whole okra
¼ cup chopped celery leaves
1 onion, sliced into thin rings
1 bay leaf
½ teaspoon celery seed
½ teaspoon Italian seasoning
½ cup cider vinegar
2 tablespoons low-calorie Italian dressing

1. Cook okra and celery leaves according to package directions on okra. Drain and cool.
2. Combine onion, spices, vinegar, and Italian dressing.
3. Add okra and celery leaves.
4. Cover and chill overnight.

Yield: 4 servings

1 serving contains:

Cal	Prot	Fat	Carb	Sat	Mono	Poly	Chol	Na
43	2	0.5	10	0.1	0.1	0.3	0	73

Exchanges: 1 serving = 2 vegetables
Recommended for: The Living Heart; Low Calorie; Diabetic; Types IIa, IIb, III, IV, and V Diets

Pickled Mushroom Salad

1 can (8 ounces) whole mushrooms, undrained
¼ cup chopped celery leaves
1 onion, sliced into thin rings
⅓ cup cider vinegar
1 bay leaf
½ teaspoon salt
¼ teaspoon celery seed
1 teaspoon low-calorie Italian dressing

1. Combine all ingredients.
2. Cover and chill in refrigerator overnight.
3. Serve on a lettuce leaf, if desired.

Yield: 4 servings

Abbreviations: **Cal,** calories; **Prot,** protein; **Carb,** carbohydrate; **Sat,** saturated fat; **Mono,** monounsaturated fat; **Poly,** polyunsaturated fat; **Chol,** cholesterol; **Na,** sodium. Protein, fat, carbohydrate, saturated fat, monounsaturated fat, and polyunsaturated fat are expressed in *grams.* Cholesterol and sodium are expressed in *milligrams.*

Hot German Potato Salad

3   potatoes, boiled in jackets
2   tablespoons imitation bacon bits
3   tablespoons finely chopped onion
2   tablespoons chopped green pepper
1   tablespoon chopped pimento
½   teaspoon salt
½   teaspoon pepper
1   tablespoon chopped fresh parsley
½   teaspoon celery seed
½   teaspoon granular beef bouillon
¼   cup boiling water
¼   cup cider vinegar

1. Peel potatoes and slice into bowl.
2. Add bacon bits, onion, green pepper, pimento, salt, pepper, parsley, and celery seed.
3. Dissolve the bouillon in the boiling water. Add to vinegar. Pour over potato mixture.
4. Toss lightly and serve warm.

Yield: 6 servings

1 serving contains:

Cal	Prot	Fat	Carb	Sat	Mono	Poly	Chol	Na
92	4	0.7	19	0.1	0.2	0.3	0	392

Exchanges: 1 serving = 1 bread, 1 vegetable
Recommended for: The Living Heart; Low Calorie; Diabetic; Types IIa, IIb, III, IV, and V Diets

Picnic Potato Salad

4   cups cubed boiled potatoes
½   cup chopped onion
½   cup chopped celery
½   cup chopped green pepper
½   cup grated carrots
1   cucumber, chopped
1   dill pickle, finely chopped
2   teaspoons prepared mustard
½   teaspoon salt
1   teaspoon garlic powder
½   cup mayonnaise
     paprika

1. Combine vegetables, mustard, and seasonings.

2. Toss lightly with mayonnaise. Sprinkle with paprika.

Yield: 12 servings

½ cup contains:

Cal	Prot	Fat	Carb	Sat	Mono	Poly	Chol	Na
112	2	7.5	10	1.3	1.6	3.9	6	330

Exchanges: ½ cup = 1 bread, 1 fat
Recommended for: The Living Heart; Low Calorie; Diabetic; Types IIa, IIb, III, and IV Diets

Herbed Potato Salad

4   potatoes, boiled and chopped
¼   cup chopped onion
¼   cup chopped celery
¼   cup chopped green pepper
¼   cup chopped pimento
¼   cup low-calorie Herbed French Dressing (see recipe, page 169)
     salt

1. Combine all ingredients.
2. Toss lightly.

Yield: 4 servings

1 serving contains:

Cal	Prot	Fat	Carb	Sat	Mono	Poly	Chol	Na
131	3	0.9	28	0.1	0.1	0.6	0	750

Exchanges: 1 serving = 1½ breads, 1 vegetable
Recommended for: The Living Heart; Low Calorie; Diabetic; Types IIa, IIb, III, IV, and V Diets

Tangy Potato Salad

1½   teaspoons horseradish
½   teaspoon salt
¼   teaspoon prepared mustard
¼   teaspoon celery seed
½   cup plain skim milk yogurt
4   cups diced cooked potatoes
½   cup chopped celery
¼   cup chopped green pepper
¼   cup chopped onion
2   tablespoons chopped pimento

1. In a small bowl, combine horseradish, salt, mustard, and celery seed.
2. Fold in yogurt.
3. In a medium bowl, combine potatoes, celery, green pepper, onion, and pimento.
4. Add dressing to salad and toss only until blended.
5. Cover and chill.

Yield: 6 servings

1 serving contains:

Cal	Prot	Fat	Carb	Sat	Mono	Poly	Chol	Na
86	3	0.2	18	0	0	0.2	0	236

Exchanges: 1 serving = 1 bread, 1 vegetable
Recommended for: The Living Heart; Low Calorie; Diabetic; Types I, IIa, IIb, III, IV, and V Diets

Variation:

Reduce potatoes to 3 cups and add 1 can (6½ ounces) water-packed tuna, drained, or 1 cup chopped cooked chicken.

1 serving contains:

Cal	Prot	Fat	Carb	Sat	Mono	Poly	Chol	Na
123	15	0.5	14	0.1	0.1	0.3	27	253

Exchanges: 1 serving = 1 meat, ½ bread, 1 vegetable
Recommended for: The Living Heart; Low Calorie; Diabetic; Types I, IIa, IIb, III, IV, and V Diets

Rice Salad

Salad

3 cups cooked rice, cooled
¾ cup chopped green onion, including tops
½ cup chopped green pepper
½ cup chopped red bell pepper
½ cup chopped celery
½ cup chopped dill pickle
½ cup chopped pimento

Dressing

1 cup mayonnaise
2 tablespoons vinegar
1 tablespoon sugar
1 tablespoon prepared mustard
1½ teaspoons salt
½ teaspoon pepper

1. Mix rice with vegetables, pickle, and pimento.
2. In separate bowl, combine ingredients for dressing.
3. Combine dressing with rice mixture.
4. Chill at least 2 hours before serving. Garnish with tomato wedges, if desired.

Yield: 12 servings

1 serving contains:

Cal	Prot	Fat	Carb	Sat	Mono	Poly	Chol	Na
203	2	14.9	17	2.6	3.2	7.6	13	831

Exchanges: 1 serving = 1 bread, 3 fats
Recommended for: The Living Heart; Diabetic; Types IIa, IIb, III, and IV Diets

Wilted Spinach Bacon Salad

1 **pound fresh spinach, washed, dried, and chilled**
⅓ **cup imitation bacon bits**
¼ **cup oil**
1 **tablespoon brown sugar**
¼ **cup sliced green onion**
½ **teaspoon salt**
¼ **cup vinegar**

1. Shred or cut spinach into a salad bowl.
2. Heat bacon bits in oil in a small skillet. Add remaining ingredients and bring to a boil.
3. Pour dressing over spinach and toss.

Yield: 6 servings

1 serving contains:

Cal	Prot	Fat	Carb	Sat	Mono	Poly	Chol	Na
148	6	10.9	9	1.3	2.8	6.0	0	540

Exchanges: 1 serving = ½ meat, 1 vegetable, 2 fats
Recommended for: The Living Heart; Diabetic; Types IIa, IIb, III, and IV Diets

Abbreviations: **Cal**, calories; **Prot**, protein; **Carb**, carbohydrate; **Sat**, saturated fat; **Mono**, monounsaturated fat; **Poly**, polyunsaturated fat; **Chol**, cholesterol; **Na**, sodium. Protein, fat, carbohydrate, saturated fat, monounsaturated fat, and polyunsaturated fat are expressed in *grams*. Cholesterol and sodium are expressed in *milligrams*.

FRUIT SALADS

Cinnamon Salad

- ¼ cup cinnamon candies (red-hots)
- 1 package (3 ounces) cherry-flavored sweetened gelatin
- 1½ cups boiling water
- ½ cup chopped apple
- ½ cup chopped celery
- ½ cup chopped walnuts

1. Dissolve candies and gelatin in boiling water. Cool in refrigerator until partially set. Add apple, celery, and walnuts.
2. Pour into mold and chill.

Yield: 6 servings

1 serving contains:

Cal	Prot	Fat	Carb	Sat	Mono	Poly	Chol	Na
167	3	6.4	27	0.7	1.0	4.2	0	58

Exchanges: Not applicable for this recipe
Recommended for: The Living Heart and Type IIa Diets

Molded Fruit Salad

- 1 tablespoon (1 envelope) unflavored gelatin
- ½ cup orange juice
- 1¼ cups boiling water
- ¼ teaspoon salt
- 1 apple, cored and chopped
- 1 orange, sectioned and chopped

1. Soften gelatin in orange juice in medium bowl. Stir in boiling water and salt.
2. Chill until slightly thickened but not set.
3. Carefully stir in fruit and pour into mold.
4. Chill until set.

Yield: 6 servings

1 serving contains:

Cal	Prot	Fat	Carb	Sat	Mono	Poly	Chol	Na
39	1	0.2	9	0	0	0.2	0	92

Exchanges: 1 serving = 1 fruit
Recommended for: The Living Heart; Low Calorie; Diabetic; Types I, IIa, IIb, III, IV, and V Diets

Tangy Orange Salad

- 2 tablespoons (2 envelopes) unflavored gelatin
- 2 cups orange juice
- 2 cups chopped orange sections
- 2 carrots, shredded
- 1 stalk celery, chopped
- 1 cup plain skim milk yogurt

1. Dissolve gelatin in boiling orange juice.
2. Chill until partially thickened.
3. Fold in oranges, carrots, celery, and yogurt.
4. Turn into mold and chill until firm.

Yield: 8 servings

1 serving contains:

Cal	Prot	Fat	Carb	Sat	Mono	Poly	Chol	Na
82	4	0.2	17	0	0	0.2	1	38

Exchanges: 1 serving = 2 fruits
Recommended for: The Living Heart; Low Calorie; Diabetic; Types I, IIa, IIb, III, IV, and V Diets

Waldorf Fruit Salad

- 2 cups chopped apple
- 1 cup chopped celery
- ⅓ cup chopped walnuts
- ⅓ cup mayonnaise
- 1 tablespoon lemon juice

1. Combine all ingredients and toss lightly.
2. Serve on a lettuce leaf, if desired.

Yield: 4 servings

1 serving contains:

Cal	Prot	Fat	Carb	Sat	Mono	Poly	Chol	Na
230	2	21.0	11	3.3	4.1	11.6	13	147

Exchanges: 1 serving = 1 fruit, 4 fats
Recommended for: The Living Heart; Diabetic; Types IIa, IIb, III, and IV Diets

Mom's Frozen Fruit Salad

2 **teaspoons unflavored gelatin**
6 **tablespoons cold water**
2 **teaspoons confectioner's sugar**
4 **tablespoons lemon juice**
2 **tablespoons maraschino cherry juice**
1 **cup canned evaporated skim milk, chilled, undiluted**
⅔ **cup mayonnaise**
1 **banana, cubed**
1½ **cups crushed pineapple, packed in own juice, drained**
1 **cup sliced maraschino cherries**

1. Sprinkle gelatin over cold water in small saucepan. Stir over low heat until gelatin dissolves.
2. Add sugar, lemon juice, and maraschino cherry juice.
3. Whip chilled evaporated milk until soft peaks form.
4. Fold mayonnaise into whipped milk. Do this step immediately or whipped milk will get runny.
5. Fold in gelatin mixture. Fold in fruits.
6. Turn into refrigerator trays, loaf pan, or large mold and freeze.
7. Stir once before mixture is firm.
8. Freeze 4–5 hours or overnight.
9. Slice and serve on salad greens, if desired.

Yield: 8 servings

1 serving contains:

Cal	Prot	Fat	Carb	Sat	Mono	Poly	Chol	Na
285	4	14.9	37	2.7	3.2	7.6	14	147

Exchanges: Not applicable for this recipe
Recommended for: The Living Heart and Type IIa Diets

MAIN DISH SALADS

Garden Rice Salad

2 **cloves garlic, minced**
1 **onion, chopped**
2 **carrots, chopped**
1 **stalk celery, chopped**
⅔ **cup fresh parsley, chopped**
2 **teaspoons dried sweet basil**
1 **teaspoon dried oregano**
2 **tomatoes, chopped**
1 **can (16 ounces) vegetarian baked beans**
5 **cups cooked rice**
1 **cup vinegar**
2 **teaspoons salt**
¾ **teaspoon pepper**

1. Sauté garlic, onion, carrot, celery, parsley, basil, and oregano in a small amount of water until vegetables are tender. Add tomatoes, beans, and rice.
2. Combine vinegar, salt, and pepper, and toss with vegetables.
3. Chill overnight before serving.

Yield: 12 servings

1 serving contains:

Cal	Prot	Fat	Carb	Sat	Mono	Poly	Chol	Na
150	5	0.5	33	0.1	0.1	0.3	0	700

Exchanges: 1 serving = 2 breads, 1 vegetable
Recommended for: The Living Heart; Low Calorie; Diabetic; Types I, IIa, IIb, III, IV, and V Diets

Abbreviations: **Cal,** calories; **Prot,** protein; **Carb,** carbohydrate; **Sat,** saturated fat; **Mono,** monounsaturated fat; **Poly,** polyunsaturated fat; **Chol,** cholesterol; **Na,** sodium. Protein, fat, carbohydrate, saturated fat, monounsaturated fat, and polyunsaturated fat are expressed in *grams.* Cholesterol and sodium are expressed in *milligrams.*

Chicken and Rice Salad

2 cups cooked rice, cooled
2 cups chopped cooked chicken
1 can (16 ounces) peas, drained
1½ cups chopped celery
½ cup chopped green pepper
2 tablespoons finely chopped onion
¾ cup mayonnaise
½ teaspoon salt
¼ teaspoon pepper
2 tablespoons lemon juice
2 tablespoons chopped fresh parsley

1. Combine rice, chicken, peas, celery, green pepper, and onion.
2. Combine remaining ingredients.
3. Toss chicken mixture with salad dressing.
4. Chill well before serving.

Yield: 8 servings

1 serving contains:

Cal	Prot	Fat	Carb	Sat	Mono	Poly	Chol	Na
311	14	19.0	22	3.6	4.3	9.1	47	613

Exchanges: 1 serving = 1 meat, 1½ breads, 3 fats
Recommended for: The Living Heart; Diabetic; Types IIa, IIb, III, and IV Diets

Luncheon Tuna Salad

1 can (6½ ounces) water-packed tuna, drained
1 can (8 ounces) peas, drained
½ cup finely chopped celery
2 tablespoons pickle relish
1 tablespoon lemon juice
¼ cup mayonnaise

1. Toss all ingredients together and chill.
2. Serve on lettuce leaf, if desired.

Yield: 4 servings

1 serving contains:

Cal	Prot	Fat	Carb	Sat	Mono	Poly	Chol	Na
234	15	14.3	11	3.0	3.3	6.6	39	620

Exchanges: 1 serving = 1½ meats, 2 vegetables, 2 fats
Recommended for: The Living Heart; Diabetic; Types IIa, IIb, III, and IV Diets

Turkey Macaroni Salad

2 cups chopped cooked turkey
2 cups cooked elbow macaroni, cooled
2 stalks celery, chopped
½ onion, chopped
½ cup mayonnaise
1 teaspoon prepared mustard
1 teaspoon lemon juice
¼ teaspoon salt
⅛ teaspoon pepper

1. Mix all ingredients together and chill.
2. Serve on lettuce leaf, if desired.

Yield: 6 servings

1 serving contains:

Cal	Prot	Fat	Carb	Sat	Mono	Poly	Chol	Na
273	15	17.9	12	3.5	4.1	8.2	56	270

Exchanges: 1 serving = 2 meats, 1 bread, 2 fats
Recommended for: The Living Heart; Diabetic; Types IIa, IIb, III, and IV Diets

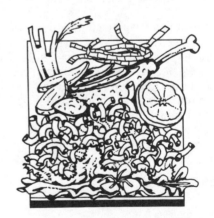

DRESSINGS

C'est La Vie Dressing

¼ **cup plain skim milk yogurt**
¼ **cup catsup**
   wine vinegar or fresh lemon juice to taste
   salt and pepper to taste
⅛ **teaspoon red pepper sauce**
⅛ **teaspoon garlic powder**
⅛ **teaspoon Worcestershire sauce**

1. Combine all ingredients.
2. Chill before serving on tossed greens.

Yield: ½ cup

1 tablespoon contains:

Cal	Prot	Fat	Carb	Sat	Mono	Poly	Chol	Na
13	1	0	3	0	0	0	0	164

Exchanges: 1–2 tablespoons = free; 3 tablespoons = ½ bread
Recommended for: The Living Heart; Low Calorie; Diabetic; Types I, IIa, IIb, III, IV, and V Diets

Avocado Dressing

1 **avocado, peeled and mashed**
1 **tomato, peeled and chopped**
2 **teaspoons chopped, seeded jalapeño pepper**
2 **tablespoons finely chopped onion**
2 **tablespoons Basic Oil and Vinegar Dressing (see recipe, this page)**
½ **teaspoon salt**

1. Mix all ingredients together.
2. Refrigerate until serving time in a covered bowl with the avocado seed resting in the dressing to prevent discoloration.

Yield: 1½ cups

1 tablespoon contains:

Cal	Prot	Fat	Carb	Sat	Mono	Poly	Chol	Na
24	0	2.3	1	0.4	0.8	0.6	0	74

Exchanges: 1 tablespoon = ½ fat
Recommended for: The Living Heart; Diabetic; Types IIa, IIb, III, and IV Diets

Basic Oil and Vinegar Dressing

½ **cup oil**
¼ **cup vinegar**
1 **teaspoon salt**
¼ **teaspoon pepper**
⅛ **teaspoon dry mustard**

1. Combine all ingredients in bottle or jar. Cover tightly and shake well.
2. Store in refrigerator. Shake before serving.

Yield: ¾ cup

Variations:

Add 1 teaspoon sesame, celery, or poppy seeds.

1 tablespoon contains:

Cal	Prot	Fat	Carb	Sat	Mono	Poly	Chol	Na
81	0	9.1	0	1.2	2.2	5.3	0	183

Exchanges: 1 tablespoon = 2 fats
Recommended for: The Living Heart; Diabetic; Types IIa, IIb, III, and IV Diets

Abbreviations: **Cal,** calories; **Prot,** protein; **Carb,** carbohydrate; **Sat,** saturated fat; **Mono,** monounsaturated fat; **Poly,** polyunsaturated fat; **Chol,** cholesterol; **Na,** sodium. Protein, fat, carbohydrate, saturated fat, monounsaturated fat, and polyunsaturated fat are expressed in *grams.* Cholesterol and sodium are expressed in *milligrams.*

Creamy Buttermilk Dressing

2 tablespoons cornstarch
2 tablespoons sugar
1 teaspoon dry mustard
½ teaspoon seasoned salt
½ cup water
1 tablespoon vinegar
3 tablespoons oil
⅔ cup buttermilk

1. Mix cornstarch, sugar, dry mustard, and salt in a saucepan.
2. Stir in water and cook over medium heat, stirring constantly, until thickened. Remove from heat.
3. Add vinegar and oil.
4. Gradually add buttermilk, stirring until smooth and creamy.
5. Store in refrigerator. Shake before serving.

Yield: 1½ cups

Variations:

Add 1 teaspoon coarsely ground black pepper and 1 clove minced garlic.
or
Add 3 tablespoons horseradish and 1 teaspoon caraway seeds.

1 tablespoon contains:

Cal	Prot	Fat	Carb	Sat	Mono	Poly	Chol	Na
24	0	1.8	2	0.3	0.4	1.0	0	33

Exchanges: 1 tablespoon = free; 2 tablespoons = 1 fat
Recommended for: The Living Heart; Low Calorie; Types IIa, IIb, III, and IV Diets

Tangy Buttermilk Dressing

¾ cup buttermilk
2 tablespoons horseradish
1 tablespoon lemon juice
1 tablespoon honey
½ teaspoon seasoned salt
½ teaspoon prepared mustard or 1 tablespoon chili sauce

1. Blend all ingredients together and chill.
2. Serve with potato salad, cole slaw, or vegetable salad.

Yield: 1 cup

1 tablespoon contains:

Cal	Prot	Fat	Carb	Sat	Mono	Poly	Chol	Na
9	0	0	2	0	0	0	0	57

Exchanges: 1–2 tablespoons = free; 3 tablespoons = ½ bread
Recommended for: The Living Heart; Low Calorie; Diabetic; Types IIa, IIb, III, IV, and V Diets

Caesar Salad Dressing

½ cup liquid egg substitute
½ cup low-calorie Italian dressing
⅛ teaspoon Worcestershire sauce
⅛ teaspoon garlic powder

1. Combine all ingredients.
2. Toss with romaine lettuce.

Yield: 1 cup

1 tablespoon contains:

Cal	Prot	Fat	Carb	Sat	Mono	Poly	Chol	Na
12	1	0.8	0	0.1	0.2	0.5	0	74

Exchanges: 1–2 tablespoons = free; 3 tablespoons = ½ fat
Recommended for: The Living Heart; Low Calorie; Diabetic; Types I, IIa, IIb, III, IV, and V Diets

Celery Seed Dressing

⅓ cup sugar
1 teaspoon salt
1 tablespoon paprika
½ teaspoon dry mustard
½ cup wine or cider vinegar
½ cup oil
1 onion, thinly sliced
1 tablespoon celery seed

1. Place all ingredients in blender. Blend for 30 seconds.
2. Store in refrigerator. Shake well before serving.

Yield: 1½ cups

1 tablespoon contains:

Cal	Prot	Fat	Carb	Sat	Mono	Poly	Chol	Na
53	0	4.6	3	0.6	1.1	2.7	0	92

Exchanges: 1 tablespoon = 1 fat
Recommended for: The Living Heart and Type IIa Diets

Cole Slaw Dressing

1 package ranch style salad dressing mix
1 quart buttermilk

1. Combine ingredients.
2. Cover and chill.

Yield: 1 quart

1 tablespoon contains:

Cal	Prot	Fat	Carb	Sat	Mono	Poly	Chol	Na
6	1	0.1	1	0.1	0	0	1	196

Exchanges: 1–4 tablespoons = free; 6 tablespoons = ½ dairy
Recommended for: The Living Heart; Low Calorie; Diabetic; Types IIa, IIb, III, IV, and V Diets

Zesty French Dressing

1 cup tomato juice
½ cup oil
¼ cup vinegar
1 tablespoon sugar
1 teaspoon dry mustard
½ teaspoon paprika
1 teaspoon salt
1 teaspoon Worcestershire sauce
1 clove garlic, minced

1. Combine all ingredients in bottle or jar. Cover tightly and shake well.
2. Store in refrigerator. Shake before serving.

Yield: 2 cups

1 tablespoon contains:

Cal	Prot	Fat	Carb	Sat	Mono	Poly	Chol	Na
33	0	3.4	1	0.4	0.8	2.0	0	87

Exchanges: 1½ tablespoons = 1 fat
Recommended for: The Living Heart; Diabetic; Types IIa, IIb, III, and IV Diets

Herbed French Dressing

¾ cup wine vinegar
1 can (10¾ ounces) condensed tomato soup, undiluted
1 clove garlic, minced
2 tablespoons finely chopped dill pickle
2 tablespoons finely chopped celery
2 tablespoons finely chopped fresh parsley
1 tablespoon Worcestershire sauce
1 teaspoon paprika
½ teaspoon dry mustard

1. Combine all ingredients in a large jar. Cover tightly and shake well.
2. Store in refrigerator. Shake well before serving.

Yield: about 2½ cups

1 tablespoon contains:

Cal	Prot	Fat	Carb	Sat	Mono	Poly	Chol	Na
7	0	0.1	1	0	0	0.1	0	94

Exchanges: 1–4 tablespoons = free; 5 tablespoons = ½ bread
Recommended for: The Living Heart; Low Calorie; Diabetic; Types I, IIa, IIb, III, IV, and V Diets

Abbreviations: **Cal,** calories; **Prot,** protein; **Carb,** carbohydrate; **Sat,** saturated fat; **Mono,** monounsaturated fat; **Poly,** polyunsaturated fat; **Chol,** cholesterol; **Na,** sodium. Protein, fat, carbohydrate, saturated fat, monounsaturated fat, and polyunsaturated fat are expressed in *grams*. Cholesterol and sodium are expressed in *milligrams*.

Merry-Berry Fruit Salad Dressing

1 **cup plain skim milk yogurt**
1 **cup fresh or frozen unsweetened berries of your choice**
¼ **teaspoon ground cinnamon**
1–2 **drops vanilla extract**

1. Blend all ingredients in blender until berries are puréed.
2. Chill well before serving over fruit salad.

Yield: about 1¾ cups

1 tablespoon contains:

Cal	Prot	Fat	Carb	Sat	Mono	Poly	Chol	Na
7	1	0	1	0	0	0	0	6

Exchanges: 1–2 tablespoons = free; 3 tablespoons = ½ fruit
Recommended for: The Living Heart; Low Calorie; Diabetic; Types I, IIa, IIb, III, IV, and V Diets

Thousand Island Dressing

½ **cup plain skim milk yogurt**
1½ **tablespoons chili sauce**
1 **tablespoon chopped dill pickle**
1–2 **tablespoons finely chopped celery**
1 **tablespoon finely chopped fresh parsley**
  salt and pepper to taste
⅛ **teaspoon cayenne pepper**
⅛ **teaspoon dry mustard**

1. Combine all ingredients.
2. Chill before serving on tossed greens.

Yield: about 1 cup

1 tablespoon contains:

Cal	Prot	Fat	Carb	Sat	Mono	Poly	Chol	Na
6	0	0	1	0	0	0	0	150

Exchanges: 1–4 tablespoons = free; 5 tablespoons = ½ bread
Recommended for: The Living Heart; Low Calorie; Diabetic; Types I, IIa, III, IV, and V Diets

Tomato Dressing

1 **can (10¾ ounces) condensed tomato soup, undiluted**
¼ **cup water**
1 **tablespoon lime juice**
1 **tablespoon lemon juice**
2 **teaspoons grated onion**
½ **teaspoon prepared mustard**
¼ **teaspoon salt**
¼ **teaspoon pepper**

1. Combine all ingredients in a tightly covered container. Shake until blended.
2. Chill well before serving over crisp salad greens.

Yield: about 2 cups

1 tablespoon contains:

Cal	Prot	Fat	Carb	Sat	Mono	Poly	Chol	Na
7	0	0.2	1	0	0	0.1	0	100

Exchanges: 1–3 tablespoons = free; 4 tablespoons = ½ bread
Recommended for: The Living Heart; Low Calorie; Diabetic; Types I, IIa, IIb, III, IV, and V Diets

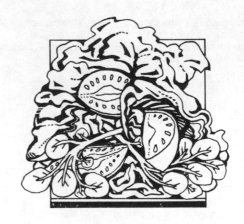

Tofu Mayonnaise

6 ounces tofu, drained
1 tablespoon lemon juice
2 teaspoons soy sauce
⅛ teaspoon pepper
¼ teaspoon dry mustard

Combine all ingredients in blender for about 30 seconds or until smooth.

Yield: about 1 cup

Variations:

Curry Tofu Mayonnaise: Add ½ teaspoon curry powder and 2 tablespoons minced onion.
Garlic Tofu Mayonnaise: Add ¼–½ teaspoon garlic powder.
Herb Tofu Mayonnaise: Add ½ teaspoon dried herbs, such as dill, oregano, rosemary, or marjoram.
Onion Tofu Mayonnaise: Add ¼ cup finely chopped onion.

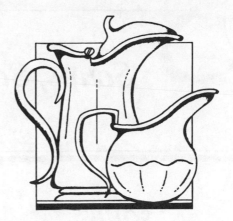

1 tablespoon contains:

Cal	Prot	Fat	Carb	Sat	Mono	Poly	Chol	Na
9	1	0.5	0	0.1	0.1	0.2	0	56

Exchanges: 1 tablespoon = free; ¼ cup = ½ meat
Recommended for: The Living Heart; Low Calorie; Diabetic; Types I, IIa, IIb, III, IV, and V Diets

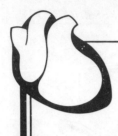

Soups, Sauces, Gravies

SOUPS

Hearty Corn Chowder

1½ onions, finely chopped
2 tablespoons oil
1 cup water
3 potatoes, peeled and chopped
1½ teaspoons salt
¼ teaspoon pepper
1 can (16 ounces) corn, drained
2 cups skim milk

1. Sauté onion in oil.
2. Add water, potatoes, and seasonings. Cook until potatoes are tender, about 15 minutes.
3. Mash potatoes slightly.
4. Add corn and milk. Heat until simmering. Be careful soup does not boil.
5. Serve with parsley garnish, if desired.

Yield: 4 servings

1 serving contains:

Cal	Prot	Fat	Carb	Sat	Mono	Poly	Chol	Na
235	8	7.8	36	1.2	1.8	4.4	2	1086

Exchanges: 1 serving = 2½ breads, 1½ fats
Recommended for: The Living Heart; Diabetic; Types IIa, IIb, III, and IV Diets

Autumn Vegetable Beef Soup

½ pound very lean ground beef
¾ cup chopped onion
2 cups hot water
¾ cup chopped celery
¾ cup diced potato
1 teaspoon salt
¼ teaspoon pepper
½ bay leaf, crumbled
⅛ teaspoon dried sweet basil
¼ teaspoon chives
⅛ teaspoon garlic powder
⅛ teaspoon dried thyme
1 jalapeño pepper, seeded (optional)
1 can (16 ounces) tomatoes, undrained
2 carrots, thinly sliced

1. Brown ground beef and onion in large saucepan. Drain off fat.
2. Add remaining ingredients.
3. Bring to a boil and simmer, covered, 30 minutes or until vegetables are tender.

Yield: 4 servings

1 serving contains:

Cal	Prot	Fat	Carb	Sat	Mono	Poly	Chol	Na
165	15	4.8	16	1.7	1.6	0.7	39	776

Exchanges: 1 serving = 1½ meats, 1 bread
Recommended for: The Living Heart; Low Calorie; Diabetic; Types IIa, IIb, III, IV, and V Diets

Chicken Vegetable Soup

1 cup chopped celery
½ cup chopped onion
2 tablespoons tub margarine
2 cups chopped cooked chicken
1 cup chopped potato
1 cup chopped carrots
½ teaspoon salt
⅛ teaspoon pepper
1 teaspoon dried thyme
2 cups chicken bouillon or broth
1½ cups water
1 can (8 ounces) peas, undrained

1. Sauté celery and onion in margarine until tender.
2. Add remaining ingredients except peas.
3. Simmer about 20 minutes until potatoes and carrots are tender.
4. Add peas and heat through.

Yield: 6 servings

1 serving contains:

Cal	Prot	Fat	Carb	Sat	Mono	Poly	Chol	Na
177	16	7.1	12	1.6	2.3	2.6	43	690

Exchanges: 1 serving = 1½ meats, 1 bread, ½ fat
Recommended for: The Living Heart; Low Calorie; Diabetic; Types IIa, IIb, III, and IV Diets

Hearty Vegetable Soup

1 package (10 ounces) frozen corn
½ package (10 ounces) frozen French cut green beans
½ cup rice, uncooked
⅓ cup dried kidney beans (⅔ cup cooked)
½ cup dried garbanzo beans (1 cup cooked)
1 can (8 ounces) whole tomatoes, undrained
½ cup chopped celery
¾ cup chopped onion
1 tablespoon dried parsley flakes
1½ teaspoons salt
½ teaspoon pepper
¾ teaspoon dried sweet basil
¼ teaspoon dried rosemary
¼ teaspoon celery salt

⅛ teaspoon cayenne pepper
1 tablespoon brown sugar, firmly packed
½ teaspoon red pepper sauce
3 cups water

1. Combine all ingredients and cover.
2. Simmer for 4–5 hours adding more water if needed.
3. Refrigerate 24 hours to allow flavors to blend. Reheat before serving.

Yield: 2 quarts

1 cup contains:

Cal	Prot	Fat	Carb	Sat	Mono	Poly	Chol	Na
136	5	0.5	29	0.1	0.1	0.3	0	81

Exchanges: 1 cup = 1½ breads, ½ meat
Recommended for: The Living Heart; Low Calorie; Diabetic; Types I, IIa, IIb, III, IV, and V Diets

Oriental Soup

6 cups chicken bouillon
½ cup sliced water chestnuts
¼ cup sliced green onion
½ cup bean sprouts
¼ cup chopped watercress
egg substitute equivalent to 1 egg

1. Bring chicken bouillon to a boil.
2. Add water chestnuts and boil 1 minute.
3. Add onion, bean sprouts, and watercress.
4. Slowly add egg substitute, turning off heat immediately.
5. Mix a few times and serve immediately.

Yield: 6 cups

1 cup contains:

Cal	Prot	Fat	Carb	Sat	Mono	Poly	Chol	Na
32	3	0.8	4	0.2	0.2	0.4	0	984

Exchanges: 1 cup = 1 vegetable
Recommended for: The Living Heart; Low Calorie; Diabetic; Types IIa, IIb, III, and IV Diets

Abbreviations: **Cal,** calories; **Prot,** protein; **Carb,** carbohydrate; **Sat,** saturated fat; **Mono,** monounsaturated fat; **Poly,** polyunsaturated fat; **Chol,** cholesterol; **Na,** sodium. Protein, fat, carbohydrate, saturated fat, monounsaturated fat, and polyunsaturated fat are expressed in *grams.* Cholesterol and sodium are expressed in *milligrams.*

Old-Fashioned Mushroom Soup

1 pound fresh mushrooms, sliced
2 tablespoons tub margarine
2 cups sliced carrot
2 cups chopped celery
1 cup chopped onion
2 cloves garlic, minced
2 cans (10¾ ounces each) condensed beef broth, undiluted
4 cups water
3 tablespoons tomato paste
¼ teaspoon salt
⅛ teaspoon pepper
¼ teaspoon Worcestershire sauce
2 tablespoons chopped fresh parsley
2 tablespoons chopped celery leaves
2 bay leaves
¼ cup dry sherry

1. Sauté one-half of the mushrooms in 1 table-spoon of the margarine in large saucepan.
2. Add carrots, celery, onion, and garlic and sauté until tender.
3. Stir in remaining ingredients except mush-rooms, margarine, and sherry.
4. Cover and simmer for 45 minutes.
5. Briefly purée in blender or run through a food mill. Return to pan.
6. Sauté remaining sliced mushrooms in re-maining margarine.
7. Add mushrooms and sherry to soup. Briefly reheat.

Yield: 8 servings

1 serving contains:

Cal	Prot	Fat	Carb	Sat	Mono	Poly	Chol	Na
98	6	3.2	11	0.5	1.0	1.6	0	667

Exchanges: 1 serving = 1 bread, ½ fat
Recommended for: The Living Heart; Low Calorie; Diabetic; Types IIa, IIb, III, and IV Diets

Oyster Bisque

4 cups skim milk
1 tablespoon grated onion
1 bay leaf
½ cup chopped celery
½ cup tub margarine
⅓ cup flour
1 teaspoon salt
⅛ teaspoon pepper
⅛ teaspoon paprika
1 pint oysters with liquid

1. Combine milk, onion, and bay leaf in saucepan and scald. Remove from heat.
2. Sauté celery in margarine until tender.
3. Stir in flour, salt, pepper, and paprika.
4. Add scalded milk. Remove bay leaf.
5. Cook over medium heat, stirring constantly, until thickened.
6. Add oysters and liquid. Heat through.

Yield: 10 servings

1 serving contains:

Cal	Prot	Fat	Carb	Sat	Mono	Poly	Chol	Na
164	8	10.3	10	2.1	3.4	4.3	26	424

Exchanges: 1 serving = 1 meat, ½ bread, 1½ fats
Recommended for: The Living Heart; Diabetic; Types IIa, IIb, III, and IV Diets

Gazpacho

3 tomatoes
1 green pepper
1 onion
1 cucumber, peeled
1¼ cups tomato juice
2 cloves garlic
1 teaspoon salt
½ teaspoon pepper
½ teaspoon dried oregano
½ teaspoon dried sweet basil
1 tablespoon oil

1. Chop three-fourths of the vegetables into large chunks. Chop remaining vegetables into small pieces and reserve.
2. Place half of the tomato juice, half of the chunk-sized vegetables, and garlic in blender container and blend at low speed until finely chopped. Repeat process with remaining tomato juice and chunk-sized vegetables.
3. Stir blenderized mixture, small-sized vegetables, salt, pepper, oregano, basil, and oil together.
4. Cover and chill.

Yield: 6 servings

1 serving contains:

Cal	Prot	Fat	Carb	Sat	Mono	Poly	Chol	Na
68	2	2.6	11	0.3	0.6	1.7	0	478

Exchanges: 1 serving = 2 vegetables, ½ fat
Recommended for: The Living Heart; Low Calorie; Diabetic; Types IIa, IIb, III, and IV Diets

Clam-Mushroom Bisque

½ **pound mushrooms, chopped**
2 **tablespoons tub margarine**
2 **tablespoons flour**
2 **cans (6½ ounces each) minced clams, undrained**
½ **cup evaporated skim milk, undiluted**
¼ **teaspoon salt**
⅛ **teaspoon pepper**

1. Sauté mushrooms in margarine.
2. Stir in flour. Add clams. Simmer 5 minutes.
3. Add milk, salt, pepper, and heat through.

Yield: 4 servings

1 serving contains:

Cal	Prot	Fat	Carb	Sat	Mono	Poly	Chol	Na
196	20	7.5	11	1.5	2.3	3.2	64	373

Exchanges: 1 serving = 1 meat, 1 dairy, 1 fat
Recommended for: The Living Heart; Diabetic; Types IIa, IIb, III, and IV Diets

SAUCES AND GRAVIES

Creole Sauce

⅓ **cup chopped green pepper**
¼ **cup chopped onion**
⅓ **cup chopped fresh mushrooms**
2 **tablespoons tub margarine**
1½ **cups finely chopped fresh tomato**
¼ **teaspoon salt**
⅛ **teaspoon pepper**
½ **teaspoon dried sweet basil**
2 **drops red pepper sauce**

1. Sauté green pepper, onion, and mushrooms in margarine until lightly browned.
2. Add tomato and spices.
3. Simmer 10–15 minutes or until thoroughly heated.
4. Serve over fish or poultry.

Yield: 2 cups

1 tablespoon contains:

Cal	Prot	Fat	Carb	Sat	Mono	Poly	Chol	Na
11	0	0.8	1	0.1	0.3	0.4	0	27

Exchanges: 1–2 tablespoons = free; ⅓ cup = 1 vegetable, ½ fat
Recommended for: The Living Heart; Low Calorie; Diabetic; Types IIa, IIb, III, IV, and V Diets

Abbreviations: **Cal,** calories; **Prot,** protein; **Carb,** carbohydrate; **Sat,** saturated fat; **Mono,** monounsaturated fat; **Poly,** polyunsaturated fat; **Chol,** cholesterol; **Na,** sodium. Protein, fat, carbohydrate, saturated fat, monounsaturated fat, and polyunsaturated fat are expressed in *grams.* Cholesterol and sodium are expressed in *milligrams.*

Seafood Cocktail Sauce

1 can (8 ounces) tomato sauce
1 teaspoon horseradish
1 tablespoon lemon juice
1 teaspoon Worcestershire sauce
½ teaspoon onion salt
1 teaspoon chopped fresh parsley
⅛ teaspoon garlic powder

1. Combine all ingredients and simmer briefly.
2. Serve with cooked fish or over a seafood cocktail.

Yield: 1¼ cups

1 tablespoon contains:

Cal	Prot	Fat	Carb	Sat	Mono	Poly	Chol	Na
4	0	0	1	0	0	0	0	89

Exchanges: 1–5 tablespoons = free
Recommended for: The Living Heart; Low Calorie; Diabetic; Types I, IIa, IIb, III, IV, and V Diets

Texas Barbecue Sauce

1 can (8 ounces) tomato sauce
2 tablespoons vinegar
1 teaspoon Worcestershire sauce
1 teaspoon dry mustard
2 teaspoons chopped fresh parsley
¼ teaspoon salt
⅛ teaspoon pepper
¼ teaspoon garlic powder

1. Combine all ingredients.
2. Serve over chicken, pork chops, or beef.

Yield: 1 cup

¼ cup contains:

Cal	Prot	Fat	Carb	Sat	Mono	Poly	Chol	Na
22	1	0	5	0	0	0	0	387

Exchanges: ¼ cup = free; ½ cup = ½ bread
Recommended for: The Living Heart; Low Calorie; Diabetic; Types I, IIa, IIb, III, IV, and V Diets

Zippy Barbecue Sauce

1 onion, quartered
1 clove garlic
1 can (8 ounces) tomato sauce
1 teaspoon dried oregano
2 tablespoons lemon juice
2 tablespoons oil
1 teaspoon salt
1 teaspoon dry mustard
1 tablespoon Worcestershire sauce
2 tablespoons brown sugar, firmly packed
3 drops red pepper sauce
¼ cup wine or water

1. Combine all ingredients in a blender for 10 seconds.
2. Use to baste chicken or other meat while baking or broiling.

Yield: 1¾ cups

¼ cup contains:

Cal	Prot	Fat	Carb	Sat	Mono	Poly	Chol	Na
68	1	4.0	8	0.5	1.0	2.3	0	484

Exchanges: ¼ cup = 1 vegetable, 1 fat
Recommended for: The Living Heart and Type IIa Diets

Mint Sauce

2 tablespoons confectioner's sugar
⅛ teaspoon salt
3 tablespoons hot water
⅓ cup finely chopped mint leaves
½ cup vinegar

1. Dissolve confectioner's sugar and salt in hot water. Add mint leaves and vinegar. Strain, if desired.
2. Serve with lamb.

Yield: ¾ cup

¼ cup contains:

Cal	Prot	Fat	Carb	Sat	Mono	Poly	Chol	Na
25	0	0	7	0	0	0	0	88

Exchanges: ¼ cup = free; ⅓ cup = ½ bread
Recommended for: The Living Heart; Low Calorie; Types I and IIa Diets

Tomato and Garlic Sauce

2 tablespoons oil
1 cup chopped onion
1 teaspoon garlic powder
1 can (16 ounces) whole tomatoes, undrained
1 can (6 ounces) tomato paste
1 teaspoon dried sweet basil
1 tablespoon dried oregano
1 teaspoon salt
¼ teaspoon pepper
½ teaspoon sugar

1. Heat oil in large saucepan and cook onions until tender and transparent.
2. Stir in garlic powder and cook 1 minute.
3. Coarsely chop tomatoes in blender and add, along with remaining ingredients, to saucepan.
4. Simmer 30 minutes, stirring occasionally.

Yield: 3 cups

1 tablespoon contains:

Cal	Prot	Fat	Carb	Sat	Mono	Poly	Chol	Na
12	0	0.6	2	0.1	0.1	0.4	0	61

Exchanges: 1 tablespoon = free; ¼ cup = ½ fat, 1 vegetable
Recommended for: The Living Heart; Low Calorie; Diabetic; Types I, IIa, IIb, III, IV, and V Diets

White Sauce

2 tablespoons tub margarine
2 tablespoons flour
¼ teaspoon salt
1 cup skim milk

1. Melt margarine in saucepan. Remove from heat.
2. Stir in flour and salt to a smooth paste.
3. Add milk slowly, stirring constantly over medium heat until thickened.

Yield: 1 cup

Variations:

Mushroom Sauce: Add 1 can (6 ounces) drained mushrooms. Serve with chicken or vegetables.

Parsley Sauce: Add 3–4 tablespoons finely chopped fresh parsley. Serve with fish or vegetables.
Pimento Sauce: Add ¼ cup chopped pimento and ¼ cup chopped green pepper. Serve with fish, chicken, or vegetables.
Curry Sauce: Add ¼–½ teaspoon curry powder with dry ingredients. Serve with chicken, lamb, fish, or rice.
Mustard Sauce: Add 1 tablespoon prepared mustard and ⅛ teaspoon pepper. Serve with beef or vegetables.
Cheese Sauce: Add ½–1 cup cubed low-fat cheese. Serve with macaroni or vegetables.

1 tablespoon White Sauce contains:

Cal	Prot	Fat	Carb	Sat	Mono	Poly	Chol	Na
22	1	1.5	1	0.3	0.5	0.6	0	60

Exchanges: 1 tablespoon White, Parsley, Pimento, Curry, or Mustard Sauce = free; 2 tablespoons = 1 fat; 3 tablespoons Cheese Sauce = ½ dairy, 1 fat (93 calories); ¼ cup Mushroom Sauce = 1 fat (48 calories)
Recommended for: The Living Heart; Diabetic; Types IIa, IIb, III, and IV Diets

Orange Syrup

1 cup honey
6 tablespoons orange juice concentrate
2 tablespoons tub margarine
⅛ teaspoon salt

1. Heat all ingredients together until margarine melts.
2. Serve over Orange Griddlecakes (see recipe, page 188).

Yield: about 1½ cups

1 tablespoon contains:

Cal	Prot	Fat	Carb	Sat	Mono	Poly	Chol	Na
59	0	1.0	13	0.2	0.3	0.4	0	23

Exchanges: Not applicable for this recipe
Recommended for: The Living Heart and Type IIa Diets

Abbreviations: **Cal,** calories; **Prot,** protein; **Carb,** carbohydrate; **Sat,** saturated fat; **Mono,** monounsaturated fat; **Poly,** polyunsaturated fat; **Chol,** cholesterol; **Na,** sodium. Protein, fat, carbohydrate, saturated fat, monounsaturated fat, and polyunsaturated fat are expressed in *grams.* Cholesterol and sodium are expressed in *milligrams.*

Gravy from Meat Drippings

skim milk, bouillon, water, or vegetable stock meat drippings with fat removed*
2 tablespoons flour
¼ cup cold skim milk, bouillon, water, or vegetable stock
salt to taste
pepper to taste

1. Add liquid to the drippings to make a total of ¾ cup.
2. Mix flour with ¼ cup cold liquid. Stir into drippings mixture.
3. Heat, stirring constantly, until thickened.
4. Season to taste with salt and pepper.

Yield: 1 cup

*To remove fat from drippings:
Pour drippings into a container. Chill in refrigerator. This may be chilled quickly by putting in the freezer or adding ice cubes to the drippings. Remove solid fat that forms at top. Store extra drippings in refrigerator or freezer for later use.

1 tablespoon (bouillon, water, stock) contains:

Cal	Prot	Fat	Carb	Sat	Mono	Poly	Chol	Na
4	0	0	1	0	0	0	0	92

Exchanges: ¼ cup = free; ½ cup = ½ bread; 1–3 tablespoons with skim milk = free; ¼ cup = ½ dairy (8 calories per tablespoon)
Recommended for: The Living Heart; Low Calorie; Diabetic; Types IIa, IIb, III, IV, and V Diets

Bouillon Gravy

¼ cup oil
¼ cup flour or 2 tablespoons cornstarch
2 cups beef bouillon
½ teaspoon Kitchen Bouquet (optional)
⅛ teaspoon pepper

1. Combine oil, flour, and bouillon in saucepan.
2. Bring to boil and stir until thickened. (Add Kitchen Bouquet if darker color is desired.)
3. Add pepper and serve.

Yield: 2 cups

1 tablespoon contains:

Cal	Prot	Fat	Carb	Sat	Mono	Poly	Chol	Na
19	0	1.7	1	0.2	0.4	1.0	0	60

Exchanges: 1 tablespoon = free; 3 tablespoons = 1 fat
Recommended for: The Living Heart; Low Calorie; Diabetic; Types IIa, IIb, III, and IV Diets

Mushroom Gravy

1 can (8 ounces) mushroom pieces, drained, or ⅓ pound fresh mushrooms, finely chopped
2 tablespoons oil
⅛ teaspoon butter flavoring
1 cup plus 2 tablespoons water
2 beef bouillon cubes
1 tablespoon cornstarch
¼ cup white wine (optional)
¼ teaspoon salt
¼ teaspoon pepper

1. Sauté mushrooms in oil for 5 minutes. Remove from heat. Add butter flavoring and set aside.
2. Dissolve bouillon cubes in 1 cup hot water in a separate pan.
3. Combine cornstarch with 2 tablespoons cold water. Stir into bouillon and simmer until thickened.
4. Add mushrooms and wine, simmering 2–3 minutes longer.
5. Season with salt and pepper.

Yield: 1¼ cups

1 tablespoon contains:

Cal	Prot	Fat	Carb	Sat	Mono	Poly	Chol	Na
16	0	1.4	1	0.2	0.3	0.8	0	175

Exchanges: 1 tablespoon = free; 2 tablespoons = ½ fat
Recommended for: The Living Heart; Low Calorie; Diabetic; Types IIa, IIb, III, and IV Diets

Yeast Breads, Rolls, Biscuits, Quick Breads, Cereals

Casserole Cheese Bread

4½ cups enriched, all-purpose flour
2 packages active dry yeast
3 tablespoons sugar
2 teaspoons salt
⅓ cup nonfat dry milk powder
2 tablespoons tub margarine
1¾ cups hot water (120–130°F)
    egg substitute equivalent to 1 egg
1 cup shredded low-fat cheese
1 cup dry oatmeal

1. Combine 2 cups flour, yeast, sugar, salt, and milk powder in a large bowl.
2. Add margarine and water, mixing well with electric mixer, about 2 minutes.
3. Add egg substitute, cheese, and ½ cup flour, mixing at high speed 2 minutes.
4. Stir in oatmeal and remaining flour to make a stiff batter, beating until blended.
5. Cover and let rise in a warm place 45 minutes.
6. Stir batter down, beating vigorously 30 seconds and turn into oiled casserole.
7. Bake immediately in a preheated 325°F oven for 50–55 minutes.

Yield: 1 round loaf (20 slices)

1 slice contains:

Cal	Prot	Fat	Carb	Sat	Mono	Poly	Chol	Na
155	6	2.3	28	0.6	0.7	0.9	2	332

Exchanges: 1 slice = 2 breads, ½ fat
Recommended for: The Living Heart; Diabetic; Types IIa, IIb, III, and IV Diets

French Bread

2½ cups plus 1 tablespoon water
2 packages active dry yeast
1 tablespoon salt
1 tablespoon tub margarine, melted
7 cups enriched, all-purpose flour
    cornmeal
1 egg white

1. Mix 2½ cups warm water (105–115°F) and yeast in mixing bowl until dissolved.
2. Add salt and melted margarine.
3. Stir in 4–5 cups of flour.
4. Work in remaining flour until well blended, using hands if necessary. Dough will be sticky.
5. Turn onto lightly floured board and knead 8–10 minutes.
6. Place dough in an oiled bowl. Turn once to oil surface.
7. Cover and let rise in a warm place until double, about 1 hour.
8. Divide dough in half.
9. Roll one-half at a time on a lightly floured board and into a rectangle about 10 × 15 inches.
10. Roll up like a jelly roll and tuck in ends.
11. Sprinkle a small amount of cornmeal on an oiled baking sheet.
12. Place roll on sheet seam side down and let rise until double, about 30 minutes.

Abbreviations: **Cal,** calories; **Prot,** protein; **Carb,** carbohydrate; **Sat,** saturated fat; **Mono,** monounsaturated fat; **Poly,** polyunsaturated fat; **Chol,** cholesterol; **Na,** sodium. Protein, fat, carbohydrate, saturated fat, monounsaturated fat, and polyunsaturated fat are expressed in *grams*. Cholesterol and sodium are expressed in *milligrams*.

13. Bake in a preheated 375°F oven for 30 minutes.
14. Remove and brush with mixture of egg white and 1 tablespoon water.
15. Bake 10 minutes more.

Yield: 2 loaves (15 slices each)

1 slice contains:

Cal	Prot	Fat	Carb	Sat	Mono	Poly	Chol	Na
111	3	0.7	22	0.1	0.2	0.4	0	227

Exchanges: 1 slice = 1½ breads
Recommended for: The Living Heart; Low Calorie; Diabetic; Types I, IIa, IIb, III, IV, and V Diets

Whole Wheat Oatmeal Bread

  1 **package active dry yeast**
1½ **cups warm water (105–115°F)**
  3 **tablespoons honey**
½ **cup nonfat dry milk powder**
  1 **teaspoon salt**
2½ **cups whole wheat flour**
  1 **cup enriched, all-purpose flour**
¼ **cup oil**
1¼ **cups dry oatmeal**

1. Dissolve yeast in water.
2. Stir in honey, milk powder, and salt.
3. Add 1 cup whole wheat flour and 1 cup flour until a thick batter is formed.
4. Let batter rest 10 minutes.
5. Fold in oil.
6. Stir in remaining whole wheat flour and oatmeal.
7. Turn onto lightly floured board and knead 10–15 minutes until dough is smooth.
8. Place in an oiled bowl. Turn once to oil surface.
9. Cover and let rise until almost double, about 50 minutes.
10. Punch down, cover, and let rise 40 minutes. (This rising may be omitted, but loaf will be slightly heavier.)
11. Shape into loaf and place in an oiled 9 × 5-inch loaf pan.
12. Let rise until double, about 35 minutes.
13. Bake in a preheated 350°F oven for 60 minutes.

Yield: 1 loaf (20 slices)

1 slice contains:

Cal	Prot	Fat	Carb	Sat	Mono	Poly	Chol	Na
133	4	3.5	22	0.5	0.8	2.0	0	120

Exchanges: 1 slice = 1½ breads, ½ fat
Recommended for: The Living Heart; Diabetic; Types IIa, IIb, III, and IV Diets

Wheat Bread

4–5 **cups enriched, all-purpose flour**
  3 **tablespoons sugar**
  1 **tablespoon salt**
  2 **packages active dry yeast**
1½ **cups water**
½ **cup skim milk**
  3 **tablespoons tub margarine**
  2 **cups whole wheat flour**

1. Mix 2 cups all-purpose flour, sugar, salt, and yeast in a large bowl.
2. Heat water, milk, and margarine in a saucepan until hot (120–130°F).
3. Gradually add liquid to dry ingredients and beat 2 minutes with electric mixer.
4. Stir in whole wheat flour until well blended.
5. Work in additional flour to form a soft dough.
6. Turn onto a lightly floured board and knead 8–10 minutes.
7. Place in an oiled bowl. Turn once to oil surface.
8. Cover and let rise in a warm place until double, about 60 minutes.
9. Punch dough down, divide in half, and let rest a few minutes.
10. Shape into two loaves and place in oiled 9 × 5-inch loaf pans.
11. Let rise until double, about 60 minutes.
12. Bake in a preheated 400°F oven for 30 minutes.

Yield: 2 loaves (20 slices each)

1 slice contains:

Cal	Prot	Fat	Carb	Sat	Mono	Poly	Chol	Na
90	3	1.2	17	0.2	0.3	0.6	0	178

Exchanges: 1 slice = 1½ breads
Recommended for: The Living Heart; Low Calorie; Diabetic; Types IIa, IIb, III, and IV Diets

Garlic Bread Sticks

3 cups enriched, all-purpose flour
½ teaspoon sugar
1½ teaspoons salt
2 teaspoons garlic powder
2 packages active dry yeast
1¼ cups plus 1 tablespoon water
1 tablespoon tub margarine
1 egg white, beaten
½ cup sesame or poppy seeds

1. Combine 1 cup of the flour, sugar, salt, garlic powder, and yeast.
2. Add 1¼ cups warm (105–115°F) water and mix until well combined.
3. Mix in margarine and 1 more cup flour.
4. Stir in remaining flour to make a soft dough.
5. Turn onto lightly floured board and divide into 16 equal portions.
6. Roll each portion into a rope about 18 inches long.
7. Cut each rope in three 6-inch pieces.
8. Place on ungreased baking sheet, cover, and let rise at room temperature about 45 minutes or until double in size.
9. Mix egg white with 1 tablespoon cold water. Brush over dough and sprinkle with seeds.
10. Bake in a preheated 375°F oven for 20 minutes.

Yield: 48 bread sticks

Note: Unbaked bread sticks may be frozen up to 4 weeks. Place on a greased baking sheet and cover with plastic wrap to freeze. Transfer to plastic bag when frozen solid. To use: allow bread sticks to come to room temperature and rise for 45 minutes. Proceed with step nine.

1 bread stick contains:

Cal	Prot	Fat	Carb	Sat	Mono	Poly	Chol	Na
40	1	1.1	6	0.2	0.4	0.5	0	73

Exchanges: 1 bread stick = ½ bread
Recommended for: The Living Heart; Low Calorie; Diabetic; Types IIa, IIb, III, and IV Diets

Monk's Bread

2 packages active dry yeast
2 cups warm water (105–115°F)
6 cups enriched, all-purpose flour
1 tablespoon salt
1 tablespoon sugar
¼ cup oil

1. Dissolve yeast in warm water.
2. Combine flour, salt, and sugar and mix in dissolved yeast and oil.
3. Turn onto lightly floured board and knead 8–10 minutes.
4. Place in an oiled bowl. Turn once to oil surface.
5. Cover and let rise in a warm place until doubled, about 45 minutes.
6. Punch down, divide dough in half, and shape into two loaves.
7. Place in two oiled 9 × 5-inch loaf pans.
8. Let rise until almost doubled, about 60 minutes.
9. Bake in a preheated 400°F oven for 45 minutes.

Yield: 2 loaves (20 slices each)

Note: This bread may also be made using 4 cups whole wheat flour and 2 cups white flour.

1 slice contains:

Cal	Prot	Fat	Carb	Sat	Mono	Poly	Chol	Na
81	2	1.6	14	0.2	0.4	0.9	0	165

Exchanges: 1 slice = 1 bread, ½ fat
Recommended for: The Living Heart; Low Calorie; Diabetic; Types IIa, IIb, III, and IV Diets

Abbreviations: **Cal,** calories; **Prot,** protein; **Carb,** carbohydrate; **Sat,** saturated fat; **Mono,** monounsaturated fat; **Poly,** polyunsaturated fat; **Chol,** cholesterol; **Na,** sodium. Protein, fat, carbohydrate, saturated fat, monounsaturated fat, and polyunsaturated fat are expressed in *grams.* Cholesterol and sodium are expressed in *milligrams.*

Party Surprise Loaf

5½ cups enriched, all-purpose flour
2 packages active dry yeast
⅓ cup sugar
2 teaspoons salt
½ cup tub margarine
1½ cups hot water (120–130°F)
    egg substitute equivalent to 2 eggs
1½ cups dry oatmeal
12 dried apricot halves
12 pitted prunes
16 walnut halves
⅓ cup tub margarine, melted
¾ cup brown sugar, firmly packed

1. Combine 2 cups flour, yeast, sugar, and salt in a large bowl.
2. Add margarine and water and mix well with electric mixer.
3. Add egg substitute and 1 cup flour, beating 1 minute on high speed.
4. Stir in oatmeal and enough of the remaining flour to make a soft dough.
5. Turn onto lightly floured board and knead 8–10 minutes.
6. Cover with towel and let rest 20 minutes.
7. Punch dough down and divide into 40 pieces.
8. Shape each piece around one apricot, prune, or walnut and seal.
9. Dip each roll into melted margarine and coat with brown sugar.
10. Arrange rolls in two layers in an oiled 10-inch tube pan. Cover and let rise in a warm place until double, about 45 minutes.
11. Bake in a preheated 350°F oven for 45–50 minutes.

Yield: 1 loaf (40 servings)

1 serving contains:

Cal	Prot	Fat	Carb	Sat	Mono	Poly	Chol	Na
150	3	4.9	24	0.9	1.6	2.3	0	164

Exchanges: Not applicable for this recipe
Recommended for: The Living Heart and Type IIa Diets

Whole Wheat Rusks

1 package active dry yeast
¼ cup warm water (105–115°F)
¼ cup tub margarine
1 tablespoon honey
1 cup skim milk
½ teaspoon salt
2 cups whole wheat flour
1–1½ cups enriched, all-purpose flour

1. Dissolve yeast in warm water.
2. Melt margarine in saucepan.
3. Add honey and milk and heat to lukewarm.
4. Combine salt, whole wheat flour, and ½ cup all-purpose flour in mixing bowl.
5. Add yeast and heated liquids, blending well with a wooden spoon.
6. Let rise in a warm place 30 minutes.
7. Turn onto lightly floured board and, using remaining all-purpose flour, knead 8–10 minutes.
8. Divide dough and shape into two rolls.
9. Cut each roll into 10 pieces and shape each piece into a small oblong bun tapered at ends.
10. Place on baking sheets and let rise in warm place about 30 minutes.
11. Bake in a preheated 400°F oven 10 minutes or until browned.
12. Place on rack, cover with towel, and cool.
13. Split with fork into two halves and place on a baking sheet, split side up.
14. Toast at 400°F for 7–8 minutes.
15. Let dry at 200°F for 2 hours or longer with oven door slightly ajar.
16. Store tightly covered in a cool dry place.

Yield: 40 pieces

1 rusk contains:

Cal	Prot	Fat	Carb	Sat	Mono	Poly	Chol	Na
52	2	1.3	9	0.3	0.4	0.6	0	45

Exchanges: 1 rusk = ½ bread
Recommended for: The Living Heart; Low Calorie; Diabetic; Types IIa, IIb, III, and IV Diets

Yeast Biscuits

1 **package active dry yeast**
2 **tablespoons warm water (105–115°F)**
6 **cups enriched, all-purpose flour**
¼ **cup sugar**
1 **teaspoon baking soda**
1 **teaspoon salt**
1 **tablespoon baking powder**
½ **cup oil**
2½ **cups buttermilk**

1. Dissolve yeast in warm water.
2. Combine dry ingredients in a bowl.
3. Combine oil, buttermilk, and dissolved yeast in a separate bowl.
4. Add dry mixture to liquid mixture.
5. Cover bowl with plastic wrap and store in refrigerator. (Dough will keep for about 1 week.)
6. To use: drop from a tablespoon onto an ungreased baking sheet. Bake in a preheated 425°F oven for 12–15 minutes.

Yield: 3½ dozen

1 biscuit contains:

Cal	Prot	Fat	Carb	Sat	Mono	Poly	Chol	Na
99	2	2.9	16	0.5	0.7	1.6	1	122

Exchanges: 1 biscuit = 1 bread, ½ fat
Recommended for: The Living Heart; Low Calorie; Diabetic; Types IIa, IIb, III, and IV Diets

Banana Nut Bread

½ **cup tub margarine**
½ **cup sugar**
½ **cup honey**
egg substitute equivalent to 2 eggs
1½ **cups mashed bananas**
1 **teaspoon lemon juice**
2 **cups enriched, all-purpose flour**
1 **tablespoon baking powder**
½ **teaspoon salt**
1 **cup chopped walnuts**

1. Preheat oven to 375°F.
2. Cream margarine, sugar, and honey.

3. Add egg substitute and beat 3–5 minutes.
4. Stir in bananas and lemon juice.
5. Blend in flour, baking powder, and salt.
6. Stir in walnuts and pour into an oiled 9 × 5-inch loaf pan.
7. Bake for 75 minutes.

Yield: 1 loaf (20 slices)

1 slice contains:

Cal	Prot	Fat	Carb	Sat	Mono	Poly	Chol	Na
192	3	8.9	26	1.3	2.3	4.8	0	166

Exchanges: Not applicable for this recipe
Recommended for: The Living Heart and Type IIa Diets

Quick Bran Bread

1 **cup enriched, all-purpose flour**
1 **cup unprocessed bran**
½ **cup sugar**
4 **teaspoons baking powder**
½ **teaspoon salt**
egg substitute equivalent to 1 egg
1 **cup skim milk**
¼ **cup tub margarine**

1. Preheat oven to 425°F.
2. Sift dry ingredients in a bowl.
3. Add egg substitute, milk, and margarine.
4. Beat until smooth, about 1 minute.
5. Bake in an oiled 8 × 8-inch pan for 20–25 minutes.

Yield: 16 servings

1 serving contains:

Cal	Prot	Fat	Carb	Sat	Mono	Poly	Chol	Na
94	2	3.2	14	0.6	1.1	1.5	0	191

Exchanges: 1 serving = 1 bread, ½ fat
Recommended for: The Living Heart; Low Calorie; Diabetic; Types IIa, IIb, III, and IV Diets

Abbreviations: **Cal,** calories; **Prot,** protein; **Carb,** carbohydrate; **Sat,** saturated fat; **Mono,** monounsaturated fat; **Poly,** polyunsaturated fat; **Chol,** cholesterol; **Na,** sodium. Protein, fat, carbohydrate, saturated fat, monounsaturated fat, and polyunsaturated fat are expressed in *grams.* Cholesterol and sodium are expressed in *milligrams.*

Honey Wheat Loaf

2½ cups whole wheat flour
1½ cups wheat germ
⅓ cup brown sugar, firmly packed
½ teaspoon salt
1 cup raisins
2 teaspoons baking soda
1¾ cups buttermilk
⅓ cup honey

1. Preheat oven to 350°F.
2. Combine flour, wheat germ, brown sugar, salt, and raisins in a large bowl.
3. Combine soda, buttermilk, and honey in a separate bowl.
4. When mixture begins to bubble, stir into dry ingredients immediately. Dough will be stiff.
5. Spoon into an oiled 9 × 5-inch loaf pan.
6. Bake for 60 minutes or until lightly browned.

Yield: 1 loaf (20 slices)

1 slice contains:

Cal	Prot	Fat	Carb	Sat	Mono	Poly	Chol	Na
138	5	1.3	29	0.4	0.2	0.7	1	219

Exchanges: 1 slice = 2 breads
Recommended for: The Living Heart; Low Calorie; Diabetic; Types IIa, IIb, III, and IV Diets

Jalapeño Cornbread

1 can (16 ounces) cream style corn
2 cups cornbread mix
½ cup oil
   egg substitute equivalent to 4 eggs
2 cups plain skim milk yogurt
1½ cups cubed low-fat cheese
1 can (4 ounces) jalapeño peppers, seeded and chopped

1. Preheat oven to 350°F.
2. Combine all ingredients and pour into an oiled 9 × 13-inch pan.
3. Bake for 60 minutes.

Yield: 24 servings

1 serving contains:

Cal	Prot	Fat	Carb	Sat	Mono	Poly	Chol	Na
130	5	5.8	15	1.1	1.5	3.1	4	307

Exchanges: 1 serving = 1 bread, ½ meat, ½ fat
Recommended for: The Living Heart; Diabetic; Types IIa, IIb, III, and IV Diets

Cornbread

1 cup yellow cornmeal
1 cup enriched, all-purpose flour
3 tablespoons sugar
1 tablespoon baking powder
¼ teaspoon salt
¼ cup oil
1 cup skim milk
   egg substitute equivalent to 2 eggs

1. Preheat oven to 425°F.
2. Combine dry ingredients in a bowl.
3. Stir in oil, milk, and egg substitute only until flour is moistened. Do not overmix.
4. Pour into an oiled 8 × 8-inch pan.
5. Bake for 20–25 minutes.

Yield: 16 servings

1 serving contains:

Cal	Prot	Fat	Carb	Sat	Mono	Poly	Chol	Na
113	3	4.1	16	0.6	1.0	2.4	0	110

Exchanges: 1 serving = 1 bread, 1 fat
Recommended for: The Living Heart; Diabetic; Types IIa, IIb, III, and IV Diets

Variation:

Cornbread Muffins: Place paper liners in muffin tins and fill about ⅔ full. Bake 20 minutes.

Yield: 12 muffins

1 muffin contains:

Cal	Prot	Fat	Carb	Sat	Mono	Poly	Chol	Na
150	4	5.4	21	0.8	1.3	3.1	0	147

Exchanges: 1 muffin = 1½ breads, 1 fat
Recommended for: The Living Heart; Diabetic; Types IIa, IIb, III, and IV Diets

Date Nut Loaf

1 package (8 ounces) pitted dates, chopped
1 tablespoon tub margarine
1½ cups boiling water
1 cup sugar
2¾ cups enriched, all-purpose flour
2 teaspoons baking soda
½ teaspoon salt
1 tablespoon vanilla extract
2 egg whites or egg substitute equivalent to 1 egg
1 cup chopped pecans or walnuts

1. Preheat oven to 325°F.
2. Combine chopped dates, margarine, and boiling water in a large mixing bowl.
3. Mix in sugar, flour, baking soda, salt, and vanilla until well blended.
4. Stir in egg whites or egg substitute and nuts.
5. Pour into a 9 × 5-inch loaf pan greased with margarine.
6. Bake for 80 minutes or until toothpick comes out clean.

Yield: 1 loaf (20 slices)

1 slice contains:

Cal	Prot	Fat	Carb	Sat	Mono	Poly	Chol	Na
173	3	4.8	31	0.6	0.9	3.0	0	206

Exchanges: Not applicable for this recipe
Recommended for: The Living Heart and Type IIa Diets

Onion Bread Squares

2 cups sliced onions
3 tablespoons tub margarine
2 cups enriched, all-purpose flour
2 teaspoons baking powder
1 teaspoon salt
¼ cup oil
2 tablespoons chopped fresh parsley
1 cup skim milk
⅓ cup "Help Your Heart" Sour Cream (see recipe, page 89)

1. Preheat oven to 425°F.
2. Sauté onions in margarine until tender. Set aside.
3. Combine flour, baking powder, and salt.
4. Cut in oil with fork until mixture resembles coarse meal.
5. Add parsley and milk, mixing until flour is just moistened.
6. Pour into an oiled and floured 8 × 8-inch baking pan.
7. Spread sautéed onions over top and cover with "Help Your Heart" Sour Cream.
8. Bake for 20 minutes. Serve immediately.

Yield: 16 servings

1 serving contains:

Cal	Prot	Fat	Carb	Sat	Mono	Poly	Chol	Na
123	3	5.8	15	0.9	1.7	3.0	1	233

Exchanges: 1 serving = 1 bread, 1 fat
Recommended for: The Living Heart; Low Calorie; Diabetic; Types IIa, IIb, III, and IV Diets

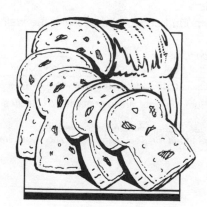

Abbreviations: **Cal,** calories; **Prot,** protein; **Carb,** carbohydrate; **Sat,** saturated fat; **Mono,** monounsaturated fat; **Poly,** polyunsaturated fat; **Chol,** cholesterol; **Na,** sodium. Protein, fat, carbohydrate, saturated fat, monounsaturated fat, and polyunsaturated fat are expressed in *grams.* Cholesterol and sodium are expressed in *milligrams.*

Pumpkin Bread

3 cups enriched, all-purpose flour
2 cups sugar
1 cup brown sugar, firmly packed
2 teaspoons baking soda
1½ teaspoons salt
1 teaspoon ground cinnamon
½ teaspoon ground nutmeg
1 cup oil
1 can (16 ounces) cooked pumpkin
⅔ cup water
½ cup chopped walnuts

1. Preheat oven to 350°F.
2. Combine dry ingredients. Make a well in the center and add oil, pumpkin, and water, mixing well. Stir in walnuts and pour into two oiled and floured 9 × 5-inch loaf pans.
3. Bake for 60 minutes.

Yield: 2 loaves (20 slices each)

Variation:

Add ½ pound chopped dates with the walnuts.

1 slice contains:

Cal	Prot	Fat	Carb	Sat	Mono	Poly	Chol	Na
155	1	6.5	24	0.8	1.5	3.9	0	154

1 slice Pumpkin Date Bread contains 170 calories.

Exchanges: Not applicable for this recipe.
Recommended for: The Living Heart and Types IIa Diets

Bran Muffins

egg substitute equivalent to 1 egg
1 cup skim milk
3 tablespoons oil
1½ cups bran cereal (bud type)
1 cup enriched, all-purpose flour
2½ teaspoons baking powder
½ teaspoon salt
¼ cup brown sugar, firmly packed

1. Preheat oven to 400°F.
2. Beat egg substitute, milk, and oil together.
3. Stir in bran and let stand 5 minutes.
4. Blend flour, baking powder, salt, and brown sugar in a separate bowl.
5. Add bran mixture and stir until just combined. Do *not* overmix.
6. Fill oiled muffin tins ⅔ full.
7. Bake for 20 minutes or until done.

Yield: 12 muffins

Variations:

Date Bran Muffins: Add ½ cup chopped dates with the bran mixture.
Raisin Bran Muffins: Add ½ cup raisins with the bran mixture.
Spice Bran Muffins: Add 1½ tablespoons molasses with the liquid ingredients and 1¼ teaspoons ground cinnamon with the dry ingredients.

1 muffin contains:

Cal	Prot	Fat	Carb	Sat	Mono	Poly	Chol	Na
116	3	4.1	19	0.6	1.0	2.4	0	235

Exchanges: 1 plain or spice muffin = 1 bread, 1 fat; 1 date or raisin muffin = 1 bread, ½ fruit, 1 fat (137 calories)
Recommended for: The Living Heart; Low Calorie; Diabetic; Types IIa, IIb, III, and IV Diets

Light Muffins

2　cups enriched, all-purpose flour
3　tablespoons sugar
3　teaspoons baking powder
¾　teaspoon salt
¼　cup oil
1　cup skim milk
1　egg white

1. Preheat oven to 425°F.
2. Combine dry ingredients in a bowl.
3. Combine oil and milk.
4. Add liquid to dry ingredients, stirring until flour is just moistened.
5. Beat egg white until stiff and fold in.
6. Fill oiled muffin tins ⅔ full.
7. Bake for 20 minutes.

Yield: 12 muffins

1 muffin contains:

Cal	Prot	Fat	Carb	Sat	Mono	Poly	Chol	Na
137	3	4.8	20	0.6	1.2	2.8	0	225

Exchanges: 1 muffin = 1½ breads, 1 fat
Recommended for: The Living Heart; Diabetic; Types IIa, IIb, III, and IV Diets

Biscuits

2　cups enriched, all-purpose flour
1　tablespoon baking powder
1　teaspoon salt
¼　cup tub margarine
¾　cup skim milk

1. Preheat oven to 400°F.
2. Combine dry ingredients and cut in margarine until mixture resembles coarse meal.
3. Add milk and mix well.
4. Roll out ½ inch thick on lightly floured board.
5. Cut with 2-inch biscuit cutter and place on an ungreased baking sheet.
6. Bake for 10–12 minutes.

Yield: 18 biscuits

Variations:

Drop Biscuits: Increase milk to 1 cup.
Herb Biscuits: Add ¼ teaspoon dried oregano and ¼ teaspoon dried thyme with flour.
Onion Biscuits: Add 1 tablespoon finely chopped onion with milk.
Bacon Biscuits: Add ¼ cup imitation bacon bits with milk.
Buttermilk Biscuits: Substitute buttermilk for skim milk. Use only 2 teaspoons baking powder and add ¼ teaspoon baking soda.
Tomato Biscuits: Substitute ¾ cup tomato juice for skim milk. Use only 2 teaspoons baking powder and add ¼ teaspoon baking soda.
Cheese Biscuits: Add ¼ cup shredded low-fat cheese to flour and margarine mixture. Use only 2 tablespoons margarine.

1 biscuit (except bacon) contains:

Cal	Prot	Fat	Carb	Sat	Mono	Poly	Chol	Na
77	2	2.7	11	0.5	0.9	1.2	0	207

Exchanges: 1 biscuit (except bacon) = 1 bread; 1 bacon biscuit = 1 bread, ½ fat (87 calories)
Recommended for: The Living Heart; Low Calorie; Diabetic; Types IIa, IIb, III, and IV Diets

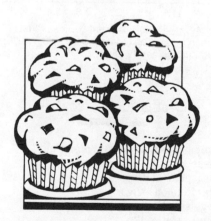

Abbreviations: **Cal,** calories; **Prot,** protein; **Carb,** carbohydrate; **Sat,** saturated fat; **Mono,** monounsaturated fat; **Poly,** polyunsaturated fat; **Chol,** cholesterol; **Na,** sodium. Protein, fat, carbohydrate, saturated fat, monounsaturated fat, and polyunsaturated fat are expressed in *grams.* Cholesterol and sodium are expressed in *milligrams.*

Breakfast Puff

  egg substitute equivalent to 3 eggs
½ cup enriched, all-purpose flour
½ teaspoon salt
½ cup skim milk
  3 tablespoons tub margarine, melted

1. Chill an 8-inch iron skillet in the freezer.
2. Preheat oven to 450°F.
3. Place egg substitute and flour in blender and blend at low speed. Add salt and milk and blend again. Coat cold iron skillet with margarine and add batter.
4. Bake until the crust is brown, about 30 minutes.
5. Serve immediately. Top with stewed fruit, jam, or maple syrup, if desired.

Yield: 4 servings

Note: When doubling recipe, use a 12-inch skillet.

1 serving contains:

Cal	Prot	Fat	Carb	Sat	Mono	Poly	Chol	Na
193	7	11.6	15	2.1	3.8	5.4	1	477

Exchanges: 1 serving = 1 meat, 1 bread, 2 fats
Recommended for: The Living Heart; Low Calorie; Diabetic; Types IIa, IIb, III, and IV Diets

Orange Griddlecakes

1½ cups enriched, all-purpose flour
  2 teaspoons baking powder
¾ teaspoon salt
  2 tablespoons sugar
  egg substitute equivalent to 1 egg
  1 cup skim milk
  6 tablespoons orange juice concentrate
  3 tablespoons oil

1. Combine flour, baking powder, salt, and sugar in a bowl.
2. Mix egg substitute, milk, orange juice concentrate, and oil together.
3. Add liquid ingredients to dry ingredients, stirring only until blended. Batter will be slightly lumpy.

4. Using about 3 tablespoons batter for each griddlecake, bake on a preheated oiled griddle until browned.

Yield: 15 3-inch griddlecakes

1 griddlecake contains:

Cal	Prot	Fat	Carb	Sat	Mono	Poly	Chol	Na
98	2	3.1	15	0.4	0.8	1.8	0	165

Exchanges: 1 griddlecake = 1 bread, ½ fat
Recommended for: The Living Heart; Diabetic; Types IIa, IIb, III, and IV Diets

Buttermilk Pancakes

1¼ cups enriched, all-purpose flour
  2 teaspoons baking powder
½ teaspoon baking soda
  1 tablespoon sugar
½ teaspoon salt
  egg substitute equivalent to 1 egg
  1 cup buttermilk
  2 tablespoons oil

1. Sift dry ingredients in a bowl.
2. Combine egg substitute, milk, and oil, and add to dry ingredients, stirring until just moistened and batter is lumpy.
3. Bake on hot griddle.

Yield: eight 4-inch pancakes

1 pancake contains:

Cal	Prot	Fat	Carb	Sat	Mono	Poly	Chol	Na
128	4	4.3	18	0.7	1.1	2.4	1	342

Exchanges: 1 pancake = 1 bread, 1 fat
Recommended for: The Living Heart; Diabetic; Types IIa, IIb, III, and IV Diets

Master Mix

⅓ **cup baking powder**
1½ **tablespoons salt**
¼ **cup sugar**
1 **teaspoon cream of tartar**
9 **cups enriched, all-purpose flour**
1¼ **cups oil**

1. Sift baking powder, salt, sugar, and cream of tartar into flour.
2. Sift together twice into a large mixing bowl.
3. Slowly add oil, cutting in with pastry blender until mix is consistency of cornmeal.
4. Store in tightly covered container at room temperature or in refrigerator.
5. This mix will keep for 6 weeks.
6. To measure Master Mix, pile it lightly into a cup and level with a spatula.

Yield: 12 cups

1 cup contains:

Cal	Prot	Fat	Carb	Sat	Mono	Poly	Chol	Na
561	10	23.6	76	3.1	5.7	13.8	0	1209

Exchanges: Not applicable for this recipe.
This recipe is part of other recipes.

Master Mix Drop Biscuits

1 **cup skim milk**
3 **cups Master Mix (see recipe, this page)**

1. Preheat oven to 425°F.
2. Add milk all at once to the Master Mix, stirring until flour is moistened.
3. Drop from a tablespoon onto an oiled baking sheet.
4. Bake for 10–12 minutes.

Yield: 12 biscuits

1 biscuit contains:

Cal	Prot	Fat	Carb	Sat	Mono	Poly	Chol	Na
118	3	4.8	16	0.6	1.1	2.8	0	250

Exchanges: 1 biscuit = 1 bread, 1 fat
Recommended for: The Living Heart; Low Calorie; Diabetic; Types IIa, IIb, III, and IV Diets

Master Mix Biscuits

⅔ **cup skim milk**
3 **cups Master Mix (see recipe, this page)**

1. Preheat oven to 425°F.
2. Add milk all at once to the Master Mix, stirring until flour is moistened.
3. Knead 15 times on a lightly floured board.
4. Roll out ½ inch thick and cut with a 2-inch biscuit cutter.
5. Bake for 10–12 minutes or until lightly browned.

Yield: 12 biscuits

1 biscuit contains:

Cal	Prot	Fat	Carb	Sat	Mono	Poly	Chol	Na
116	2	4.7	16	0.6	1.1	2.8	0	247

Exchanges: 1 biscuit = 1 bread, 1 fat
Recommended for: The Living Heart; Low Calorie; Diabetic; Types IIa, IIb, III, and IV Diets

Master Mix Beer Rolls

4 **cups Master Mix (see recipe, this page)**
¼ **cup sugar**
1 **can (12 ounces) beer**

1. Preheat oven to 400°F.
2. Combine all ingredients, stirring until flour is just moistened.
3. Fill oiled muffin tins ⅔ full.
4. Bake for 15 minutes.

Yield: 15 rolls

1 roll contains:

Cal	Prot	Fat	Carb	Sat	Mono	Poly	Chol	Na
166	3	6.3	25	0.8	1.5	3.7	0	322

Exchanges: 1 roll = 1½ breads, 1½ fats
Recommended for: The Living Heart; Diabetic; Types IIa, IIb, III, and IV Diets

Abbreviations: **Cal,** calories; **Prot,** protein; **Carb,** carbohydrate; **Sat,** saturated fat; **Mono,** monounsaturated fat; **Poly,** polyunsaturated fat; **Chol,** cholesterol; **Na,** sodium. Protein, fat, carbohydrate, saturated fat, monounsaturated fat, and polyunsaturated fat are expressed in *grams.* Cholesterol and sodium are expressed in *milligrams.*

Master Mix Pancakes or Waffles

1½ cups skim milk
2 egg whites
3 cups Master Mix (see recipe, page 189)

1. Preheat griddle or waffle iron.
2. Blend milk and egg whites.
3. Add to Master Mix, stirring until just moistened.
4. Bake on hot griddle or waffle iron.

Yield: 20 pancakes or four 9-inch waffles

1 pancake contains:

Cal	Prot	Fat	Carb	Sat	Mono	Poly	Chol	Na
92	2	3.6	12	0.5	0.9	2.1	0	196

Exchanges: 1 pancake = 1 bread, ½ fat
Recommended for: The Living Heart; Diabetic; Types IIa, IIb, III, and IV Diets

¼ of 1 waffle contains:

Cal	Prot	Fat	Carb	Sat	Mono	Poly	Chol	Na
115	3	4.5	16	0.6	1.1	2.6	0	245

Exchanges: ¼ of 1 waffle = 1 bread, 1 fat
Recommended for: The Living Heart; Diabetic; Types IIa, IIb, III, and IV Diets

Master Mix Muffins

2 tablespoons sugar
3 cups Master Mix (see recipe, page 189)
1 cup skim milk
2 egg whites

1. Preheat oven to 425°F.
2. Add sugar to Master Mix.
3. Combine milk and egg whites.
4. Add to Master Mix, stirring until flour is just moistened.
5. Fill oiled muffin tins ⅔ full.
6. Bake for 20 minutes.

Yield: 12 muffins

1 muffin contains:

Cal	Prot	Fat	Carb	Sat	Mono	Poly	Chol	Na
158	4	5.9	22	0.8	1.4	3.4	0	321

Exchanges: 1 muffin = 1½ breads, 1 fat
Recommended for: The Living Heart; Diabetic; Types IIa, IIb, III, and IV Diets

Master Mix Quick Supper Bread

1½ cups Master Mix (see recipe, page 189)
1 tablespoon sugar
3 tablespoons finely chopped onion
egg substitute equivalent to 1 egg
¼ cup skim milk
¼ cup white wine or apple juice
½ teaspoon dried oregano
1 tablespoon tub margarine, melted
1 teaspoon poppy seeds or sesame seeds

1. Preheat oven to 400°F.
2. Combine Master Mix, sugar, onion, egg substitute, milk, wine or apple juice, and oregano with a fork until a soft dough forms.
3. Spread in an oiled 9-inch round pan.
4. Sprinkle with melted margarine and seeds.
5. Bake for 20–25 minutes.

Yield: 8 servings

1 serving contains:

Cal	Prot	Fat	Carb	Sat	Mono	Poly	Chol	Na
145	3	6.6	17	1.0	1.8	3.5	0	264

Exchanges: 1 serving = 1 bread, 1½ fats
Recommended for: The Living Heart; Diabetic; Types IIa, IIb, III, and IV Diets

Master Mix Banana Bread

2 cups Master Mix (see recipe, page 189)
¾ cup sugar
¼ teaspoon baking soda
¼ cup tub margarine
2 bananas, mashed
4 egg whites, stiffly beaten
½ cup chopped walnuts

1. Preheat oven to 350°F.
2. Combine Master Mix, sugar, and baking soda in large bowl.
3. Blend in margarine and bananas until smooth.
4. Fold in beaten egg whites and walnuts.
5. Turn into a 9 × 5-inch loaf pan that has been brushed with margarine.
6. Bake for 50–60 minutes or until cake tester inserted in center of loaf comes out clean.
7. Cool 10 minutes, turn onto rack, and cool completely.

Yield: 1 loaf (20 slices)

1 slice contains:

Cal	Prot	Fat	Carb	Sat	Mono	Poly	Chol	Na
140	2	6.6	19	0.9	1.7	3.7	0	176

Exchanges: Not applicable for this recipe
Recommended for: The Living Heart and Type IIa Diets

Master Mix Coffee Cake

Cake
½ cup sugar
3 cups Master Mix (see recipe, page 189)
¾ cup plus 2 tablespoons skim milk
2 egg whites or egg substitute equivalent to 1 egg

Topping
¼ cup enriched, all-purpose flour
¼ teaspoon ground cinnamon
3 tablespoons brown sugar, firmly packed
¼ cup tub margarine

1. Preheat oven to 400°F.
2. Add sugar to Master Mix.
3. Combine milk and egg whites and stir into Master Mix until flour is just moistened.

4. Pour into an oiled 9-inch round baking pan.
5. Combine topping ingredients and sprinkle over batter.
6. Bake for 35 minutes.

Yield: 12 servings

1 serving contains:

Cal	Prot	Fat	Carb	Sat	Mono	Poly	Chol	Na
237	4	9.8	34	1.5	2.8	5.1	0	368

Exchanges: Not applicable for this recipe
Recommended for: The Living Heart and Type IIa Diets

Master Mix Shortcake

2⅓ cups Master Mix (see recipe, page 189)
5 tablespoons sugar
3 tablespoons margarine
½ cup skim milk

1. Preheat oven to 400°F.
2. Combine Master Mix, 3 tablespoons sugar, margarine, and milk with a fork until a soft dough is formed.
3. Form into six round shortcakes and place on an oiled baking sheet.
4. Bake 15 minutes or until browned.
5. Sprinkle with remaining sugar while still warm.

Yield: 6 servings

1 serving contains:

Cal	Prot	Fat	Carb	Sat	Mono	Poly	Chol	Na
316	5	15.0	41	2.3	4.3	7.9	0	550

Exchanges: Not applicable for this recipe
Recommended for: The Living Heart and Type IIa Diets

Abbreviations: **Cal,** calories; **Prot,** protein; **Carb,** carbohydrate; **Sat,** saturated fat; **Mono,** monounsaturated fat; **Poly,** polyunsaturated fat; **Chol,** cholesterol; **Na,** sodium. Protein, fat, carbohydrate, saturated fat, monounsaturated fat, and polyunsaturated fat are expressed in *grams.* Cholesterol and sodium are expressed in *milligrams.*

Cornmeal Master Mix

6 cups cornmeal
2 cups enriched, all-purpose flour
1¼ cups nonfat dry milk powder
3½ tablespoons baking powder
4 teaspoons salt
¾ teaspoon cream of tartar
1 cup oil

1. Sift dry ingredients together several times.
2. Slowly add oil, cutting in with pastry blender until mix is very fine.
3. Store in covered container at room temperature or in refrigerator. This mix will keep for 6 weeks.

Yield: 10½ cups

1 cup contains:

Cal	Prot	Fat	Carb	Sat	Mono	Poly	Chol	Na
588	12	22.0	85	3.0	5.3	12.8	1	1172

Exchanges: Not applicable for this recipe.
This recipe is part of other recipes.

Cornmeal Master Mix Muffins

⅓ cup water
2 egg whites
1½ cups Cornmeal Master Mix (see recipe, this page)

1. Preheat oven to 425°F.
2. Blend water and egg whites together.
3. Add to Cornmeal Master Mix, stirring until moistened.
4. Fill oiled muffin tins ⅔ full.
5. Bake for 20 minutes or until brown.

Yield: 6 muffins

1 muffin contains:

Cal	Prot	Fat	Carb	Sat	Mono	Poly	Chol	Na
152	4	5.5	21	0.8	1.3	3.2	0	310

Exchanges: 1 muffin = 1½ breads, 1 fat
Recommended for: The Living Heart; Diabetic; Types IIa, IIb, III, and IV Diets

Cornmeal Master Mix Pancakes

⅔ cup water
2 egg whites
2 cups Cornmeal Master Mix (see recipe, this page)

1. Blend water and egg whites together.
2. Stir into Cornmeal Master Mix.
3. Bake on a hot griddle.

Yield: 8 pancakes

1 pancake contains:

Cal	Prot	Fat	Carb	Sat	Mono	Poly	Chol	Na
151	4	5.5	21	0.8	1.3	3.2	0	306

Exchanges: 1 pancake = 1½ breads, 1 fat
Recommended for: The Living Heart; Diabetic; Types IIa, IIb, III, and IV Diets

Honey Apple Oatmeal

4 teaspoons tub margarine
3 tablespoons honey
2 teaspoons lemon juice
1½ cups sliced apples
3 cups hot cooked oatmeal

1. Heat margarine, honey, and lemon juice in a skillet.
2. Add apples, stirring until well coated.
3. Cover and simmer for 3–4 minutes or until apples are tender.
4. Spoon topping onto bowls of hot oatmeal.
5. Serve with skim milk, if desired.

Yield: 6 servings

1 serving contains:

Cal	Prot	Fat	Carb	Sat	Mono	Poly	Chol	Na
136	3	3.8	24	0.7	1.3	1.7	0	293

Exchanges: 1 serving = 1 bread, 1 fruit, ½ fat
Recommended for: The Living Heart; Low Calorie; Type IIa Diets

Raisin and Spice Oatmeal

2½ cups water
¾ teaspoon salt
1½ teaspoons ground cinnamon
¼ teaspoon ground nutmeg
⅓ cup raisins
1¼ cups quick cooking oatmeal, uncooked

1. Bring water, salt, cinnamon, nutmeg, and raisins to a boil.
2. Stir in oatmeal and cook 1 minute, stirring occasionally.
3. Cover pan, remove from heat, and let stand for a few minutes.
4. Serve with skim milk, if desired.

Yield: 6 servings

1 serving contains:

Cal	Prot	Fat	Carb	Sat	Mono	Poly	Chol	Na
90	3	1.3	18	0.2	0.4	0.5	0	277

Exchanges: 1 serving = 1 bread, ½ fruit
Recommended for: The Living Heart; Low Calorie; Diabetic; Types IIa, IIb, III, IV, and V Diets

Crunchy Granola

3 cups dry oatmeal
¼ cup oil
½ cup honey
½ cup brown sugar, firmly packed
1 teaspoon vanilla extract
½ cup sunflower seeds (optional)
½ cup chopped walnuts (optional)
½ cup wheat germ
½ cup raisins

1. Preheat oven to 350°F.
2. Place oatmeal in a 9 × 13-inch baking pan and toast for 10 minutes.
3. Combine oil, honey, brown sugar, and vanilla. Add mixture, seeds, and walnuts to toasted oatmeal.
4. Bake 20–30 minutes, stirring every 10 minutes. Cool.
5. Add wheat germ and raisins.
6. Store in a covered container in the refrigerator.

Yield: 5–6 cups

¼ cup contains:

Cal	Prot	Fat	Carb	Sat	Mono	Poly	Chol	Na
161	4	6.8	23	0.9	1.5	4.1	0	4

Exchanges: Not applicable for this recipe
Recommended for: The Living Heart and Type IIa Diets

Abbreviations: **Cal,** calories; **Prot,** protein; **Carb,** carbohydrate; **Sat,** saturated fat; **Mono,** monounsaturated fat; **Poly,** polyunsaturated fat; **Chol,** cholesterol; **Na,** sodium. Protein, fat, carbohydrate, saturated fat, monounsaturated fat, and polyunsaturated fat are expressed in *grams*. Cholesterol and sodium are expressed in *milligrams*.

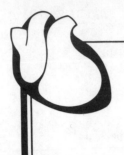

Desserts

FRUIT-TYPE DESSERTS, PUDDINGS, DESSERT SAUCES

Apple Orange Crumb

4 apples, pared, cored, and sliced
½ cup orange juice
¼ teaspoon ground cinnamon
⅓ cup dry oatmeal
2 tablespoons enriched, all-purpose flour
2 tablespoons tub margarine, melted

1. Preheat oven to 400°F.
2. Combine apples and orange juice in a 9 × 9-inch baking pan.
3. Mix remaining ingredients together until crumbly and sprinkle over apple mixture.
4. Bake 35–40 minutes or until apples are tender.

Yield: 9 servings

1 serving contains:

Cal	Prot	Fat	Carb	Sat	Mono	Poly	Chol	Na
94	1	3.0	17	0.5	1.0	1.4	0	32

Exchanges: 1 serving = 1½ fruits, ½ fat
Recommended for: The Living Heart; Low Calorie; Diabetic; Types IIa, IIb, III, and IV Diets

Apple-Bread Pudding

4 slices bread
¼ cup tub margarine
2 apples, peeled, cored, and chopped
    egg substitute equivalent to 2 eggs
½ cup sugar
⅛ teaspoon salt
1 cup evaporated skim milk, undiluted
1 cup boiling water
1 teaspoon vanilla extract
1 teaspoon ground cinnamon

1. Spread bread with margarine and toast in oven.
2. Cut toasted bread into cubes and place in an 8 × 8-inch baking pan greased with margarine. Add apples.
3. Mix egg substitute, ¼ cup sugar, salt, milk, and water together in a separate bowl.
4. Pour mixture over apples and let set 10 minutes.
5. Stir in vanilla.
6. Combine remaining sugar and cinnamon and sprinkle over top.
7. Bake in a preheated 350°F oven 40 minutes or until knife inserted in center comes out clean.

Yield: 9 servings

1 serving contains:

Cal	Prot	Fat	Carb	Sat	Mono	Poly	Chol	Na
169	5	6.4	24	1.2	2.2	2.8	1	205

Exchanges: Not applicable for this recipe
Recommended for: The Living Heart and Type IIa Diets

Apple Fluff

2 tablespoons (2 envelopes) unflavored gelatin
2 cups apple juice
4 apples, peeled, cored, and sliced
4 tablespoons lemon juice
¼ teaspoon ground cinnamon
¼ teaspoon ground nutmeg
½ cup nonfat dry milk powder
½ cup ice water

1. In blender, sprinkle gelatin over ½ cup apple juice and let stand until softened.
2. Heat remaining apple juice to boiling and pour into blender. Cover and blend at low speed until gelatin is dissolved, about 2 minutes.
3. Add apples, 3 tablespoons lemon juice, cinnamon, and nutmeg, and blend at high speed.
4. Pour into large bowl and chill, stirring occasionally, until mixture mounds when dropped from a spoon.
5. In a small bowl, beat milk powder with ice water and 1 tablespoon lemon juice until soft peaks form.
6. Fold into apple mixture and turn into a mold. Chill until firm.

Yield: 8 servings

1 serving contains:

Cal	Prot	Fat	Carb	Sat	Mono	Poly	Chol	Na
82	3	0.2	18	0	0	0.2	1	24

Exchanges: 1 serving = 2 fruits
Recommended for: The Living Heart; Low Calorie; Diabetic; Types I, IIa, IIb, III, IV, and V Diets

Applesauce Mousse

1 tablespoon (1 envelope) unflavored gelatin
1 cup cold water
1 teaspoon grated lemon peel
2 tablespoons lemon juice
2 cups unsweetened applesauce
cinnamon

1. Sprinkle gelatin over ½ cup cold water in a saucepan. Stir over low heat until gelatin dissolves. Remove from heat.

2. Stir in remaining ½ cup water, lemon peel, lemon juice, and applesauce.
3. Chill, stirring occasionally, until mixture mounds slightly when dropped from a spoon.
4. Beat with a rotary or electric beater until soft and creamy.
5. Sprinkle with cinnamon.

Yield: 4 servings

1 serving contains:

Cal	Prot	Fat	Carb	Sat	Mono	Poly	Chol	Na
58	2	0.3	14	0	0	0.3	0	3

Exchanges: 1 serving = 1½ fruits
Recommended for: The Living Heart; Low Calorie; Diabetic; Types I, IIa, IIb, III, IV, and V Diets

Apple Crisp

7 apples, peeled, cored, and sliced
4 teaspoons lemon juice
1 cup brown sugar, firmly packed
½ teaspoon ground cinnamon
1 cup dry oatmeal
½ cup tub margarine

1. Preheat oven to 400°F.
2. Layer sliced apples in an 8 × 8-inch baking pan and sprinkle with lemon juice.
3. Combine brown sugar, cinnamon, and oatmeal in a bowl. Cut in margarine until mixture looks crumbly and sprinkle over apples.
4. Bake for 45 minutes or until apples are tender.

Yield: 16 servings

1 serving contains:

Cal	Prot	Fat	Carb	Sat	Mono	Poly	Chol	Na
148	1	6.3	24	1.1	2.2	2.8	0	75

Exchanges: Not applicable for this recipe
Recommended for: The Living Heart and Type IIa Diets

Abbreviations: **Cal,** calories; **Prot,** protein; **Carb,** carbohydrate; **Sat,** saturated fat; **Mono,** monounsaturated fat; **Poly,** polyunsaturated fat; **Chol,** cholesterol; **Na,** sodium. Protein, fat, carbohydrate, saturated fat, monounsaturated fat, and polyunsaturated fat are expressed in *grams.* Cholesterol and sodium are expressed in *milligrams.*

Baked Apples

¼ **cup brown sugar, firmly packed**
4 **teaspoons tub margarine**
2 **teaspoons ground cinnamon**
4 **baking apples, cored**

1. Preheat oven to 350°F.
2. Mix brown sugar, margarine, and cinnamon.
3. Place mixture in centers of cored apples.
4. Put apples in casserole and add water to depth of ¼ inch.
5. Cover and bake 30 minutes.

Yield: 4 servings

Variations:

Cranberry Baked Apples: Add ¼ cup chopped fresh cranberries and substitute white sugar for brown sugar.
Maple Baked Apples: Baste with maple syrup several times while baking.
Raisin Baked Apples: Add ¼ cup raisins to margarine mixture.

1 apple or cranberry apple contains:

Cal	Prot	Fat	Carb	Sat	Mono	Poly	Chol	Na
168	0	4.7	34	0.7	1.4	2.5	0	52

1 Maple Baked Apple contains 218 calories.
1 Raisin Baked Apple contains 195 calories.
Recommended for: The Living Heart and Type IIa Diets
For Low Calorie Diets, substitute 2 tablespoons raisins for brown sugar.
Count as 2 fruits, 1 fat (130 calories).

Broiled Grapefruit

1 **grapefruit**
2 **tablespoons honey**
⅛ **teaspoon ground cinnamon**
⅛ **teaspoon ground nutmeg**

1. Cut grapefruit in half and loosen sections with knife.
2. Spread honey over grapefruit and sprinkle with spices.

3. Broil 6 inches from heat for 10 minutes or until thoroughly heated.

Yield: 2 servings

1 serving contains:

Cal	Prot	Fat	Carb	Sat	Mono	Poly	Chol	Na
105	1	0.1	28	0	0	0.1	0	2

Exchanges: Not applicable for this recipe
Recommended for: The Living Heart; Types I and IIa Diets

Full-of-Berries Gelatin

1 **tablespoon (1 envelope) unflavored gelatin**
1 **cup orange juice**
⅓ **cup skim milk**
⅛ **teaspoon salt**
4 **teaspoons lemon juice**
1 **cup unsweetened fresh or frozen straw-berries**

1. Soften gelatin in ¼ cup orange juice.
2. Heat remaining juice to boiling. Remove from heat.
3. Stir in softened gelatin until dissolved.
4. Add milk, salt, and lemon juice, beating until blended.
5. Chill until firm.
6. Blend fruit and jelled mixture in blender until desired consistency is reached.
7. Chill until firm.

Yield: 6 servings

Variation:

Substitute unsweetened fresh or frozen blackberries for strawberries.

1 serving contains:

Cal	Prot	Fat	Carb	Sat	Mono	Poly	Chol	Na
39	2	0.2	8	0	0	0.2	0	51

Exchanges: 1 serving = 1 fruit
Recommended for: The Living Heart; Low Calorie; Diabetic; Types I, IIa, IIb, III, IV, and V Diets

Fruit Poached in Wine

2 cups red or white wine
¾ cup sugar
  sliced peel of ½ fresh lemon
2 tablespoons lemon juice
1 cinnamon stick
4 pieces fresh fruit of choice, such as pears, peaches, or nectarines, peeled and cored

1. Place wine, sugar, lemon peel, lemon juice, and cinnamon stick in a saucepan.
2. Stir over medium heat until sugar is dissolved and mixture comes to a boil.
3. Reduce heat and simmer 5 minutes.
4. Add fruit and simmer until tender, occasionally basting with juice. Do not allow liquid to boil.
5. Let set in juice 20 minutes before serving.
6. Serve with 1 tablespoon regular Dessert Topping (see recipe, page 216) or skim milk, if desired.

Yield: 4 servings

1 serving contains:

Cal	Prot	Fat	Carb	Sat	Mono	Poly	Chol	Na
264	1	0.7	68	0	0	0.7	0	4

Exchanges: Not applicable for this recipe
Recommended for: The Living Heart; Types I and IIa Diets

Baked Pears

4 pears, peeled, halved, and cored
¾ cup pear nectar
¾ cup water
2 teaspoons lemon juice
1 teaspoon vanilla extract
1 teaspoon rum extract
1 cinnamon stick
¼ teaspoon ground mace

1. Preheat oven to 350°F.
2. Arrange pears in a large casserole.
3. Mix together remaining ingredients and pour over pears.
4. Cover and bake 30 minutes.
5. Turn pears gently and bake uncovered 30

minutes longer, or until tender. Baste every 10 minutes.
6. Remove from oven, cover, and cool. Baste every few minutes as the pears cool.

Yield: 4 servings

1 serving contains:

Cal	Prot	Fat	Carb	Sat	Mono	Poly	Chol	Na
63	1	0.4	16	0	0	0.4	0	2

Exchanges: 1 serving = 1½ fruits
Recommended for: The Living Heart; Low Calorie; Diabetic; Types I, IIa, IIb, III, IV, and V Diets

Master Mix Peach Cobbler

2 cans (29 ounces each) peach slices, undrained
½ teaspoon almond extract
2⅓ cups Master Mix (see recipe, page 189)
5 tablespoons sugar
3 tablespoons tub margarine, melted
½ cup skim milk

1. Preheat oven to 400°F.
2. Place peaches and almond extract in a 9 × 13-inch baking pan and heat in oven 15 minutes.
3. Combine Master Mix, 3 tablespoons sugar, margarine, and milk with a fork until a soft dough is formed.
4. Drop dough from a tablespoon onto hot peaches.
5. Sprinkle with 2 tablespoons sugar.
6. Bake, uncovered, 15–20 minutes or until browned.

Yield: 8 servings

1 serving contains:

Cal	Prot	Fat	Carb	Sat	Mono	Poly	Chol	Na
327	3	11.4	54	1.7	3.2	6.0	0	415

Exchanges: Not applicable for this recipe
Recommended for: The Living Heart and Type IIa Diets

Abbreviations: **Cal,** calories; **Prot,** protein; **Carb,** carbohydrate; **Sat,** saturated fat; **Mono,** monounsaturated fat; **Poly,** polyunsaturated fat; **Chol,** cholesterol; **Na,** sodium. Protein, fat, carbohydrate, saturated fat, monounsaturated fat, and polyunsaturated fat are expressed in *grams.* Cholesterol and sodium are expressed in *milligrams.*

Pineapple Deep-Dish Dessert

5 apples, peeled, cored, and sliced
1 can (8 ounces) crushed pineapple, packed in its own juice, undrained
¾ cup brown sugar, firmly packed
3 tablespoons cornstarch
½ teaspoon salt
¼ teaspoon ground cinnamon
1 tablespoon tub margarine

1. Preheat oven to 350°F.
2. Place layers of sliced apples and pineapple in baking dish greased with margarine.
3. Combine sugar, cornstarch, salt, and cinnamon. Sprinkle over apples and dot with margarine.
4. Bake for 35–40 minutes.

Yield: 6 servings

Note: May be packaged for freezing before baking, if desired. Bake at 350°F 60 minutes from frozen state.

1 serving contains:

Cal	Prot	Fat	Carb	Sat	Mono	Poly	Chol	Na
207	0	2.2	49	0.4	0.7	1.1	0	216

Exchanges: Not applicable for this recipe
Recommended for: The Living Heart and Type IIa Diets

Rhubarb Crisp

2 cups cut fresh or frozen unsweetened rhubarb
½ cup sugar
¼ cup plus 2 tablespoons enriched, all-purpose flour
⅓ cup brown sugar, firmly packed
3 tablespoons dry oatmeal
¼ cup tub margarine, melted

1. Preheat oven to 325°F.
2. Put rhubarb in baking dish greased with margarine.
3. Mix sugar with 2 tablespoons flour and sprinkle over rhubarb.

4. Combine brown sugar, oatmeal, remaining flour, and melted margarine. Sprinkle over top.
5. Bake for 40 minutes.

Yield: 6 servings

1 serving contains:

Cal	Prot	Fat	Carb	Sat	Mono	Poly	Chol	Na
222	1	8.0	37	1.5	2.8	3.5	0	98

Exchanges: Not applicable for this recipe
Recommended for: The Living Heart and Type IIa Diets

Baked Custard

1½ cups skim milk
⅓ cup sugar
¼ teaspoon salt
2 tablespoons tub margarine
egg substitute equivalent to 4 eggs
1 teaspoon vanilla extract
nutmeg

1. Preheat oven to 350°F.
2. Scald milk and remove from heat. Add sugar, salt, and margarine, stirring until margarine is melted.
3. Beat egg substitute in separate bowl for 5 minutes.
4. Add milk mixture and vanilla slowly to beaten egg substitute, stirring constantly. Pour into custard cups and sprinkle with nutmeg.
5. Place cups in a pan of hot water and bake for 35–40 minutes or until knife inserted in center comes out clean.

Yield: 6 servings

1 serving contains:

Cal	Prot	Fat	Carb	Sat	Mono	Poly	Chol	Na
141	6	6.4	15	1.2	2.0	3.0	1	242

Exchanges: Not applicable for this recipe
Recommended for: The Living Heart and Type IIa Diets

Master Mix Brownie Pudding

1½ cups Master Mix (see recipe, page 189)
½ cup sugar
2 tablespoons cocoa powder
½ cup skim milk
1 teaspoon vanilla extract
¾ cup chopped walnuts

Topping
¼ cup cocoa powder
¾ cup brown sugar, firmly packed
1½ cups hot water

1. Preheat oven to 350°F.
2. Combine Master Mix, sugar, and cocoa. Mix in milk and vanilla, then stir in walnuts. Pour into an oiled 8 × 8-inch baking pan.
3. Mix topping ingredients together and gently pour over batter in pan.
4. Bake for 40 minutes.

Yield: 16 servings

1 serving contains:

Cal	Prot	Fat	Carb	Sat	Mono	Poly	Chol	Na
160	2	6.2	0.6	0.9	1.2	3.7	0	121

Exchanges: Not applicable for this recipe
Recommended for: The Living Heart and Type IIa Diets

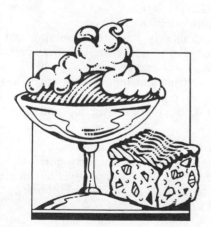

Butterscotch Pudding

½ cup brown sugar, firmly packed
3 tablespoons cornstarch
½ teaspoon salt
2 cups skim milk
1 teaspoon vanilla extract
1 tablespoon tub margarine
¼ teaspoon butter flavoring
10 drops yellow food coloring (optional)
2 drops red food coloring (optional)

1. Combine sugar, cornstarch, and salt in saucepan.
2. Gradually add milk, stirring until smooth.
3. Heat to boiling, stirring constantly. Boil 2 minutes. Remove from heat.
4. Stir in vanilla, margarine, butter flavoring, and food colorings.
5. Pour into serving dishes.

Yield: 4 servings

1 serving contains:

Cal	Prot	Fat	Carb	Sat	Mono	Poly	Chol	Na
193	4	3.1	38	0.7	1.1	1.3	2	381

Exchanges: Not applicable for this recipe
Recommended for: The Living Heart and Type IIa Diets

Variation:

Butterscotch Cream Pie: Make 1½ recipes of pudding and pour into a baked 9-inch pie shell (see recipe, page 215). Top with Meringue for 9-inch pie (see recipe, page 215).

⅛ pie contains:

Cal	Prot	Fat	Carb	Sat	Mono	Poly	Chol	Na
311	6	10.1	50	1.9	3.5	4.3	2	534

Exchanges: Not applicable for this recipe
Recommended for: The Living Heart and Type IIa Diets

Abbreviations: **Cal,** calories; **Prot,** protein; **Carb,** carbohydrate; **Sat,** saturated fat; **Mono,** monounsaturated fat; **Poly,** polyunsaturated fat; **Chol,** cholesterol; **Na,** sodium. Protein, fat, carbohydrate, saturated fat, monounsaturated fat, and polyunsaturated fat are expressed in *grams.* Cholesterol and sodium are expressed in *milligrams.*

Chocolate Fondue

2 cups sugar
¾ cup cocoa powder
2 tablespoons cornstarch
½ teaspoon salt
4 cups cold skim milk
3 tablespoons tub margarine
1½ teaspoons vanilla extract
¼ teaspoon butter flavoring

1. Mix sugar, cocoa, cornstarch, and salt together in saucepan.
2. Add skim milk, stirring well.
3. Cook over medium heat to a boil.
4. Lower heat and simmer 20 minutes. (This can be done in a fondue pot.)
5. Add margarine, vanilla, and flavoring.
6. Dip angel food cake squares, marshmallows, fresh strawberries, banana slices, pineapple cubes, and other fruits.

Yield: 5 cups

⅓ cup contains:

Cal	Prot	Fat	Carb	Sat	Mono	Poly	Chol	Na
161	3	3.2	33	1.0	1.2	1.0	1	135

Exchanges: Not applicable for this recipe
Recommended for: The Living Heart and Type IIa Diets

Chocolate Pudding

⅔ cup sugar
2 tablespoons cornstarch
½ teaspoon salt
2 tablespoons cocoa powder
2 cups skim milk
1 teaspoon vanilla extract
2 teaspoons tub margarine

1. Combine sugar, cornstarch, salt, and cocoa in saucepan.
2. Gradually add milk, stirring until smooth.
3. Heat to a boil, stirring constantly. Boil 2 minutes. Remove from heat.
4. Stir in vanilla and margarine.

5. Pour into serving dishes. May be served warm or chilled.

Yield: 4 servings

1 serving contains:

Cal	Prot	Fat	Carb	Sat	Mono	Poly	Chol	Na
159	5	2.7	31	0.8	0.9	0.9	2	361

Exchanges: Not applicable for this recipe
Recommended for: The Living Heart and Type IIa Diets

Layered Fruit Yogurt Pudding

Bottom Layer
1½ tablespoons unflavored gelatin
6 tablespoons cold water
2 cups cranberry juice
¾ cup orange juice
1½ cups sliced bananas
1 can (16 ounces) pineapple chunks, drained
½ cup chopped walnuts

Top Layer
1½ teaspoons unflavored gelatin
2 tablespoons cranberry juice
2 tablespoons sugar
1 cup plain skim milk yogurt

Bottom Layer
1. Soften gelatin in cold water.
2. Heat cranberry juice to simmering and add softened gelatin. Stir over low heat until dissolved and add orange juice.
3. Spread fruit and nuts in bottom of 8 × 8-inch baking pan.
4. Pour juice mixture over top and chill until set.

Top Layer
1. Soften gelatin in cranberry juice in small saucepan. Add sugar and stir over low heat until gelatin and sugar are dissolved. Remove from heat and blend in yogurt.
2. Cool to room temperature and pour over bottom layer. Chill several hours.

Yield: 12 servings

1 serving contains:

Cal	Prot	Fat	Carb	Sat	Mono	Poly	Chol	Na
124	3	3.3	22	0.4	0.5	2.2	0	16

Exchanges: Not applicable for this recipe
Recommended for: The Living Heart and Type IIa Diets

Orange Tapioca Pudding

2 cups orange juice
2 tablespoons quick-cooking tapioca
¼ teaspoon salt
egg substitute equivalent to 1 egg
½ teaspoon vanilla extract

1. Combine orange juice, tapioca, and salt. Let stand 5 minutes.
2. Add egg substitute.
3. Bring to a boil over medium heat, stirring constantly. Remove from heat.
4. Add vanilla and pour into individual serving dishes.
5. Chill until firm.

Yield: 6 servings

1 serving contains:

Cal	Prot	Fat	Carb	Sat	Mono	Poly	Chol	Na
62	2	0.8	12	0.1	0.2	0.5	0	110

Exchanges: 1 serving = 1½ fruits
Recommended for: The Living Heart; Low Calorie; Diabetic; Types I, IIa, IIb, III, IV, and V Diets

Lemon Sauce

1 cup sugar
2 tablespoons cornstarch
2 cups water
2 tablespoons tub margarine
2 tablespoons lemon juice
2 tablespoons grated lemon peel

1. Mix sugar and cornstarch in saucepan. Stir in water.
2. Bring to a boil and boil 1 minute, stirring constantly. Remove from heat.

3. Stir in margarine and flavoring.
4. Serve over pound cake or other dessert.

Yield: about 2 cups

¼ cup contains:

Cal	Prot	Fat	Carb	Sat	Mono	Poly	Chol	Na
130	0	2.9	27	0.5	1.0	1.3	0	35

Exchanges: Not applicable for this recipe
Recommended for: The Living Heart and Type IIa Diets

Peachy Dessert Sauce

2 cups sliced fresh or frozen peaches
1 tablespoon lemon juice
sugar to taste

1. Combine all ingredients in blender until smooth.
2. Serve over cake or sherbet

Yield: 2 cups

Variation:
May use any fresh or frozen fruit.

¼ cup contains:

Cal	Prot	Fat	Carb	Sat	Mono	Poly	Chol	Na
23	0	0.1	6	0	0	0.1	0	1

Exchanges: ¼ cup = free; ½ cup = 1 fruit
Recommended for: The Living Heart; Low Calorie; Types I and IIa Diets

Abbreviations: **Cal,** calories; **Prot,** protein; **Carb,** carbohydrate; **Sat,** saturated fat; **Mono,** monounsaturated fat; **Poly,** polyunsaturated fat; **Chol,** cholesterol; **Na,** sodium. Protein, fat, carbohydrate, saturated fat, monounsaturated fat, and polyunsaturated fat are expressed in *grams.* Cholesterol and sodium are expressed in *milligrams.*

CAKES AND FROSTINGS

Spicy Applesauce Cake

½ cup tub margarine
1 cup sugar
  egg substitute equivalent to 1 egg
2 cups sifted enriched, all-purpose flour
1½ teaspoons baking powder
½ teaspoon baking soda
1 teaspoon salt
1 teaspoon ground cinnamon
¼ teaspoon ground cloves
¼ teaspoon ground allspice
1 cup applesauce
1 cup chopped walnuts
1 cup raisins
¼ cup confectioner's sugar (optional)

1. Preheat oven to 350°F.
2. Cream margarine and sugar together.
3. Add egg substitute and beat 3–5 minutes.
4. Combine flour, baking powder, baking soda, salt, and spices in a separate bowl.
5. Add dry ingredients and applesauce to creamed mixture alternately in three additions, mixing well after each addition.
6. Stir in walnuts and raisins.
7. Bake in an oiled and floured 9 × 9-inch baking pan for 45–50 minutes.
8. Sprinkle with confectioner's sugar, if desired.

Yield: 16 servings

1 serving contains:

Cal	Prot	Fat	Carb	Sat	Mono	Poly	Chol	Na
253	3	10.9	37	1.7	2.9	5.9	0	288

Exchanges: Not applicable for this recipe
Recommended for: The Living Heart and Type IIa Diets

Eggless Applesauce Cake

1 cup tub margarine
2 cups brown sugar, firmly packed
1 can (16 ounces) applesauce
3 cups sifted enriched, all-purpose flour
2 teaspoons baking soda
2 teaspoons salt
2 teaspoons ground cinnamon
1 teaspoon ground cloves
2 cups raisins

1. Preheat oven to 350°F.
2. Cream margarine and brown sugar together.
3. Mix in applesauce.
4. Add remaining ingredients and mix well.
5. Pour into an oiled and floured 9 × 13-inch pan.
6. Bake for 55 minutes.

Yield: 24 servings

1 serving contains:

Cal	Prot	Fat	Carb	Sat	Mono	Poly	Chol	Na
248	2	7.9	44	1.4	2.8	3.5	0	401

Exchanges: Not applicable for this recipe
Recommended for: The Living Heart and Type IIa Diets

Carrot Cake

  egg substitute equivalent to 4 eggs
2 cups sugar
1½ cups oil
1 teaspoon vanilla extract
2 cups enriched, all-purpose flour
1 teaspoon baking soda
½ teaspoon salt
1 teaspoon ground cinnamon
1 cup chopped walnuts
3 cups grated carrots

1. Preheat oven to 350°F.
2. Beat egg substitute for 5 minutes.
3. Mix in sugar, oil, and vanilla.
4. Add flour, soda, salt, and cinnamon, and mix well.
5. Stir in nuts and carrots until well blended.

6. Pour into an oiled and floured 9 × 13-inch pan.
7. Bake for 40–45 minutes.
8. Top with Mock Cream Cheese Frosting (see recipe, page 208), if desired.

Yield: 24 servings

1 serving contains:

Cal	Prot	Fat	Carb	Sat	Mono	Poly	Chol	Na
271	3	17.5	27	2.2	4.0	10.4	0	128

Exchanges: Not applicable for this recipe
Recommended for: The Living Heart and Type IIa Diets

Gingerbread

2½ **cups enriched, all-purpose flour**
¾ **cup sugar**
1 **teaspoon baking soda**
½ **teaspoon baking powder**
2 **teaspoons ground ginger**
1 **teaspoon ground cinnamon**
½ **teaspoon ground cloves**
¼ **teaspoon salt**
¾ **cup tub margarine**
¾ **cup water**
½ **cup molasses**

1. Preheat oven to 350°F.
2. Mix flour, sugar, soda, baking powder, ginger, cinnamon, cloves, and salt.
3. Blend in margarine, water, and molasses until smooth.
4. Pour into an oiled and floured 9 × 9-inch baking pan.
5. Bake for 45 minutes or until gingerbread springs back when lightly touched in center.
6. Allow to cool slightly before serving.
7. Serve with Lemon Sauce (see recipe, page 201), if desired.

Yield: 16 servings

1 serving contains:

Cal	Prot	Fat	Carb	Sat	Mono	Poly	Chol	Na
211	2	8.8	31	1.6	3.1	3.9	0	237

Exchanges: Not applicable for this recipe
Recommended for: The Living Heart and Type IIa Diets

Million-Dollar Pound Cake

3 **cups sugar**
2 **cups tub margarine**
   egg substitute equivalent to 6 eggs
½ **teaspoon lemon extract**
1 **teaspoon vanilla extract**
1 **teaspoon butter flavoring**
¼ **cup skim milk**
4 **cups enriched, all-purpose flour**
⅛ **teaspoon salt**

Glaze (optional)
1½ **cups confectioner's sugar**
¼ **cup lemon juice**

1. Preheat oven to 325°F.
2. Cream sugar and margarine together.
3. Add egg substitute a small amount at a time, beating well after each addition.
4. Continue beating until batter is very light and fluffy.
5. Add lemon extract, vanilla, butter flavoring, milk, flour, and salt, mixing well.
6. Bake in a greased and floured bundt pan for 80 minutes.
7. Cool cake in pan for 10 minutes before removing.
8. While cake is baking, combine confectioner's sugar and lemon juice.
9. Pour glaze over warm cake immediately after removing from pan.

Yield: 32 servings

1 serving without glaze contains:

Cal	Prot	Fat	Carb	Sat	Mono	Poly	Chol	Na
244	3	12.4	31	2.3	4.3	5.5	0	170

Exchanges: Not applicable for this recipe
Recommended for: The Living Heart and Type IIa Diets

Abbreviations: **Cal,** calories; **Prot,** protein; **Carb,** carbohydrate; **Sat,** saturated fat; **Mono,** monounsaturated fat; **Poly,** polyunsaturated fat; **Chol,** cholesterol; **Na,** sodium. Protein, fat, carbohydrate, saturated fat, monounsaturated fat, and polyunsaturated fat are expressed in *grams.* Cholesterol and sodium are expressed in *milligrams.*

Golden Loaf Cake

2 cups enriched, all-purpose flour
1¼ cups sugar
1½ teaspoons baking powder
½ teaspoon salt
⅔ cup tub margarine
2 egg whites
¾ cup skim milk
1 teaspoon vanilla extract
3–4 drops yellow food coloring

1. Preheat oven to 325°F.
2. Mix flour, sugar, baking powder, and salt together in a mixing bowl.
3. Add margarine, egg whites, and ¼ cup milk. Beat 2 minutes with electric mixer.
4. Add remaining milk, vanilla, and food coloring. Beat 2 minutes more.
5. Pour batter into an oiled and floured 9 × 5-inch loaf pan.
6. Bake 60 minutes or until cake springs back when lightly touched. (Cake will have a crack on top.)
7. Allow to cool before cutting. Serve with Lemon Sauce (see recipe, page 201).

Yield: 14 servings

1 serving contains:

Cal	Prot	Fat	Carb	Sat	Mono	Poly	Chol	Na
219	3	9.0	32	1.7	3.2	3.9	0	231

Exchanges: Not applicable for this recipe
Recommended for: The Living Heart and Type IIa Diets

Peanut Butter Loaf Cake

1 cup brown sugar, firmly packed
⅓ cup crunchy peanut butter
  egg substitute equivalent to 1 egg
1 teaspoon baking soda
1 teaspoon salt
1¾ cups enriched, all-purpose flour
1 cup buttermilk

1. Preheat oven to 350°F.
2. Blend sugar and peanut butter together.

3. Add egg substitute and beat well.
4. Mix in baking soda, salt, and ¾ cup flour.
5. Add buttermilk and remaining flour alternately, mixing well after each addition.
6. Pour into an oiled and floured 9 × 5-inch loaf pan.
7. Bake for 60 minutes.

Yield: 14 servings

1 serving contains:

Cal	Prot	Fat	Carb	Sat	Mono	Poly	Chol	Na
163	4	3.7	29	0.8	1.6	1.2	1	323

Exchanges: Not applicable for this recipe
Recommended for: The Living Heart and Type IIa Diets

Strawberry Cheesecake

  egg substitute equivalent to 1 egg
¼ cup sugar
1 tablespoon cornstarch
¼ teaspoon salt
1 cup skim milk
2 tablespoons (2 envelopes) unflavored gelatin
¼ cup cold water
1 teaspoon grated lemon peel
2 tablespoons lemon juice
1 teaspoon vanilla extract
3 cups low-fat cottage cheese, puréed in blender or food processor
2 egg whites
⅓ cup sugar
⅓ cup evaporated skim milk, undiluted
1 Graham Cracker Crumb Crust (see recipe, page 215)
10 fresh strawberries

1. Beat egg substitute for 5 minutes and set aside.
2. Combine sugar, cornstarch, and salt in a saucepan.
3. Slowly add skim milk and heat to boiling, stirring constantly. Remove from heat and allow to set for 3 minutes.
4. Stir in egg substitute.
5. Soften gelatin in cold water.
6. Add gelatin, lemon peel, lemon juice, and vanilla, and let stand at room temperature until mixture begins to set.

7. Fold cottage cheese into thickened gelatin mixture. Add sugar-cornstarch mixture.
8. Beat egg whites, gradually adding sugar, until soft peaks form.
9. Whip chilled milk until soft peaks form.
10. Fold egg whites and whipped milk into gelatin mixture.
11. Spoon into crust in spring-form pan and refrigerate until firm.
12. Unmold and arrange strawberries on top.

Yield: 10 servings

1 serving contains:

Cal	Prot	Fat	Carb	Sat	Mono	Poly	Chol	Na
219	14	5.1	30	1.6	1.8	1.6	7	445

Exchanges: Not applicable for this recipe
Recommended for: The Living Heart and Type IIa Diets

Pumpkin Spice Cake

½ **cup tub margarine**
½ **cup brown sugar, firmly packed**
   egg substitute equivalent to 2 eggs
¾ **cup buttermilk**
½ **cup pumpkin**
½ **cup molasses**
2½ **cups enriched, all-purpose flour**
2 **teaspoons grated orange peel**
1 **teaspoon baking soda**
½ **teaspoon salt**
1 **teaspoon ground cinnamon**
½ **teaspoon ground nutmeg**
   confectioner's sugar (optional)

1. Preheat oven to 350°F.
2. Cream margarine and brown sugar together.
3. Add egg substitute and beat 3–5 minutes.
4. Combine buttermilk, pumpkin, and molasses.
5. Combine dry ingredients in a separate bowl.
6. Add liquid mixture and dry mixture alternately to creamed mixture, beating well after each addition.
7. Bake in a greased and floured 9 × 13-inch baking pan 30–35 minutes.
8. Sprinkle with confectioner's sugar, if desired.

Yield: 24 servings

1 serving contains:

Cal	Prot	Fat	Carb	Sat	Mono	Poly	Chol	Na
126	2	4.4	20	0.8	1.5	1.9	0	170

Exchanges: Not applicable for this recipe
Recommended for: The Living Heart and Type IIa Diets

Yogurt Spice Cake

½ **cup tub margarine**
1 **cup brown sugar, firmly packed**
   egg substitute equivalent to 1 egg
1⅔ **cups enriched, all-purpose flour**
3 **tablespoons cocoa powder**
½ **teaspoon salt**
1 **teaspoon baking soda**
1 **teaspoon ground cinnamon**
½ **teaspoon ground nutmeg**
¼ **teaspoon ground cloves**
¾ **cup chopped walnuts**
1 **cup raisins**
¾ **cup plain skim milk yogurt**

1. Preheat oven to 350°F.
2. Cream margarine and brown sugar together.
3. Add egg substitute and beat 3–5 minutes.
4. Combine flour, cocoa, salt, soda, spices, walnuts, and raisins.
5. Add dry ingredients alternately with yogurt to creamed mixture, stirring by hand just to blend ingredients.
6. Pour into an oiled and floured 8 × 8-inch baking pan.
7. Bake for 35–40 minutes.

Yield: 16 servings

1 serving contains:

Cal	Prot	Fat	Carb	Sat	Mono	Poly	Chol	Na
226	4	9.9	33	1.6	2.8	5.1	0	247

Exchanges: Not applicable for this recipe
Recommended for: The Living Heart and Type IIa Diets

Abbreviations: **Cal,** calories; **Prot,** protein; **Carb,** carbohydrate; **Sat,** saturated fat; **Mono,** monounsaturated fat; **Poly,** polyunsaturated fat; **Chol,** cholesterol; **Na,** sodium. Protein, fat, carbohydrate, saturated fat, monounsaturated fat, and polyunsaturated fat are expressed in *grams*. Cholesterol and sodium are expressed in *milligrams*.

Basic White Cake

```
2  cups sifted enriched, all-purpose flour
1  teaspoon salt
1  tablespoon baking powder
1¼ cups sugar
½  cup oil
1  cup skim milk
1  teaspoon vanilla extract
¼  teaspoon butter flavoring
¼  teaspoon almond extract
4  egg whites
```

1. Preheat oven to 350°F.
2. Sift flour, salt, baking powder and 1 cup sugar into large mixing bowl.
3. Add oil, milk, and flavorings.
4. Mix with electric mixer on low speed 30 seconds, scraping sides of bowl. Beat on high speed 1 minute.
5. In medium-size bowl, beat egg whites until frothy. Gradually add remaining ¼ cup sugar to egg whites. Beat at high speed to stiff peak stage, about 4–5 minutes.
6. Gently fold whites into batter, about 30–35 strokes.
7. Bake in oiled and floured 10-inch tube pan 35–40 minutes. *Or* use two 9-inch round pans, oiled, floured, and lined with waxed paper and bake 25–30 minutes.
8. Cool 5 minutes before removing from pan.

Yield: 24 servings

Variations:
Chocolate Cake: Decrease flour to 1¾ cups. Add ½ cup cocoa powder with dry ingredients.
Buttermilk Cake: Add ½ teaspoon baking soda with dry ingredients. Decrease baking powder to 1 teaspoon. Substitute 1 cup buttermilk for skim milk.
Lemon Cake: Substitute 2 teaspoons lemon extract, 2 tablespoons grated lemon peel, and ¼ teaspoon yellow food coloring for flavorings.

1 serving contains:

Cal	Prot	Fat	Carb	Sat	Mono	Poly	Chol	Na
122	2	4.7	18	0.6	1.1	2.7	0	142

Exchanges: Not applicable for this recipe
Recommended for: The Living Heart and Type IIa Diets

One-Pan Snack Cake

```
1½ cups enriched, all-purpose flour
1  cup sugar
1  teaspoon baking soda
6  tablespoons cocoa powder
1  cup cold water
1  teaspoon vanilla extract
6  tablespoons oil
1  tablespoon vinegar
```

1. Preheat oven to 375°F.
2. Combine dry ingredients in an ungreased 8 × 8-inch baking pan.
3. Add liquid ingredients and stir with a fork until completely mixed.
4. Bake for 25 minutes.

Yield: 16 servings

1 serving contains:

Cal	Prot	Fat	Carb	Sat	Mono	Poly	Chol	Na
141	2	5.6	22	0.9	1.4	3.0	0	87

Exchanges: Not applicable for this recipe
Recommended for: The Living Heart and Type IIa Diets

Quick Snack Cake

```
2½ cups enriched, all-purpose flour
¾  cup sugar
1  cup brown sugar, firmly packed
1  teaspoon salt
1  teaspoon ground cinnamon
¾  cup oil
1  cup chopped walnuts
   egg substitute equivalent to 1 egg
1  teaspoon baking soda
1  teaspoon baking powder
1  cup skim milk
```

1. Preheat oven to 350°F.
2. Mix flour, sugars, salt, cinnamon, oil, and ½ cup nuts. Set aside 1 cup of the mixture for topping.
3. To mixture, add remaining ingredients, mixing well.
4. Pour into an oiled 9 × 13-inch baking pan.

5. Add remaining ½ cup walnuts to topping mixture and sprinkle on batter.
6. Bake for 30 minutes.

Yield: 24 servings

1 serving contains:

Cal	Prot	Fat	Carb	Sat	Mono	Poly	Chol	Na
205	3	10.3	26	1.3	2.2	6.2	0	174

Exchanges: Not applicable for this recipe
Recommended for: The Living Heart and Type IIa Diets

Souper Cake

1 can (10¾ ounces) condensed tomato soup, undiluted
1 cup sugar
1½ cups enriched, all-purpose flour
1 teaspoon baking soda
½ teaspoon ground cloves
1 teaspoon ground cinnamon
1 cup chopped dates
1 cup chopped walnuts

1. Preheat oven to 350°F.
2. Combine soup and sugar. Thoroughly mix in flour, baking soda, cloves, and cinnamon by hand.
3. Stir in dates and walnuts.
4. Pour into an oiled and floured 9 × 5-inch loaf pan.
5. Bake for 45–50 minutes.

Yield: 14 servings

1 serving contains:

Cal	Prot	Fat	Carb	Sat	Mono	Poly	Chol	Na
210	3	6.0	38	0.7	0.9	3.9	0	273

Exchanges: Not applicable for this recipe
Recommended for: The Living Heart and Type IIa Diets

Easy Vanilla Frosting

3 cups confectioner's sugar
3 tablespoons skim milk
2 tablespoons oil
½ teaspoon butter flavoring
½ teaspoon vanilla extract

Combine all ingredients.

Yield: frosting for a two-layer cake

Variations:

Easy Lemon or Orange Frosting: Substitute 1 teaspoon lemon or orange extract for vanilla extract.
Easy Coffee Frosting: Dissolve 1 teaspoon instant coffee in milk before mixing with other ingredients.
Easy Mocha Frosting: Dissolve 1 teaspoon instant coffee in milk before mixing with other ingredients. Add 1 tablespoon cocoa powder to confectioner's sugar.

1/24 recipe contains:

Cal	Prot	Fat	Carb	Sat	Mono	Poly	Chol	Na
68	0	1.1	15	0.1	0.3	0.7	0	1

Exchanges: Not applicable for this recipe
Recommended for: The Living Heart and Type IIa Diets

Abbreviations: **Cal,** calories; **Prot,** protein; **Carb,** carbohydrate; **Sat,** saturated fat; **Mono,** monounsaturated fat; **Poly,** polyunsaturated fat; **Chol,** cholesterol; **Na,** sodium. Protein, fat, carbohydrate, saturated fat, monounsaturated fat, and polyunsaturated fat are expressed in *grams.* Cholesterol and sodium are expressed in *milligrams.*

Mock Cream Cheese Frosting

1 cup Mock Cream Cheese (see recipe, page 90)
¼ cup tub margarine
1½ teaspoons vanilla extract
4 cups (1 pound) confectioner's sugar

1. Cream cheese and margarine together.
2. Add vanilla.
3. Beat in sugar a little at a time until of spreading consistency.

Yield: frosting for a two-layer cake

1/24 recipe contains:

Cal	Prot	Fat	Carb	Sat	Mono	Poly	Chol	Na
119	1	4.0	20	0.8	1.4	1.4	1	85

Exchanges: Not applicable for this recipe
Recommended for: The Living Heart and Type IIa Diets

Chocolate Cheese Frosting

1 cup dry curd cottage cheese
½ cup tub margarine
9 tablespoons cocoa powder
3 tablespoons skim milk
½ teaspoon salt
½ teaspoon vanilla extract
4 cups sifted confectioner's sugar

1. Blend cottage cheese and margarine thoroughly in blender.
2. Mix cottage cheese mixture, cocoa, skim milk, salt, and vanilla in a bowl.
3. Gradually stir in confectioner's sugar.

Yield: frosting for a two-layer cake or a 9 × 13-inch sheet cake

1/24 recipe contains:

Cal	Prot	Fat	Carb	Sat	Mono	Poly	Chol	Na
109	1	4.2	18	0.9	1.5	1.7	0	94

Exchanges: Not applicable for this recipe
Recommended for: The Living Heart and Type IIa Diets

Mexicali Chocolate Frosting

2 tablespoons cocoa powder
2 tablespoons oil
1½ teaspoons vanilla extract
⅛ teaspoon salt
½ teaspoon ground cinnamon
¼ teaspoon butter flavoring
2½ cups confectioner's sugar
2–3 tablespoons skim milk

1. Combine cocoa, oil, vanilla, salt, cinnamon, and flavoring.
2. Gradually stir in confectioner's sugar and enough milk to make a good spreading consistency.

Yield: frosting for a 9 × 13-inch cake

1/24 recipe contains:

Cal	Prot	Fat	Carb	Sat	Mono	Poly	Chol	Na
60	0	1.2	13	0.2	0.3	0.7	0	12

Exchanges: Not applicable for this recipe
Recommended for: The Living Heart and Type IIa Diets

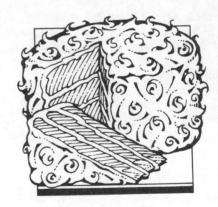

COOKIES

Sugared Almond Crescents

1 cup tub margarine
⅓ cup sugar
⅔ cup ground blanched almonds
1⅔ cups enriched, all-purpose flour
¼ teaspoon salt
½ cup confectioner's sugar
½ teaspoon ground cinnamon

1. Preheat oven to 325°F.
2. Mix margarine, sugar, and almonds thoroughly.
3. Work in the flour and salt.
4. Chill dough 2–3 hours.
5. Roll dough, a small portion at a time, with hands until pencil thick.
6. Cut into 2½-inch lengths and shape in crescents on an ungreased baking sheet.
7. Bake for 15 minutes or until set but not browned.
8. Cool on baking sheet for a few minutes.
9. While still warm, carefully dip in mixture of confectioner's sugar and cinnamon.

Yield: 48 cookies

1 cookie contains:

Cal	Prot	Fat	Carb	Sat	Mono	Poly	Chol	Na
80	1	5.7	7	0.9	2.6	2.0	0	58

Exchanges: Not applicable for this recipe
Recommended for: The Living Heart and Type IIa Diets

Banana Oatmeal Cookies

1½ cups enriched, all-purpose flour
1 cup sugar
½ teaspoon baking soda
1 teaspoon salt
¼ teaspoon ground nutmeg
¾ teaspoon ground cinnamon
¾ cup tub margarine
   egg substitute equivalent to 1 egg
1 cup mashed bananas
1¾ cups dry oatmeal
½ cup chopped walnuts

1. Preheat oven to 400°F.
2. Sift flour, sugar, baking soda, salt, nutmeg, and cinnamon into a large mixing bowl.
3. Add margarine, egg substitute, and bananas, beating well.
4. Mix in oatmeal and walnuts until thoroughly blended.
5. Drop from a teaspoon onto an ungreased baking sheet.
6. Bake for 12–15 minutes. Remove from pan immediately.

Yield: 54 cookies

Variation:

Banana Oatmeal Raisin Cookies: Add ½ cup raisins with nuts.

1 cookie without raisins contains:

Cal	Prot	Fat	Carb	Sat	Mono	Poly	Chol	Na
74	1	3.6	10	0.6	1.1	1.7	0	87

One cookie with raisins contains 78 calories
Exchanges: Not applicable for this recipe.
Recommended for: The Living Heart and Type IIa Diets

Abbreviations: **Cal,** calories; **Prot,** protein; **Carb,** carbohydrate; **Sat,** saturated fat; **Mono,** monounsaturated fat; **Poly,** polyunsaturated fat; **Chol,** cholesterol; **Na,** sodium. Protein, fat, carbohydrate, saturated fat, monounsaturated fat, and polyunsaturated fat are expressed in *grams.* Cholesterol and sodium are expressed in *milligrams.*

Black Raspberry Bars

¾ **cup tub margarine**
1 **cup brown sugar, firmly packed**
1¾ **cups enriched, all-purpose flour**
1 **teaspoon salt**
½ **teaspoon baking soda**
1½ **cups dry oatmeal**
1 **can (16 ounces) black raspberries, drained**

1. Preheat oven to 400°F.
2. Cream margarine and sugar.
3. Mix in flour, salt, and soda until well blended.
4. Stir in oatmeal.
5. Press half of mixture into a 9 × 13-inch baking pan greased with margarine.
6. Spread raspberries over mixture and sprinkle with remaining oatmeal mixture.
7. Bake for 25 minutes. Cool 5 minutes before cutting into bars.

Yield: 24 servings

1 bar contains:

Cal	Prot	Fat	Carb	Sat	Mono	Poly	Chol	Na
158	2	6.3	24	1.1	2.2	2.7	0	194

Exchanges: Not applicable for this recipe
Recommended for: The Living Heart and Type IIa Diets

Brownies

1¼ **cups tub margarine**
⅔ **cup cocoa powder**
2 **cups sugar**
egg substitute equivalent to 4 eggs
2 **teaspoons vanilla extract**
1½ **cups enriched, all-purpose flour**
1 **cup chopped walnuts**
confectioner's sugar (optional)

1. Preheat oven to 350°F.
2. Heat margarine and cocoa in saucepan until melted.
3. Place in bowl with sugar and mix well.
4. Add egg substitute gradually, beating very well after each addition.
5. Add vanilla, flour, and nuts and mix thoroughly.

6. Spread in 9 × 13-inch baking pan greased with margarine.
7. Bake for 35 minutes. Be careful not to over-bake.
8. Cool before cutting. Sprinkle with confectioner's sugar, if desired.

Yield: 24 brownies

1 brownie contains:

Cal	Prot	Fat	Carb	Sat	Mono	Poly	Chol	Na
227	3	13.9	25	2.5	4.2	6.7	0	135

Exchanges: Not applicable for this recipe
Recommended for: The Living Heart and Type IIa Diets

Sugar Cookies

1½ **cups confectioner's sugar, sifted**
1 **cup tub margarine**
¼ **cup skim milk**
1 **teaspoon vanilla extract**
½ **teaspoon almond extract**
2½ **cups enriched, all-purpose flour**
1 **teaspoon cream of tartar**
1 **teaspoon baking soda**

1. Cream sugar and margarine together.
2. Mix in milk and flavorings.
3. Stir in remaining ingredients and mix well.
4. Refrigerate 2–3 hours.
5. Preheat oven to 350°F.
6. Divide dough in half and roll each half out to ¼ inch thick on lightly floured board. (The best cookies are achieved when the dough is worked with very little.)
7. Cut into desired shapes with cookie cutter and place on lightly oiled baking sheet.
8. Bake for 8 minutes or until golden.
9. Let cool 3–4 minutes before removing from baking sheet.

Yield: 36 cookies

1 cookie contains:

Cal	Prot	Fat	Carb	Sat	Mono	Poly	Chol	Na
93	1	5.2	11	1.0	1.8	2.3	0	102

Exchanges: Not applicable for this recipe
Recommended for: The Living Heart and Type IIa Diets

Shortbread

1 **cup tub margarine**
½ **cup sugar**
2½ **cups enriched, all-purpose flour**
½ **teaspoon butter flavoring**

1. Cream margarine and sugar together.
2. Mix in flour and flavoring until well blended.
3. Refrigerate 4–6 hours.
4. Roll dough about ⅓ inch thick on lightly floured board.
5. Cut with 2-inch round cutter.
6. Bake on ungreased baking sheet in a preheated 300°F oven for 25 minutes.

Yield: 4 dozen cookies

1 cookie contains:

Cal	Prot	Fat	Carb	Sat	Mono	Poly	Chol	Na
65	1	3.9	7	0.7	1.4	1.7	0	47

Exchanges: 1 cookie = ½ bread, ½ fat
Recommended for: The Living Heart; Low Calorie; and Type IIa Diets

Peanut Butter Cookies

1 **cup tub margarine**
1 **cup sugar**
1 **cup brown sugar, firmly packed**
5 **tablespoons evaporated skim milk, undiluted**
1 **teaspoon vanilla extract**
1 **cup peanut butter**
2 **cups enriched, all-purpose flour**
2 **teaspoons baking soda**
½ **teaspoon salt**

1. Preheat oven to 350°F.
2. Thoroughly cream margarine, sugars, milk, and vanilla.
3. Stir in peanut butter and add dry ingredients.
4. Drop from a teaspoon onto an ungreased baking sheet.
5. Press with back of floured fork to make criss-cross pattern.
6. Bake for 15 minutes.

Yield: 72 cookies

1 cookie contains:

Cal	Prot	Fat	Carb	Sat	Mono	Poly	Chol	Na
79	1	4.4	9	0.9	1.8	1.7	0	109

Exchanges: Not applicable for this recipe
Recommended for: The Living Heart and Type IIa Diets

Molasses Spice Cookies

½ **cup oil**
¾ **cup sugar**
1 **cup molasses**
4⅓ **cups whole wheat flour**
1 **teaspoon baking soda**
½ **teaspoon salt**
1½ **teaspoons ground ginger**
¾ **teaspoon ground cloves**
¾ **teaspoon ground nutmeg**
¼ **teaspoon ground allspice**
⅓ **cup water**

1. Mix oil and sugar together.
2. Add molasses and beat well.
3. Combine flour, baking soda, salt, and spices.
4. Add alternately with water to sugar mixture, beating well after each addition.
5. Wrap dough in foil and chill overnight.
6. Roll dough about ¼ inch thick on a lightly floured surface.
7. Cut with floured 4-inch round cookie cutter.
8. Bake in a preheated 375°F oven 8–9 minutes or until done. Be careful not to overbake.

Yield: 36 cookies

1 cookie contains:

Cal	Prot	Fat	Carb	Sat	Mono	Poly	Chol	Na
114	2	3.3	20	0.5	0.8	1.9	0	71

Exchanges: Not applicable for this recipe
Recommended for: The Living Heart and Type IIa Diets

Abbreviations: **Cal,** calories; **Prot,** protein; **Carb,** carbohydrate; **Sat,** saturated fat; **Mono,** monounsaturated fat; **Poly,** polyunsaturated fat; **Chol,** cholesterol; **Na,** sodium. Protein, fat, carbohydrate, saturated fat, monounsaturated fat, and polyunsaturated fat are expressed in *grams.* Cholesterol and sodium are expressed in *milligrams.*

Pecan Drops

1½ cups sugar
¾ cup tub margarine
2 teaspoons vanilla extract
1 teaspoon baking soda
1 teaspoon cream of tartar
3 cups enriched, all-purpose flour
¾ cup buttermilk
½ cup chopped pecans

1. Preheat oven to 400°F.
2. Cream sugar and margarine together.
3. Add vanilla, baking soda, and cream of tartar.
4. Add flour and buttermilk alternately in three additions, mixing thoroughly after each addition.
5. Drop from a teaspoon onto a lightly oiled baking sheet.
6. Bake for 8–10 minutes.

Yield: 60 cookies

Variation:

Walnut Drops: Substitute ½ cup chopped walnuts for pecans.

1 cookie contains:

Cal	Prot	Fat	Carb	Sat	Mono	Poly	Chol	Na
70	1	3.1	10	0.5	1.3	1.2	0	54

Exchanges: Not applicable for this recipe
Recommended for: The Living Heart and Type IIa Diets

Lemon Doodle Cookies

⅔ cup tub margarine
½ cup brown sugar, firmly packed
½ teaspoon lemon extract
⅔ cup enriched, all-purpose flour
1½ cups dry oatmeal
    sugar

1. Preheat oven to 325°F.
2. Cream margarine and sugar together.
3. Add lemon extract, flour, and oatmeal, and mix well.

4. Form dough into walnut-sized balls and place on baking sheet.
5. Flatten balls with bottom of glass dipped in sugar.
6. Bake for 13–15 minutes.

Yield: 36 cookies

1 cookie contains:

Cal	Prot	Fat	Carb	Sat	Mono	Poly	Chol	Na
67	1	3.7	8	0.7	1.3	1.6	0	43

Exchanges: Not applicable for this recipe
Recommended for: The Living Heart and Type IIa Diets

Walnut Crispies

3 egg whites
⅛ teaspoon salt
1 teaspoon vanilla extract
1 cup sugar
2 cups chopped walnuts

1. Preheat oven to 350°F.
2. Beat egg whites until stiff.
3. Add salt and vanilla and gradually add sugar.
4. Fold in nuts. Drop batter from a teaspoon onto a greased baking sheet.
5. Bake for 2–3 minutes.
6. Turn off oven and leave cookies in oven for 60 minutes.

Yield: 72 cookies

1 cookie contains:

Cal	Prot	Fat	Carb	Sat	Mono	Poly	Chol	Na
33	1	2.1	3	0.2	0.3	1.4	0	6

Exchanges: Not applicable for this recipe
Recommended for: The Living Heart and Type IIa Diets

PIES AND TOPPINGS

Creamy Cocoa Pie

2 cups skim milk
¼ cup cocoa powder
¼ cup cornstarch
¾ cup sugar
2 teaspoons oil
1 tablespoon vanilla extract
1 teaspoon butter flavoring
¼ teaspoon salt
1 9-inch Graham Cracker Crumb Crust or baked pie shell of Margarine Pastry *or* Oil Pastry (see recipes, pages 214 and 215) Meringue for 9-inch pie (see recipe, page 215)

1. Scald 1½ cups skim milk.
2. While milk is heating, make a paste of the cocoa, cornstarch, ½ cup skim milk, and sugar.
3. Stir paste into hot milk until thick.
4. Remove from heat and add oil.
5. When cooled slightly, add vanilla, butter flavoring, and salt.
6. Pour into crust and chill at least 2 hours before serving.
7. Top with Meringue and brown according to recipe directions.

Yield: 8 servings

1 serving contains:

Cal	Prot	Fat	Carb	Sat	Mono	Poly	Chol	Na
292	5	9.5	48	1.9	3.2	4.1	1	349

Exchanges: Not applicable for this recipe
Recommended for: The Living Heart and Type IIa Diets

Cottage Cheese Pie

egg substitute equivalent to 2 eggs
½ cup sugar
⅛ teaspoon salt
½ teaspoon ground cinnamon
1½ tablespoons enriched, all-purpose flour
½ teaspoon vanilla extract
2 tablespoons evaporated skim milk, undiluted
2 tablespoons tub margarine, melted
1 carton (16 ounces) low-fat cottage cheese
1 9-inch unbaked pie shell of Margarine Pastry *or* Oil Pastry (see recipes, page 214 and 215) cinnamon

1. Preheat oven to 375°F.
2. Beat egg substitute 5 minutes.
3. Add sugar, salt, cinnamon, flour, and vanilla.
4. Combine milk, melted margarine, and cottage cheese in blender and purée.
5. Blend into egg mixture.
6. Pour into pie shell and sprinkle with cinnamon.
7. Bake for 45 minutes.

Yield: 8 servings

1 serving contains:

Cal	Prot	Fat	Carb	Sat	Mono	Poly	Chol	Na
274	11	12.7	29	2.8	4.3	5.2	5	559

Exchanges: Not applicable for this recipe
Recommended for: The Living Heart and Type IIa Diets

Abbreviations: **Cal,** calories; **Prot,** protein; **Carb,** carbohydrate; **Sat,** saturated fat; **Mono,** monounsaturated fat; **Poly,** polyunsaturated fat; **Chol,** cholesterol; **Na,** sodium. Protein, fat, carbohydrate, saturated fat, monounsaturated fat, and polyunsaturated fat are expressed in *grams.* Cholesterol and sodium are expressed in *milligrams.*

Honey Apple Pie

6–7 **apples, peeled, cored, and sliced**
  1 **9-inch unbaked pie shell of Margarine Pastry**
    or Oil Pastry (see recipes this page and page
    215)
  ½ **cup honey**
  ¼ **cup tub margarine**
  1 **cup whole wheat flour**
  ⅛ **teaspoon salt**
  1 **teaspoon ground cinnamon**
  ⅓ **cup sugar**

1. Preheat oven to 375°F.
2. Place apples in unbaked pie shell.
3. Drizzle with honey.
4. Combine margarine, flour, salt, cinnamon, and sugar. Sprinkle over apples.
5. Bake for 35 minutes.

Yield: 8 servings

1 serving contains:

Cal	Prot	Fat	Carb	Sat	Mono	Poly	Chol	Na
370	4	14.1	61	2.6	4.8	6.3	0	336

Exchanges: Not applicable for this recipe
Recommended for: The Living Heart and Type IIa Diets

Pumpkin Pie

   egg substitute equivalent to 2 eggs
  1 **can (16 ounces) pumpkin**
  ¾ **cup sugar**
  ½ **teaspoon salt**
  1 **teaspoon ground cinnamon**
  ½ **teaspoon ground ginger**
  ¼ **teaspoon ground cloves**
  1 **can (13 ounces) evaporated skim milk,**
    undiluted
  1 **9-inch unbaked pie shell of Margarine Pastry**
    or Oil Pastry (see recipes this page and page
    215)

1. Preheat oven to 425°F.
2. Beat egg substitute 5 minutes.
3. Mix in pumpkin, sugar, salt, spices, and milk, and pour into pie shell.
4. Bake 15 minutes.

5. Reduce temperature to 350°F and continue baking 45–50 minutes or until knife inserted in center comes out clean.

Yield: 8 servings

1 serving contains:

Cal	Prot	Fat	Carb	Sat	Mono	Poly	Chol	Na
276	8	9.0	42	1.6	3.0	4.1	2	457

Exchanges: Not applicable for this recipe
Recommended for: The Living Heart and Type IIa Diets

Margarine Pastry

  1 **cup enriched, all-purpose flour**
  ½ **teaspoon salt**
  ⅓ **cup tub margarine**
2–3 **tablespoons water**

1. Mix flour and salt.
2. Cut in margarine until coarse meal texture is obtained.
3. Sprinkle water over flour, mixing gradually with fork.
4. Form into ball and chill 10 minutes.
5. Roll out ball from center to edge until about ⅛ inch thick.
6. Fit into 9-inch pie pan and flute edges of pastry.
7. If prebaked shell is needed, bake in a preheated 425°F oven 12–15 minutes.

Yield: one 9-inch pie shell

Note: Double recipe for two-crust pie or lattice-top pie.

⅛ of single crust recipe contains:

Cal	Prot	Fat	Carb	Sat	Mono	Poly	Chol	Na
124	2	7.8	12	1.4	2.7	3.4	0	230

Exchanges: ⅛ of single crust recipe = 1 bread, 1½ fats
Recommended for: The Living Heart; Low Calorie; Diabetic; Types IIa, IIb, III, and IV Diets

Oil Pastry

1 **cup enriched, all-purpose flour**
½ **teaspoon salt**
¼ **cup oil**
2 **tablespoons cold water**

1. Mix flour and salt in bowl.
2. Blend in oil with fork.
3. Sprinkle water over mixture, mixing well.
4. Shape into ball and chill.
5. Roll out between two pieces of waxed paper.
6. Remove top layer of waxed paper and invert dough into pie pan.
7. Peel off other sheet of waxed paper and flute edges of pastry.
8. If prebaked shell is needed, bake in a preheated 450°F oven for 10–12 minutes.

Yield: one 9-inch pie shell

Note: Double recipe for two-crust pie or lattice-top pie.

⅛ of single crust recipe contains:

Cal	Prot	Fat	Carb	Sat	Mono	Poly	Chol	Na
117	2	7.0	12	0.9	1.7	4.1	0	138

Exchanges: ⅛ of single crust recipe = 1 bread, 1 fat
Recommended for: The Living Heart; Low Calorie; Diabetic; Types IIa, IIb, III, and IV Diets

Graham Cracker Crumb Crust

1 **cup graham cracker crumbs**
2 **tablespoons tub margarine, melted**
¼ **cup sugar**
⅛ **teaspoon ground nutmeg**
¼ **cup chopped pecans (optional)**

1. Preheat oven to 350°F.
2. Combine ingredients and mix well.
3. Press into a 9-inch round pan and place in oven for 1 minute.
4. Chill in refrigerator until firm.

Yield: one 9-inch round crust

⅛ recipe contains:

Cal	Prot	Fat	Carb	Sat	Mono	Poly	Chol	Na
119	1	6.7	15	1.0	3.2	2.2	1	89

Exchanges: Not applicable for this recipe
Recommended for: The Living Heart and Type IIa Diets

Meringue

3 **egg whites**
¼ **teaspoon cream of tartar**
½ **teaspoon vanilla extract**
6 **tablespoons sugar**

1. Preheat oven to 350°F.
2. Beat egg whites with cream of tartar and vanilla until soft peaks form. Gradually add sugar while beating until stiff and glossy.
3. Spread meringue on pie filling, sealing against pastry.
4. Bake for 12–15 minutes or until peaks are golden brown.

Yield: meringue for one 9-inch pie

⅛ recipe for 9-inch pie contains:

Cal	Prot	Fat	Carb	Sat	Mono	Poly	Chol	Na
42	1	0	9	0	0	0	0	19

Exchanges: Not applicable for this recipe
Recommended for: The Living Heart; Types I and IIa Diets

Note: For meringue for 8-inch pie, use 2 egg whites and decrease sugar to 4 tablespoons.

⅛ recipe for 8-inch pie contains:

Cal	Prot	Fat	Carb	Sat	Mono	Poly	Chol	Na
28	1	0	6	0	0	0	0	13

Exchanges: Not applicable for this recipe
Recommended for: The Living Heart; Types I and IIa Diets

Abbreviations: **Cal**, calories; **Prot**, protein; **Carb**, carbohydrate; **Sat**, saturated fat; **Mono**, monounsaturated fat; **Poly**, polyunsaturated fat; **Chol**, cholesterol; **Na**, sodium. Protein, fat, carbohydrate, saturated fat, monounsaturated fat, and polyunsaturated fat are expressed in *grams*. Cholesterol and sodium are expressed in *milligrams*.

Dessert Topping
(Whipped Cream Substitute)

⅓ cup evaporated skim milk, undiluted
½ teaspoon unflavored gelatin
1 tablespoon cold water
1 tablespoon sugar
½ teaspoon vanilla extract
1–2 teaspoons lemon juice

1. Chill evaporated skim milk in a small bowl.
2. Sprinkle gelatin over cold water in a small saucepan.
3. Stir over low heat until gelatin dissolves, then add to milk.
4. Beat with a rotary or electric beater until stiff.
5. Add sugar, vanilla, and lemon juice.
6. Use immediately, or chill and beat again before using.

Yield: 1 cup

1 tablespoon contains:

Cal	Prot	Fat	Carb	Sat	Mono	Poly	Chol	Na
8	0	0	1	0	0	0	0	6

Exchanges: Not applicable for this recipe
Recommended for: The Living Heart; Types I and IIa Diets

For Low Calorie, Diabetic, Types IIb, III, IV, and V Diets, omit sugar. Count 1–6 tablespoons = free; 7 tablespoons = ½ dairy (4 calories per tablespoon).

FROZEN DESSERTS

"Help Your Heart" Ice Cream

2 cans (13 ounces each) evaporated skim milk, undiluted
2½ cups sugar
egg substitute equivalent to 4 eggs
2 tablespoons cornstarch
⅛ teaspoon salt
1 tablespoon vanilla extract
8 cups skim milk

1. Scald evaporated skim milk.
2. Mix together sugar, egg substitute, cornstarch, and salt with electric mixer, beating at least 5 minutes on medium-high speed.
3. Add hot milk *gradually* to egg substitute and sugar mixture.
4. Pour into pan and heat custard mixture until it coats spoon.
5. Add vanilla extract.
6. Pour mixture into 1-gallon ice cream freezer container.
7. Add skim milk until container is ¾ full and churn according to freezer directions.

Yield: 1 gallon

Variation:

Flavored Ice Cream: Substitute half of a 3-ounce package of flavored sweetened gelatin for cornstarch. Mixture will not thicken as much on heating.

¼ cup contains:

Cal	Prot	Fat	Carb	Sat	Mono	Poly	Chol	Na
56	2	0.3	11	0.1	0.1	0.1	1	42

Exchanges: ¼ cup = 1 bread
Recommended for: The Living Heart; Low Calorie; Types I and IIa Diets

Fresh Fruit Ice

1 envelope (1 tablespoon) unflavored gelatin
½ cup cold water
1 cup orange juice
6 tablespoons lemon juice
¼ cup sugar
1 cup sliced strawberries, peaches, or other fresh or frozen unsweetened fruit
3 bananas, mashed

1. Stir gelatin into water over low heat until dissolved. Remove from heat. Mix in orange juice, lemon juice, sugar, ⅔ cup of the sliced fruit, and bananas. Place in freezer until almost set.
2. Beat with an electric mixer on high speed until fluffy.
3. Pour into individual parfait glasses and garnish with remaining fruit.
4. Cover and return to freezer.

Yield: 8 servings

1 serving contains:

Cal	Prot	Fat	Carb	Sat	Mono	Poly	Chol	Na
90	2	0.2	22	0	0	0.2	0	1

Exchanges: 1 serving = 2 fruits
Recommended for: The Living Heart; Low Calorie; Types I and IIa Diets

Banana Tropicana Sherbet

1 cup sugar
⅛ teaspoon salt
2 cups water
1 cup nonfat dry milk powder
¼ cup lemon juice
⅓ cup orange juice
1 banana, mashed

1. Dissolve sugar and salt in 1 cup water.
2. Add remaining water and milk powder and chill 1 hour.
3. Add juices and banana. (Mixture may have a curdled appearance.)
4. Pour into freezer tray and freeze until firm.

5. Turn into bowl and beat until fluffy.
6. Return to freezer tray and refreeze.

Yield: 8 servings

1 serving contains:

Cal	Prot	Fat	Carb	Sat	Mono	Poly	Chol	Na
146	3	0.1	34	0	0	0.1	2	80

Exchanges: Not applicable for this recipe
Recommended for: The Living Heart; Types I and IIa Diets

Variation:
Add ½ cup chopped walnuts in last beating or as garnish.

1 serving with walnuts contains:

Cal	Prot	Fat	Carb	Sat	Mono	Poly	Chol	Na
195	4	4.9	35	0.6	0.8	3.2	2	80

Exchanges: Not applicable for this recipe
Recommended for: The Living Heart and Type IIa Diets

Pineapple Freeze

1 can (16 ounces) crushed pineapple, packed in own juice

1. Place unopened can of pineapple in freezer until hard.
2. Place under hot running water 30 seconds and remove from can.
3. Place in blender or food processor ½ at a time and blend to slush consistency.
4. Spoon into serving dishes.

Yield: 4 servings

1 serving contains:

Cal	Prot	Fat	Carb	Sat	Mono	Poly	Chol	Na
74	1	0.2	19	0	0	0.2	0	2

Exchanges: 1 serving = 2 fruits
Recommended for: The Living Heart; Low Calorie; Diabetic; Types I, IIa, IIb, III, IV, and V Diets

Abbreviations: **Cal,** calories; **Prot,** protein; **Carb,** carbohydrate; **Sat,** saturated fat; **Mono,** monounsaturated fat; **Poly,** polyunsaturated fat; **Chol,** cholesterol; **Na,** sodium. Protein, fat, carbohydrate, saturated fat, monounsaturated fat, and polyunsaturated fat are expressed in *grams.* Cholesterol and sodium are expressed in *milligrams.*

Section II.
The Living Heart Diet:
Low-Sodium Recipes

LOW-SODIUM RECIPES

All of the recipes in this section are low in sodium. These recipes do not use ingredients which contain high levels of salt or sodium compounds and can be used by those following very restricted sodium diets. If the physician recommends a more moderate level, sodium can be increased by use of some "regular" ingredients, such as soft tub margarine in place of low-sodium corn oil margarine and regular bread instead of low-sodium bread. (Refer to Table 2 in the *Appendix* for the sodium content of specific foods.) Special ingredients used in these low-sodium recipes are listed on page 220. Some may be located in the "diet" section of the grocery store or in specialty shops. It is very important to read the label on all foods in order to know if salt or other sodium-containing ingredients have been added; a list of compounds containing sodium is given in Chapter 3.

In addition to being low in sodium, these recipes are all low in cholesterol and saturated fat. The upper level of sodium content for the recipes is as follows:

Appetizers	up to 26 milligrams per serving
Soups	up to 77 milligrams per serving
Entrées	up to 108 milligrams per serving
Vegetables	up to 29 milligrams per serving
Salads	up to 29 milligrams per serving
Sauces, gravies, salad dressings	up to 8 milligrams per serving
Breads	up to 39 milligrams per serving
Desserts	up to 23 milligrams per serving

The amount of sodium in one serving is given for each recipe in this book. Some of the recipes in the main recipe section have only small amounts of sodium and therefore can be used for sodium-restricted diets; these recipes have not been reprinted here; however they are listed below for your information:

LOW-SODIUM, LOW-CALORIE RECIPES

Exchanges are given for 1 serving of the recipe recommended for persons following a low-calorie diet. Use of the "vegetable exchange" may not be necessary if the individual is not particularly sensitive to carbohydrates and can lose weight without accounting for the calories in the nonstarchy vegetables (28 calories per ½ cup).

LOW-SODIUM RECIPES FOR DIABETICS

Exchanges are given for the low-sodium recipes recommended for diabetics. These exchanges are similar to those in the booklet *Exchange Lists for Meal Planning* published by the American Diabetes Association, Inc. and the American Dietetic Association (1976). These recipes will add variety and zest to meal plans and still allow for dietary control.

LOW-SODIUM RECIPES FOR TYPES I–V HYPERLIPOPROTEINEMIA DIETS

Each recipe identifies the hyperlipoproteinemic types for which it can be used. Some recipes which are not identified as "recommended for Type V diets" may be used by counting the fat exchanges carefully.

LOW-SODIUM, VERY LOW FAT RECIPES

Recipes recommended for the Type V diet can also be used for diets very low in fat.

PRODUCTS USED IN LOW-SODIUM RECIPES

Liquid smoke—read labels and choose brands that do not contain salt

Chili powder—read labels and choose brands that do not contain salt

Dry curd cottage cheese—uncreamed cottage cheese

Low-sodium polyunsaturated fat cheese—low-sodium cheese product that has had butterfat replaced with corn oil

Low-sodium canned vegetables, meats, condiments, and other products—packed without salt or sodium compounds

Low-sodium corn oil margarine—stick or tub

Very lean ground beef—round steak that has been trimmed and ground

Low-sodium baking powder—use 1½ times the amount called for in a regular recipe

Low-sodium bread crumbs—make using low-sodium bread

Low-Sodium Appetizers

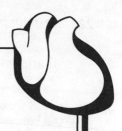

VEGETABLE APPETIZERS

Herbed Artichokes

¼ cup finely chopped onion
1 clove garlic, minced
1 cup low-sodium chicken bouillon
1 package (10 ounces) frozen artichoke hearts, thawed
2 tablespoons lemon juice
¼ teaspoon pepper
½ teaspoon dried oregano
¼ teaspoon dried sweet basil

1. Cook onion and garlic in bouillon until tender.
2. Add remaining ingredients and simmer 5 minutes.
3. Drain and chill.
4. Serve speared with toothpicks.

Yield: 4 servings

1 serving contains:

Cal	Prot	Fat	Carb	Sat	Mono	Poly	Chol	Na
20	1	0.1	5	0	0	0.1	0	11

Exchanges: 1 serving = free; 2 servings = 1 vegetable
Recommended for: The Living Heart; Low Calorie; Diabetic; Types I, IIa, IIb, III, IV, and V Diets

Pickled Beet Relish

¼ cup water
⅓ cup white vinegar
¼ cup brown sugar, firmly packed
½ teaspoon ground cinnamon
¼ teaspoon cloves
1 can (16 ounces) low-sodium beets, drained, chopped

1. Bring water, vinegar, brown sugar, cinnamon, and cloves to a boil in a saucepan. Pour over beets.
2. Let stand at least 8 hours. This will keep well in a covered jar in the refrigerator.

Yield: 2 cups

1 tablespoon contains:

Cal	Prot	Fat	Carb	Sat	Mono	Poly	Chol	Na
11	0	0	3	0	0	0	0	5

Exchanges: 1–2 tablespoons = free; 3 tablespoons = ½ bread
Recommended for: The Living Heart; Low Calorie; Types I, IIa, IIb, III, IV, and V Diets

Abbreviations: **Cal,** calories; **Prot,** protein; **Carb,** carbohydrate; **Sat,** saturated fat; **Mono,** monounsaturated fat; **Poly,** polyunsaturated fat; **Chol,** cholesterol; **Na,** sodium. Protein, fat, carbohydrate, saturated fat, monounsaturated fat, and polyunsaturated fat are expressed in *grams.* Cholesterol and sodium are expressed in *milligrams.*

Tangy Italian Mushrooms

½ pound fresh mushrooms, sliced
¾ cup low-sodium Italian Dressing (see recipe, page 261)
2 tablespoons low-sodium corn oil margarine

1. Marinate mushrooms in dressing at least 1 hour or overnight and then drain.
2. Cook mushrooms 5 minutes in skillet or chafing dish in the margarine. Serve warm with toothpicks or relish forks.

Yield: 2 cups

⅓ cup contains:

Cal	Prot	Fat	Carb	Sat	Mono	Poly	Chol	Na
28	1	2.0	2	0.4	0.8	0.7	0	6

Exchanges: ⅓ cup = 1 vegetable
Recommended for: The Living Heart; Low Calorie; Diabetic; Types IIa, IIb, III, and IV Diets

Relish Stuffed Tomatoes

3 fresh jalapeño peppers, seeded and finely chopped
½ cup finely chopped celery
3 tablespoons finely chopped green onion, including tops
2 tablespoons wine vinegar
1 teaspoon sugar
⅛ teaspoon pepper
40 cherry tomatoes

1. Combine jalapeño peppers, celery, onion, vinegar, sugar, and pepper.
2. Slice top off each tomato and scoop out insides.
3. Mix tomato insides with relish mixture and fill tomatoes.

Yield: 40 tomatoes

1 tomato contains:

Cal	Prot	Fat	Carb	Sat	Mono	Poly	Chol	Na
6	0	0.1	1	0	0	0.1	0	3

Exchanges: 1–4 tomatoes = free; 5 tomatoes = ½ bread
Recommended for: The Living Heart; Low Calorie; Diabetic; Types I, IIa, IIb, III, IV, and V Diets

Cherry Tomato Stars

1 cup dry curd cottage cheese
2 tablespoons finely chopped green pepper
2 tablespoons finely chopped celery
3 tablespoons finely chopped green onion
¼ cup low-sodium mayonnaise
30 cherry tomatoes
    paprika

1. Mix cottage cheese, green pepper, celery, onion, and mayonnaise.
2. Cut each cherry tomato into fourths almost to the base. Do *not* cut completely through the tomato.
3. Fill with cottage cheese mixture. Sprinkle with paprika.

Yield: 30 tomatoes

1 cherry tomato contains:

Cal	Prot	Fat	Carb	Sat	Mono	Poly	Chol	Na
23	1	1.5	1	0.3	0.3	0.8	2	2

Exchanges: 1 cherry tomato = free; 2 cherry tomatoes = 1 fat
Recommended for: The Living Heart; Low Calorie; Diabetic; Types IIa, IIb, III, and IV Diets

Variation:
Fill four small tomatoes and serve as salad.

1 regular tomato contains:

Cal	Prot	Fat	Carb	Sat	Mono	Poly	Chol	Na
174	9	11.6	11	2.1	2.4	6.0	12	17

Exchanges: 1 regular tomato = 1 dairy, 2 fats
Recommended for: The Living Heart; Low Calorie; Diabetic; Types IIa, IIb, III, and IV Diets

FRUIT APPETIZERS

Spicy Pineapple Pickups

1 **can (16 ounces) pineapple chunks, packed in own juice, drained, reserve liquid**
⅓ **cup vinegar**
½ **cup sugar**
2 **whole cloves**
1 **cinnamon stick**

1. To ⅓ cup of reserved pineapple juice, add vinegar, sugar, cloves, and cinnamon stick. Simmer for 8 minutes.
2. Add pineapple chunks and heat until just boiling. Chill 1–2 days.
3. Drain and serve with toothpicks.

Yield: 2 cups

¼ cup contains:

Cal	Prot	Fat	Carb	Sat	Mono	Poly	Chol	Na
49	0	0.1	13	0	0	0.1	0	1

Exchanges: ¼ cup = 1 fruit
Recommended for: The Living Heart; Low Calorie; Types I, IIa, IIb, III, IV, and V Diets

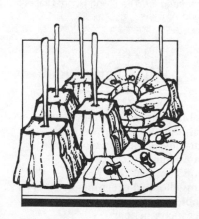

CRISPY APPETIZERS

Pastry Cheese Puffs

½ **cup low-sodium, low-fat cheese, shredded**
2 **tablespoons low-sodium corn oil margarine**
5 **tablespoons flour**
¼ **teaspoon paprika**
12 **unsalted walnut halves**

1. Preheat oven to 400°F.
2. Blend cheese with margarine. Mix in flour and paprika.
3. Wrap 1–2 teaspoons dough around each walnut half.
4. Bake on an ungreased baking sheet 15 minutes.

Yield: 12 puffs

Note: Puffs can be frozen on sheet before baking. When frozen, transfer to plastic bag. Remove from freezer and bake as above.

1 puff contains:

Cal	Prot	Fat	Carb	Sat	Mono	Poly	Chol	Na
58	2	4.3	3	0.6	1.3	2.1	0	26

Exchanges: 2 puffs = ½ bread, 1½ fats
Recommended for: The Living Heart; Diabetic; Types IIa, IIb, III, and IV Diets

Abbreviations: **Cal**, calories; **Prot**, protein; **Carb**, carbohydrate; **Sat**, saturated fat; **Mono**, monounsaturated fat; **Poly**, polyunsaturated fat; **Chol**, cholesterol; **Na**, sodium. Protein, fat, carbohydrate, saturated fat, monounsaturated fat, and polyunsaturated fat are expressed in *grams*. Cholesterol and sodium are expressed in *milligrams*.

Texas Scramble

   1   **cup small round oat cereal**
   1   **cup small square rice cereal**
   1   **cup small square wheat cereal**
   ½   **cup slivered almonds**
   ½   **cup walnut pieces**
   2   **tablespoons oil**
   ¼   **teaspoon garlic powder**
   ¼   **teaspoon onion powder**
   ½   **teaspoon natural low-sodium vegetable seasoning**

1. Preheat oven to 250°F.
2. Place cereals and nuts in small roasting pan or 9 × 13-inch baking pan.
3. Mix the oil and seasonings and sprinkle over top of cereal mixture and toss well.
4. Bake 60 minutes, stirring occasionally.

Yield: 4 cups

½ cup contains:

Cal	Prot	Fat	Carb	Sat	Mono	Poly	Chol	Na
164	3.5	12.4	11.7	1.4	3.9	6.6	0	109

Exchanges: ½ cup = 1 bread, 2 fats
Recommended for: The Living Heart; Diabetic; Types IIa, IIb, III and IV Diets

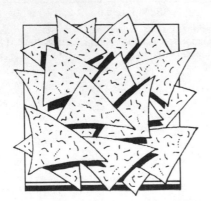

DIPS AND SPREADS

Guacamole Dip

   3   **avocados, peeled and seeded**
   1   **tomato, chopped**
   ½   **onion, chopped**
   1   **jalapeño pepper, seeded**
   ¼   **teaspoon pepper**
   ½   **teaspoon sugar**
   ¼   **cup low-sodium mayonnaise**
   ¼   **cup lemon juice**

1. Mash avocados and combine with remaining ingredients.
2. Mix with electric mixer or blender until smooth.
3. Store in covered container with avocado seed in center.
4. Dip with fresh vegetables.

Yield: approximately 2 cups

1 tablespoon contains:

Cal	Prot	Fat	Carb	Sat	Mono	Poly	Chol	Na
50	1	4.8	2	0.9	1.8	1.2	1	2

Exchanges: 1 tablespoon = 1 fat
Recommended for: The Living Heart; Diabetic; Types IIa, IIb, III, and IV Diets

Tuna Party Mold

   2   **tablespoons (2 envelopes) unflavored gelatin**
   3   **tablespoons cold water**
   1   **cup low-sodium mayonnaise**
   ¾   **cup lemon juice**
   ¾   **cup chopped celery**
   ½   **cup chopped green pepper**
   6   **tablespoons finely chopped onion**
   ¼   **teaspoon pepper**
   3   **cans (6½ ounces each) low-sodium water-packed tuna, drained**

1. Soften gelatin in cold water.
2. Dissolve softened gelatin mixture in a double-boiler over hot water. Blend into mayonnaise and add remaining ingredients.
3. Pour into 1 quart ring mold coated with mayonnaise and chill until firm.
4. Unmold, garnish with endive and radish flowers, if desired. Serve with low-sodium crackers.

Yield: 48 servings

1 tablespoon contains:

Cal	Prot	Fat	Carb	Sat	Mono	Poly	Chol	Na
25	2	1.9	0	0.3	0.4	0.9	5	4

Exchanges: 1 tablespoon = free; 2 tablespoons = ½ meat, ½ fat
Recommended for: The Living Heart; Diabetic; Types IIa, IIb, III, and IV Diets

Salmon Spread

1 **can (6½ ounces) low-sodium salmon, drained, skin and bones removed**
¼ **cup low-sodium mayonnaise**
¼ **teaspoon pepper**
¼ **teaspoon garlic powder**
2 **tablespoons finely chopped green onions**
2 **teaspoons lemon juice**

1. Combine all ingredients.
2. Serve on low-sodium crackers or bread that has been spread with low-sodium margarine, if desired.

Yield: approximately 1½ cups

1 tablespoon contains:

Cal	Prot	Fat	Carb	Sat	Mono	Poly	Chol	Na
30	2	2.3	0	0.5	0.6	1.0	4	9

Exchanges: 1 tablespoon = ½ meat
Recommended for: The Living Heart; Diabetic; Types IIa, IIb, III, IV, and V Diets

Mock Cream Cheese

1 **cup dry curd cottage cheese**
½ **cup low-sodium corn oil margarine**

Mix ingredients thoroughly in a blender, using a spatula to help cream the mixture.

Yield: about 1 cup

1 tablespoon contains:

Cal	Prot	Fat	Carb	Sat	Mono	Poly	Chol	Na
59	2	5.8	0	1.1	2.5	1.8	1	2

Exchanges: 1 tablespoon = 1 fat
Recommended for: The Living Heart; Diabetic; Types IIa, IIb, III, and IV Diets

Seasoned Margarine

1. To ¼ stick of low-sodium corn oil margarine add:
    4 **teaspoons chives and ¼ teaspoon lemon juice**
    or
    1 **teaspoon chopped fresh parsley, ¾ teaspoon chives, and ¼ teaspoon dried sweet basil**
2. Use as a spread on low-sodium crackers or bread, or as a seasoning for vegetables.

1 teaspoon contains:

Cal	Prot	Fat	Carb	Sat	Mono	Poly	Chol	Na
34	0	3.8	0	0.7	1.7	1.2	0	0

Exchanges: 1 teaspoon = 1 fat
Recommended for: The Living Heart; Low Calorie; Diabetic; Types IIa, IIb, III, and IV Diets

Abbreviations: **Cal,** calories; **Prot,** protein; **Carb,** carbohydrate; **Sat,** saturated fat; **Mono,** monounsaturated fat; **Poly,** polyunsaturated fat; **Chol,** cholesterol; **Na,** sodium. Protein, fat, carbohydrate, saturated fat, monounsaturated fat, and polyunsaturated fat are expressed in *grams.* Cholesterol and sodium are expressed in *milligrams.*

POULTRY, MEAT, EGG APPETIZERS

Barbecued Chicken Drummettes

16 chicken wings, skin and fat removed
¼ teaspoon pepper
2 tablespoons low-sodium corn oil margarine
2 tablespoons brown sugar, firmly packed
¼ cup low-sodium catsup
1 tablespoon low-sodium prepared mustard
   dash liquid smoke

1. Preheat oven to 400°F.
2. Cut off wing tips from chicken and straighten remaining sections to resemble a small drumstick.
3. Place in baking dish and season lightly with pepper.
4. Combine margarine, brown sugar, catsup, mustard, and liquid smoke. Spoon half of the sauce mixture over chicken and bake 15 minutes.
5. Turn drummettes and spoon on remaining sauce. Bake an additional 15 minutes until chicken is tender.

Yield: 16 servings

1 drummette contains:

Cal	Prot	Fat	Carb	Sat	Mono	Poly	Chol	Na
48	5	2.0	3	0.4	0.8	0.6	11	10

Exchanges: 1 drummette = 1 meat
Recommended for: The Living Heart; Low Calorie; Diabetic; Types IIa, IIb, III, IV, and V Diets

Chicken Curry Sandwiches

2 cups chopped cooked chicken
¾ teaspoon curry powder
⅓ cup finely chopped celery
¼ cup chopped unsalted walnuts
¼ cup raisins
¼ cup skim milk yogurt
¼ cup low-sodium mayonnaise
8 slices low-sodium bread, crusts removed

1. Combine all ingredients except bread.
2. Spread mixture on four slices of bread. Top with remaining bread slices.
3. Cut each sandwich in fourths.
4. Cover with plastic wrap and chill until ready to serve.

Yield: 16 servings

1 serving contains:

Cal	Prot	Fat	Carb	Sat	Mono	Poly	Chol	Na
114	7	5.5	10	1.1	1.3	2.5	18	23

Exchanges: ¼ sandwich = ½ bread, 1 meat, ½ fat
Recommended for: The Living Heart; Diabetic; Types IIa, IIb, III, and IV Diets

Chicken in Fondue Broth

1½ pounds chicken breasts, boned, skin and fat removed
3 cups low-sodium chicken bouillon
1 bay leaf
3 whole cloves
¼ teaspoon dried sweet basil
¾ cup white wine
1 pound fresh mushrooms, sliced

1. Cut chicken in ¾-inch cubes.
2. Simmer bouillon, bay leaf, cloves, basil, and wine in a saucepan 15 minutes.
3. Pour half of mixture into fondue pot. Keep remainder hot.
4. Spear chicken cube and mushroom on fork and cook in bouillon 2–3 minutes.

5. Replace broth in fondue pot as needed.

Yield: 16 servings

1 serving contains:

Cal	Prot	Fat	Carb	Sat	Mono	Poly	Chol	Na
51	9	1.0	1	0.3	0.3	0.3	22	21

Exchanges: 1 serving = 1 meat
Recommended for: The Living Heart; Low Calorie; Diabetic; Types I, IIa, IIb, III, IV, and V Diets

Sharon's Sherried Meatballs

2 pounds very lean ground beef
1 cup low-sodium catsup
1 cup sherry
2 tablespoons brown sugar, firmly packed

1. Shape ground meat into 1-inch meatballs.
2. Brown meatballs in skillet or chafing dish and drain off fat.
3. Add remaining ingredients.
4. Cook until sauce is thick, 1–2 hours.

Yield: 50 meatballs

1 meatball contains:

Cal	Prot	Fat	Carb	Sat	Mono	Poly	Chol	Na
38	4	1.4	2	0.5	0.5	0.1	12	10

Exchanges: 1 meatball = ½ meat
Recommended for: The Living Heart; Low Calorie; Diabetic; Types IIa, IIb, III, IV, and V Diets

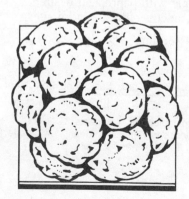

Okay Deviled Eggs*

egg substitute equivalent to 3 eggs
2 tablespoons low-sodium mayonnaise
2 teaspoons low-sodium prepared mustard
⅛ teaspoon pepper
1 teaspoon vinegar
6 eggs, hard-cooked and cooled
paprika

1. Cook egg substitute according to package directions for scrambled eggs.
2. Mash scrambled egg substitute with mayonnaise, mustard, pepper, and vinegar. Cover and refrigerate until chilled.
3. Halve hard-cooked eggs lengthwise and discard yolks.
4. Fill each egg half with chilled egg substitute mixture and sprinkle with paprika.

Yield: 12 servings

1 egg half contains:

Cal	Prot	Fat	Carb	Sat	Mono	Poly	Chol	Na
42	3	2.8	1	0.5	0.6	1.4	2	52*

Exchanges: 1 egg half = ½ meat, ½ fat
Recommended for: The Living Heart; Diabetic; Types IIa, IIb, III, and IV Diets

*Limit to 1 egg half daily due to sodium content.

Abbreviations: **Cal,** calories; **Prot,** protein; **Carb,** carbohydrate; **Sat,** saturated fat; **Mono,** monounsaturated fat; **Poly,** polyunsaturated fat; **Chol,** cholesterol; **Na,** sodium. Protein, fat, carbohydrate, saturated fat, monounsaturated fat, and polyunsaturated fat are expressed in *grams.* Cholesterol and sodium are expressed in *milligrams.*

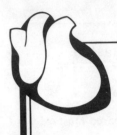

Low-Sodium Entrées

FISH ENTRÉES

Fancy Fillets Poached with Wine

¼ cup chopped onion
½ cup sliced fresh mushrooms
1 pound fish fillets
⅛ teaspoon pepper
¼ cup white wine
¼ cup water
4 tablespoons chopped fresh parsley

1. Preheat oven to 350°F.
2. Sprinkle onion and mushrooms over bottom of lightly oiled baking dish.
3. Place fillets on top of onion–mushroom mixture. Sprinkle with pepper. Cover fish with mixture of wine and water. Sprinkle on parsley.
4. Bake 20 minutes or until fish flakes easily.

Yield: 4 servings

1 serving contains:

Cal	Prot	Fat	Carb	Sat	Mono	Poly	Chol	Na
118	22	2.1	2	0.6	0.7	0.8	68	75

Exchanges: 1 serving = 2½ meats
Recommended for: The Living Heart; Low Calorie; Diabetic; Types I, IIa, IIb, III, IV, and V Diets

Scalloped Fish

1 pound fish fillets
1 tablespoon low-sodium corn oil margarine
2 tablespoons flour
1 cup skim milk
¼ teaspoon garlic powder
¼ teaspoon pepper
¼ teaspoon dried thyme
⅛ teaspoon dried oregano
¼ cup chopped green onion, including tops
paprika (optional)

1. Preheat oven to 350°F.
2. Place fish in an ungreased baking dish and dot with margarine.
3. In a saucepan over medium heat, slowly stir flour into milk. Stir until thick and then cook 1 minute longer.
4. Stir in remaining ingredients and pour sauce over fish.
5. Sprinkle with paprika, if desired.
6. Bake, uncovered, 20–25 minutes.

Yield: 4 servings

1 serving contains:

Cal	Prot	Fat	Carb	Sat	Mono	Poly	Chol	Na
175	24	5.1	7	1.2	2.0	1.7	69	105

Exchanges: 1 serving = 3 meats, ½ bread
Recommended for: The Living Heart; Low Calorie; Diabetic; Types IIa, IIb, III, IV, and V Diets

Fancy Parisian Fillets

1 tablespoon oil
1 onion, chopped
1 tablespoon chopped fresh parsley
2 pounds fish fillets
1 clove garlic, minced
1 cup white wine
1 can (16 ounces) low-sodium tomatoes, undrained
2 tablespoons lemon juice

1. Preheat oven to 350°F.
2. Place oil, half of the onion, and parsley in baking dish. Place fillets on top.
3. Combine remaining ingredients and pour over fish.
4. Bake 35–40 minutes or until fish flakes easily.

Yield: 8 servings

1 serving contains:

Cal	Prot	Fat	Carb	Sat	Mono	Poly	Chol	Na
146	22	3.9	5	0.8	1.2	1.9	68	76

Exchanges: 1 serving = 2½ meats
Recommended for: The Living Heart; Low Calorie; Diabetic; Types IIa, IIb, III, IV, and V Diets

Easy-to-Bake Fish Fillets

¾ cup chopped celery
6 tablespoons chopped onion
4 tablespoons chopped fresh parsley
¼ cup low-sodium corn oil margarine, melted
1 pound fish fillets
⅛ teaspoon pepper
  paprika

1. Preheat oven to 450°F.
2. Mix celery, onion, parsley, and margarine together. Place mixture on top of fillets in a shallow baking dish. Season with pepper and paprika.
3. Cover and bake 20 minutes or until fish flakes easily with a fork.

Yield: 4 servings

1 serving contains:

Cal	Prot	Fat	Carb	Sat	Mono	Poly	Chol	Na
222	22	13.6	2	2.7	5.7	4.4	68	100

Exchanges: 1 serving = 3 meats, 1 fat
Recommended for: The Living Heart; Diabetic; Types IIa, IIb, III, and IV Diets

Stuffed Fish Rolls

¼ cup finely chopped onion
¼ cup finely chopped celery
1 tablespoon low-sodium corn oil margarine
¼ cup sliced fresh mushrooms
4 tablespoons chopped fresh parsley
2 tablespoons lemon juice
1 pound fish fillets

1. Preheat oven to 400°F.
2. Sauté onion and celery in margarine until tender.
3. Stir in mushrooms, parsley, and lemon juice. Spread mixture over fillets.
4. Roll up fillets and secure with toothpicks. Place in lightly oiled baking dish.
5. Bake 20–25 minutes or until fish flakes easily with a fork.

Yield: 4 servings

Note: May also be baked in a microwave oven, 1 minute per roll.

1 serving contains:

Cal	Prot	Fat	Carb	Sat	Mono	Poly	Chol	Na
144	22	5.0	2	1.1	2.0	1.7	68	83

Exchanges: 1 serving = 2½ meats
Recommended for: The Living Heart; Low Calorie; Diabetic; Types IIa, IIb, III, IV, and V Diets

---

Abbreviations: **Cal,** calories; **Prot,** protein; **Carb,** carbohydrate; **Sat,** saturated fat; **Mono,** monounsaturated fat; **Poly,** polyunsaturated fat; **Chol,** cholesterol; **Na,** sodium. Protein, fat, carbohydrate, saturated fat, monounsaturated fat, and polyunsaturated fat are expressed in *grams.* Cholesterol and sodium are expressed in *milligrams.*

Oven-Fried Fillets

1   pound fish fillets
½ teaspoon pepper
½ cup fine, dry low-sodium bread crumbs
3   tablespoons low-sodium corn oil margarine

1. Preheat oven to 500°F.
2. Lightly season fillets with pepper. Roll in bread crumbs. Place in lightly oiled baking dish and dot with margarine.
3. Bake 10 minutes or until fish flakes easily with a fork.

Yield: 4 servings

1 serving contains:

Cal	Prot	Fat	Carb	Sat	Mono	Poly	Chol	Na
225	23	11.2	7	2.2	4.7	3.6	68	76

Exchanges: 1 serving = 2½ meats, ½ bread, 1 fat
Recommended for: The Living Heart; Diabetic; Types IIa, IIb, III, and IV Diets

So-Good Poached Fillets

¾ cup water
1   tablespoon lemon juice
½ onion, sliced
1   tablespoon vinegar
4   peppercorns
1   pound fish fillets or fish steaks

1. Place all ingredients except fish in saucepan and heat for 5 minutes.
2. Cut fish in serving-size pieces and add to liquid.
3. Simmer 5–10 minutes until fish flakes easily with a fork.

Yield: 4 servings

1 serving contains:

Cal	Prot	Fat	Carb	Sat	Mono	Poly	Chol	Na
115	21	2.1	1	0.6	0.7	0.8	68	74

Exchanges: 1 serving = 2½ meats
Recommended for: The Living Heart; Low Calorie; Diabetic; Types I, IIa, IIb, III, IV, and V Diets

Salmon-Broccoli Casserole

2   tablespoons low-sodium corn oil margarine
1   tablespoon flour
¼ teaspoon pepper
¼ teaspoon garlic powder
1   cup skim milk
3   fresh tomatoes, chopped
1   teaspoon lemon juice
1   package (10 ounces) frozen broccoli, thawed
1   can (6½ ounces) low-sodium salmon, drained
2   tablespoons fine, dry low-sodium bread crumbs

1. Preheat oven to 375°F.
2. Melt 1 tablespoon margarine in saucepan. Blend in flour, pepper, and garlic powder. Add milk and bring to a simmer, stirring constantly.
3. Add tomatoes and lemon juice and cook over low heat for 5 minutes.
4. Arrange broccoli on bottom of casserole. Cover with salmon and top with sauce. Sprinkle with bread crumbs and dot with 1 tablespoon margarine. Bake for 30 minutes.

Yield: 4 servings

1 serving contains:

Cal	Prot	Fat	Carb	Sat	Mono	Poly	Chol	Na
191	14	10.0	13	2.0	4.5	3.1	26	71

Exchanges: 1 serving = 1½ meats, 1 bread, ½ fat
Recommended for: The Living Heart; Diabetic; Types IIa, IIb, III, and IV Diets

Seafood Croquettes

2   tablespoons finely chopped onion
3   tablespoons low-sodium corn oil margarine
2   tablespoons flour
⅓ cup skim milk
1   can (6½ ounces) low-sodium, water-packed tuna, drained
⅛ teaspoon pepper
¼ cup fine, dry low-sodium bread or cracker crumbs

1. Sauté onion in 1 tablespoon margarine until tender. Stir in flour and cook 1 minute, stirring

constantly. Blend in milk and cook over medium heat until thick. Cool slightly.

2. Stir in tuna, pepper, and 2 tablespoons bread crumbs.

3. Shape into six patties and roll in remaining bread crumbs.

4. Sauté in 2 tablespoons margarine until browned.

Yield: 3 servings

1 serving contains:

Cal	Prot	Fat	Carb	Sat	Mono	Poly	Chol	Na
231	18	12.4	11	2.3	5.2	3.8	36	40

Exchanges: 1 serving = 1½ meats, 1 bread, 1½ fats
Recommended for: The Living Heart; Diabetic; Types IIa, IIb, III, and IV Diets

Curried Tuna

1½ cups chopped celery
½ cup slivered unsalted almonds
¼ cup low-sodium corn oil margarine
¼ cup flour
½ teaspoon curry powder
¼ teaspoon pepper
2 cups skim milk
2 cans (6½ ounces each) low-sodium, water-packed tuna, drained
1 can (13¼ ounces) pineapple chunks, packed in its own juice, drained

1. Sauté celery and almonds in margarine in a large saucepan.

2. Blend in flour, curry powder, and pepper until mixture is smooth. Remove from heat and stir in milk.

3. Return to flame and heat to boiling; stir 1 minute.

4. Add tuna and pineapple and heat thoroughly.

5. Serve over rice, if desired.

Yield: 6 servings

1 serving contains:

Cal	Prot	Fat	Carb	Sat	Mono	Poly	Chol	Na
209	7	13.2	17	1.9	6.9	3.5	5	79

Exchanges: 1 serving = 1 meat, 1 bread, 2 fats
Recommended for: The Living Heart; Diabetic; Types IIa, IIb, III, and IV Diets

Tuna Macaroni Casserole*

2 tablespoons chopped celery
¼ cup chopped onion
2 tablespoons chopped green pepper
1 tablespoon oil
1 tablespoon flour
¼ teaspoon pepper
1 cup skim milk
½ cup cubed low-sodium low-fat cheese
1 cup unsalted cooked elbow macaroni
2 fresh tomatoes, chopped
1 can (6½ ounces) low-sodium, water-packed tuna, drained
2 tablespoons chopped fresh parsley
1 tablespoon lemon juice
paprika

1. Preheat oven to 375°F.

2. Sauté celery, onion, and green pepper in oil until tender. Stir in flour and pepper until smooth.

3. Gradually stir in milk and cook, stirring constantly, until thickened. Add cheese and stir until melted.

4. Add macaroni, tomatoes, tuna, parsley, and lemon juice, and pour into casserole. Sprinkle with paprika and bake 30–35 minutes.

Yield: 4 servings

1 serving contains:

Cal	Prot	Fat	Carb	Sat	Mono	Poly	Chol	Na
225	21	8.1	17	1.1	2.0	4.5	29	154*

Exchanges: 1 serving = 2½ meats, 1 bread
Recommended for: The Living Heart; Diabetic; Types IIa, IIb, III, and IV Diets

*Limit to 1 serving daily due to sodium content.

Abbreviations: **Cal,** calories; **Prot,** protein; **Carb,** carbohydrate; **Sat,** saturated fat; **Mono,** monounsaturated fat; **Poly,** polyunsaturated fat; **Chol,** cholesterol; **Na,** sodium. Protein, fat, carbohydrate, saturated fat, monounsaturated fat, and polyunsaturated fat are expressed in *grams*. Cholesterol and sodium are expressed in *milligrams*.

POULTRY ENTRÉES

Hearty Chicken Stew with Dumplings

  1 chicken fryer (2–3 pounds), cut up, skin and fat removed
2¼ cups water
  1 can (16 ounces) low-sodium tomatoes, undrained
  2 onions, quartered
  4 stalks celery, cut into 1-inch pieces
  ½ teaspoon pepper
  ¼ teaspoon dried thyme
  1 bay leaf
  2 tablespoons cornstarch

  Dumplings
1½ cups flour
1½ tablespoons low-sodium baking powder
  2 tablespoons chopped fresh parsley
  ¾ cup skim milk

1. Simmer chicken, 2 cups water, tomatoes, onion, celery, pepper, thyme, and bay leaf in large saucepan or Dutch oven for 2 hours.
2. Remove from heat and chill.
3. Remove fat from the surface and bone chicken.
4. Combine ¼ cup cold water and cornstarch, and add to chicken mixture. Reheat to boiling.
5. Combine dumpling ingredients and drop from a tablespoon onto boiling chicken.
6. Cover and steam 20 minutes.

Yield: 6 servings

1 serving contains:

Cal	Prot	Fat	Carb	Sat	Mono	Poly	Chol	Na
271	22	4.2	36	1.1	1.1	1.2	52	100

Exchanges: 1 serving = 2½ meats, 1½ breads, 1 vegetable
Recommended for: The Living Heart; Diabetic; Types I, IIa, IIb, III, IV, and V Diets

Acapulco Chicken

  2 onions, finely chopped
  ¼ cup oil
  ½ teaspoon garlic powder
  ½ teaspoon pepper
  1 chicken fryer (2–3 pounds), cut up, skin and fat removed
  4 fresh tomatoes, chopped
  1 fresh jalapeño pepper, seeded and finely chopped
  ½ teaspoon ground cumin
  ½ teaspoon cayenne pepper
  2 cups low-sodium chicken bouillon
  1 cup rice, uncooked

1. Sauté onion in oil. Remove from pan.
2. Rub garlic powder and pepper into chicken. Brown seasoned chicken in oil.
3. Return onion to pan and add tomatoes, jalapeño, cumin, cayenne, and bouillon. Heat to boiling and simmer 20 minutes.
4. Add rice, cover, and cook until rice and chicken are tender and liquid has been absorbed.

Yield: 4 servings

1 serving contains:

Cal	Prot	Fat	Carb	Sat	Mono	Poly	Chol	Na
480	29	19.4	46	3.3	5.1	9.4	78	85

Exchanges: 1 serving = 3 meats, 3 breads, 2 fats
Recommended for: The Living Heart; Diabetic; Types IIa, IIb, III, and IV Diets

Citrus Chicken with Gravy

  ½ cup flour
  2 teaspoons grated orange peel
  1 teaspoon paprika
  ¼ teaspoon pepper
  1 chicken fryer (2–3 pounds), cut up, skin and fat removed
  1 tablespoon low-sodium corn oil margarine
  ¾ cup water
1½ cups orange juice
  1 tablespoon brown sugar, firmly packed
  ⅛ teaspoon ground ginger

1. Combine flour, orange peel, paprika, and pepper. Reserve 1–2 tablespoons for gravy and coat chicken with remaining mixture.
2. Brown chicken in margarine over low heat.
3. Add water, cover, and simmer 30 minutes. Add more water if needed.
4. Remove chicken and keep warm. Remove fat from drippings.
5. Stir reserved flour into drippings. Add orange juice, sugar, and ginger. Cook, stirring constantly, until gravy boils.

Yield: 4 servings

1 serving contains:

Cal	Prot	Fat	Carb	Sat	Mono	Poly	Chol	Na
293	26	8.6	26	2.1	2.8	2.3	78	76

Exchanges: 1 serving = 3 meats, 1 bread, 1 fruit
Recommended for: The Living Heart; Diabetic; Types IIa, IIb, III, IV, and V Diets

Chicken Italiano

 1 **chicken fryer (2–3 pounds), cut up, skin and fat removed**
 ¼ **teaspoon pepper**
 ¼ **cup flour**
 ¼ **cup oil**
 1 **medium onion, chopped**
 ½ **cup dry white wine**
 1 **can (16 ounces) low-sodium tomatoes, undrained**
 1 **clove garlic, minced**
 1 **tablespoon chopped fresh parsley**
 1 **teaspoon dried sweet basil**
 ½ **teaspoon pepper**
 1 **teaspoon dried oregano**
 ¼ **cup fresh mushrooms, sliced**

1. Season the chicken pieces with pepper and coat with flour. Brown chicken on all sides in oil.
2. Add remaining ingredients except mushrooms to pan. Cover and cook 30 minutes.
3. Add mushrooms and cook 5 minutes more or until chicken and mushrooms are tender.

Yield: 4 servings

1 serving contains:

Cal	Prot	Fat	Carb	Sat	Mono	Poly	Chol	Na
336	26	19.3	14	3.3	4.9	9.5	78	80

Exchanges: 1 serving = 3 meats, 1 bread, 2 fats
Recommended for: The Living Heart; Diabetic; Types IIa, IIb, III, and IV Diets
For Low Calorie Diets, omit flour and decrease oil to 2 tablespoons. Count as 3 meats, ½ bread, 1 fat (254 calories).

Chicken Cacciatore

 1 **chicken fryer (2–3 pounds), cut up, skin and fat removed**
 ¼ **cup flour**
 2 **tablespoons oil**
 1 **onion, chopped**
 1 **green pepper, chopped**
 1 **clove garlic, minced**
 ¼ **teaspoon pepper**
 1 **teaspoon dried oregano**
 2 **bay leaves, crushed**
 2 **tablespoons chopped fresh parsley**
 1 **can (16 ounces) low-sodium tomatoes, undrained**
 1 **can (6 ounces) low-sodium tomato paste**
 ¼ **cup dry white wine**

1. Coat chicken pieces with flour and brown in oil. Remove from pan.
2. Sauté onion, green pepper, and garlic in pan for about 3 minutes.
3. Add remaining ingredients, cover, and simmer 30 minutes or until chicken is tender.

Yield: 4 servings

1 serving contains:

Cal	Prot	Fat	Carb	Sat	Mono	Poly	Chol	Na
318	28	12.8	24	2.5	3.3	5.6	78	88

Exchanges: 1 serving = 3 meats, 1 bread, 1 vegetable, 1 fat
Recommended for: The Living Heart; Diabetic; Types IIa, IIb, III, and IV Diets

Abbreviations: **Cal,** calories; **Prot,** protein; **Carb,** carbohydrate; **Sat,** saturated fat; **Mono,** monounsaturated fat; **Poly,** polyunsaturated fat; **Chol,** cholesterol; **Na,** sodium. Protein, fat, carbohydrate, saturated fat, monounsaturated fat, and polyunsaturated fat are expressed in *grams.* Cholesterol and sodium are expressed in *milligrams.*

Jalapeño Pepper Chicken

1 **chicken fryer (2–3 pounds), cut up, skin and fat removed**
3 **tablespoons oil**
1 **onion, sliced into rings**
1½ **cups low-sodium chicken bouillon**
½ **teaspoon ground nutmeg**
¼ **teaspoon pepper**
2 **teaspoons finely chopped and seeded fresh jalapeño pepper**

1. Brown chicken pieces in oil. When browned, remove and set aside.
2. Sauté onion rings in the oil. Add bouillon and bring to a boil, stirring often.
3. Return chicken to pan and add nutmeg and pepper. Cover and simmer for 35 minutes or until chicken is tender.
4. Stir in jalapeño pepper and simmer 1 minute more.

Yield: 4 servings

1 serving contains:

Cal	Prot	Fat	Carb	Sat	Mono	Poly	Chol	Na
252	25	15.7	3	2.9	4.1	7.2	78	77

Exchanges: 1 serving = 3 meats, 1½ fats
Recommended for: The Living Heart; Diabetic; Types IIa, IIb, III, and IV Diets

Lemon Baked Chicken

1 **chicken fryer (2–3 pounds), cut up, skin and fat removed**
2 **tablespoons lemon juice**
3 **tablespoons oil**
2 **cloves garlic, minced**
¼ **teaspoon pepper**
¼ **teaspoon paprika**
¼ **teaspoon dried thyme**
3 **tablespoons chopped fresh parsley**

1. Preheat oven to 350°F.
2. Arrange chicken in a shallow baking dish.
3. Combine remaining ingredients and pour over chicken.
4. Cover and bake 40 minutes.

5. Uncover and cook an additional 20 minutes or until brown.
May be prepared ahead and frozen.

Yield: 4 servings

1 serving contains:

Cal	Prot	Fat	Carb	Sat	Mono	Poly	Chol	Na
242	24	15.6	1	2.8	4.1	7.2	78	73

Exchanges: 1 serving = 3 meats, 1½ fats
Recommended for: The Living Heart; Diabetic; Types IIa, IIb, III, and IV Diets

Crispy Corny Baked Chicken

1 **chicken fryer (2–3 pounds), cut up, skin and fat removed**
½ **teaspoon paprika**
½ **teaspoon pepper**
1 **cup skim milk**
1 **cup low-sodium cornflake crumbs**

1. Preheat oven to 400°F.
2. Season chicken pieces with paprika and pepper. Dip in milk and roll in crumbs. Place in lightly oiled baking dish. Be sure that pieces do not touch.
3. Bake 45 minutes or until tender.

Yield: 4 servings

1 serving contains:

Cal	Prot	Fat	Carb	Sat	Mono	Poly	Chol	Na
249	28	6.4	17	1.8	2.0	1.4	79	108

Exchanges: 1 serving = 3 meats, 1 bread
Recommended for: The Living Heart; Low Calorie; Diabetic; Types I, IIa, IIb, III, IV, and V Diets

Chicken Divan

2 tablespoons low-sodium corn oil margarine
2 tablespoons flour
1½ cups low-sodium chicken bouillon
⅓ cup sliced fresh mushrooms
2 tablespoons white wine
¼ teaspoon pepper
1 package (10 ounces) frozen asparagus spears, thawed
4 chicken breast halves, skin and fat removed, cooked and boned
1 tablespoon chopped fresh parsley
2 tablespoons fine, dry low-sodium bread crumbs

1. Preheat oven to 375°F.
2. Melt the margarine in a small saucepan. Stir in flour and cook 1 minute.
3. Add chicken bouillon and cook until thickened.
4. Add mushrooms, wine, and pepper.
5. Place asparagus spears in a shallow baking dish or four individual casseroles. Add chicken and top with sauce. Sprinkle with parsley and bread crumbs.
6. Bake 20 minutes.

Yield: 4 servings

1 serving contains:

Cal	Prot	Fat	Carb	Sat	Mono	Poly	Chol	Na
192	19	10.0	7	2.1	3.6	2.8	52	52

Exchanges: 1 serving = 2½ meats, ½ bread
Recommended for: The Living Heart; Low Calorie; Diabetic; Types IIa, IIb, III, IV, and V Diets

Fat-Free Fried Chicken

4 deboned split chicken breasts, skin removed
1 teaspoon natural low-sodium vegetable seasoning
½ teaspoon pepper

1. Sprinkle vegetable seasoning and pepper on both sides of chicken. Place in frying pan with non-stick surface and cover. Cook on medium heat 10 to 15 minutes.

2. Turn chicken and continue cooking on medium heat about 10 minutes.
3. Remove lid and allow moisture to evaporate and chicken to brown.

Yield: 4 servings

1 serving contains:

Cal	Prot	Fat	Carb	Sat	Mono	Poly	Chol	Na
141	27	2.9	0	0.9	0.8	0.6	67	55

Exchanges: 1 serving = 3 meats
Recommended for: The Living Heart; Low Calorie; Diabetic; Types I, IIa, IIb, III, IV, and V Diets

Chicken and Rice Salad

2 cups cooked unsalted rice, cooled
2 cups chopped cooked chicken
1 can (16 ounces) low-sodium peas, drained
1 cup chopped celery
1 cup chopped green pepper
2 tablespoons finely chopped onion
¾ cup low-sodium mayonnaise
½ teaspoon pepper
2 tablespoons lemon juice
2 tablespoons chopped fresh parsley

1. Combine rice, chicken, peas, celery, green pepper, and onion.
2. Combine remaining ingredients and toss with chicken mixture.
3. Chill well before serving.

Yield: 8 servings

1 serving contains:

Cal	Prot	Fat	Carb	Sat	Mono	Poly	Chol	Na
305	13	19.1	20	3.6	4.3	9.1	47	56

Exchanges: 1 serving = 1 meat, 1½ breads, 3 fats
Recommended for: The Living Heart; Diabetic; Types IIa, IIb, III, and IV Diets

---

Abbreviations: **Cal,** calories; **Prot,** protein; **Carb,** carbohydrate; **Sat,** saturated fat; **Mono,** monounsaturated fat; **Poly,** polyunsaturated fat; **Chol,** cholesterol; **Na,** sodium. Protein, fat, carbohydrate, saturated fat, monounsaturated fat, and polyunsaturated fat are expressed in *grams.* Cholesterol and sodium are expressed in *milligrams.*

Chicken Crêpes*

½ cup chopped onion
16 fresh mushrooms, sliced
2 tablespoons oil
6 tablespoons flour
1 low-sodium chicken bouillon cube
¼ teaspoon pepper
¼ cup chopped fresh parsley
3 cups skim milk
⅓ cup white wine
3½ cups chopped cooked chicken
9 Basic Crêpes (see recipe, page 275)

1. Preheat oven to 350°F.
2. Sauté onion and mushrooms in oil.
3. Stir in flour. Add bouillon cube, pepper, and parsley.
4. Gradually stir in milk and cook, stirring constantly, until mixture thickens.
5. Stir in wine and cook 5 minutes longer.
6. Add half of sauce mixture to chicken.
7. Place ¼ cup of the chicken mixture on each crêpe. Roll crêpes and place seam side down in a 9 × 13-inch baking dish. Top with remaining sauce.
8. Cover and bake 20–30 minutes.

Yield: 9 crêpes

1 crêpe contains:

Cal	Prot	Fat	Carb	Sat	Mono	Poly	Chol	Na
256	23	9.5	19	2.0	2.8	3.7	52	133*

Exchanges: 1 crêpe = 3 meats, 1 bread
Recommended for: The Living Heart; Low Calorie; Diabetic; Types IIa, IIb, III, IV, and V Diets

*Limit to 1 serving daily due to sodium content.

Chicken Gumbo

2 cups chopped cooked chicken
2 tablespoons oil
1 can (16 ounces) low-sodium tomatoes, undrained
1 package (10 ounces) frozen okra
½ cup low-sodium chicken bouillon
1 cup sliced onion
1 fresh jalapeño pepper, seeded
½ cup chopped fresh parsley
½ teaspoon pepper
1 bay leaf
2 cloves garlic, minced
¼ teaspoon dried thyme
1 cup water
½ cup rice, uncooked

1. Brown chicken in oil in large saucepan.
2. Add all ingredients except rice.
3. Cover and simmer 10 minutes.
4. Add rice and cook 25 minutes more until rice is tender, stirring occasionally.

Yield: 6 servings

1 serving contains:

Cal	Prot	Fat	Carb	Sat	Mono	Poly	Chol	Na
240	17	7.9	26	1.5	2.0	3.6	43	48

Exchanges: 1 serving = 1½ meats, 1½ breads, 1 fat
Recommended for: The Living Heart; Diabetic; Types IIa, IIb, III, and IV Diets

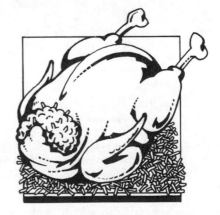

Stuffed Cornish Hens*

¼ **cup chopped celery**
¼ **cup chopped green pepper**
¼ **cup chopped onion**
¼ **cup plus 3 tablespoons low-sodium corn oil margarine**
¼ **teaspoon ground sage**
1 **clove garlic, minced**
⅛ **teaspoon pepper**
1 **tablespoon chopped fresh parsley**
1 **cup fine dry low-sodium bread crumbs**
¼ **cup chopped unsalted walnuts**
¼ **cup low-sodium low-fat cheese, cubed**
4 **Rock Cornish hens**

1. Preheat oven to 350°F.
2. Sauté celery, green pepper, and onion in 3 tablespoons margarine until celery is tender.
3. Stir in sage, garlic, pepper, parsley, and bread crumbs. Remove from heat.
4. Add walnuts and cheese, and spoon mixture into cavities of Cornish hens.
5. Brush hens with remaining margarine that has been melted.
6. Bake breast side up in a shallow pan for 60 minutes. Baste occasionally with the melted margarine.
7. Remove skin and fat before eating.

Yield: 4 servings

1 serving contains:

Cal	Prot	Fat	Carb	Sat	Mono	Poly	Chol	Na
621	60	33.6	17	6.4	11.9	12.1	135	173*

Exchanges: 1 serving = 6½ meats, 1½ breads, 2 fats
Recommended for: The Living Heart; Diabetic; Types IIa, IIb, III, and IV Diets

*Limit to 1 serving daily due to sodium content.

VEAL ENTRÉES

Veal Scallopini

2 **tablespoons flour**
¼ **teaspoon pepper**
¼ **teaspoon dried sweet basil**
¼ **teaspoon dried oregano**
1 **pound veal cutlets, well trimmed**
2 **tablespoons oil**
1 **onion, chopped**
1 **clove garlic, minced**
½ **cup white wine**
½ **pound fresh mushrooms**
¼ **cup chopped fresh parsley**
 paprika (optional)

1. Combine flour, pepper, basil, and oregano. Coat veal with flour mixture and brown in oil.
2. Add onion, garlic, and wine. Cover and cook 20 minutes.
3. Add more wine if necessary.
4. Add mushrooms and parsley, cover, and cook 5–10 minutes longer, until meat and mushrooms are tender.
5. Garnish with paprika, if desired.

Yield: 4 servings

1 serving contains:

Cal	Prot	Fat	Carb	Sat	Mono	Poly	Chol	Na
267	28	13.1	8	3.0	3.6	4.4	78	68

Exchanges: 1 serving = 3 meats, ½ bread, 1 fat
Recommended for: The Living Heart; Diabetic; Types IIa, IIb, III, and IV Diets
For Low Calorie Diets, omit flour and decrease oil to 1 tablespoon. Count as 3 meats, 1½ vegetables (221 calories).

Abbreviations: **Cal,** calories; **Prot,** protein; **Carb,** carbohydrate; **Sat,** saturated fat; **Mono,** monounsaturated fat; **Poly,** polyunsaturated fat; **Chol,** cholesterol; **Na,** sodium. Protein, fat, carbohydrate, saturated fat, monounsaturated fat, and polyunsaturated fat are expressed in *grams.* Cholesterol and sodium are expressed in *milligrams.*

Braised Veal

¼ cup flour
½ teaspoon pepper
2 pounds veal cutlets, well trimmed
2 tablespoons oil
2 onions, cut into rings
2 cloves garlic, minced
½ cup water
2 tablespoons lemon juice
1 teaspoon dried oregano
2 tablespoons chopped fresh parsley

1. Combine flour and pepper and coat veal with mixture. Brown veal on both sides in oil. Remove veal from pan.
2. Sauté onion and garlic until tender.
3. Return veal to pan and add remaining ingredients. Cover pan.
4. Simmer over low heat for 30 minutes. Add more water if needed.

Yield: 8 servings

1 serving contains:

Cal	Prot	Fat	Carb	Sat	Mono	Poly	Chol	Na
217	26	9.5	5	2.6	2.7	2.2	78	59

Exchanges: 1 serving = 3 meats, ½ bread
Recommended for: The Living Heart; Diabetic; Types IIa, IIb, III, and IV Diets

Veal Birds

⅓ cup finely chopped celery
¼ cup finely chopped unsalted walnuts
1½ pounds thinly sliced veal cutlets, well trimmed
¼ cup flour
½ teaspoon pepper
½ teaspoon garlic powder
½ teaspoon paprika
1 tablespoon low-sodium corn oil margarine
1 cup low-sodium beef bouillon
⅓ cup sliced fresh mushrooms

1. Mix celery and walnuts and place 2 tablespoons on each veal cutlet. Roll each cutlet up like a jelly roll and secure with toothpicks.

2. Mix flour and seasonings and coat rolls with seasoned flour.
3. Brown veal lightly on all sides in margarine.
4. Add bouillon. Cover and simmer until tender, about 45 minutes. Turn meat occasionally. Add water if needed.
5. Add mushrooms and heat through.

Yield: 6 servings

1 serving contains:

Cal	Prot	Fat	Carb	Sat	Mono	Poly	Chol	Na
236	27	11.2	5	2.9	3.2	3.0	78	66

Exchanges: 1 serving = 3 meats, 1 vegetable, ½ fat
Recommended for: The Living Heart; Diabetic; Types IIa, IIb, III, and IV Diets

Roast Veal

3 pound veal leg or shoulder roast, well trimmed
1 large onion cut into small chunks
2 cloves garlic, sliced
  ground ginger
  pepper
2 cups water
¼ cup lemon juice
¼ teaspoon dried marjoram

1. Preheat oven to 325°F.
2. Make small, deep cuts in veal to insert onion and garlic.
3. Rub roast with ginger and pepper. Place in baking dish.
4. Pour remaining ingredients over roast.
5. Roast 35 minutes per pound.

Yield: 8 servings

1 serving contains:

Cal	Prot	Fat	Carb	Sat	Mono	Poly	Chol	Na
188	24	8.8	2	3.4	3.3	0.5	78	58

Exchanges: 1 serving = 3 meats
Recommended for: The Living Heart; Low Calorie; Diabetic; Types I, IIa, IIb, III, IV, and V Diets

Veal Curry

1   **cup sliced onion**
½   **cup chopped celery**
1   **medium apple, cored and sliced**
3   **tablespoons low-sodium corn oil margarine**
2   **cups chopped cooked veal, well trimmed**
4   **teaspoons flour**
1   **teaspoon curry powder**
1   **cup low-sodium beef bouillon**
1   **tablespoon lemon juice**
¼   **teaspoon pepper**

1. Sauté onion, celery, and apple in margarine until tender. Remove from pan.
2. Lightly brown veal in the same pan. When browned remove from pan.
3. Stir in flour, curry powder, and bouillon until smooth. Add lemon juice and pepper.
4. Return vegetables, apple, and veal to pan, and heat thoroughly.
5. Serve over rice if desired.

Yield: 4 servings

1 serving contains:

Cal	Prot	Fat	Carb	Sat	Mono	Poly	Chol	Na
231	19	12.9	10	3.1	5.0	3.0	52	60

Exchanges: 1 serving = 2 meats, ½ bread, 1½ fats
Recommended for: The Living Heart; Diabetic; Types IIa, IIb, III, and IV Diets

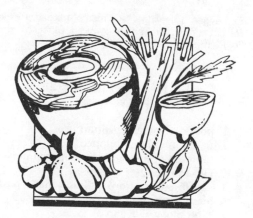

GROUND BEEF ENTRÉES

Spaghetti Sauce

1   **pound very lean ground beef**
1   **onion, chopped**
1   **green pepper, finely chopped**
1   **clove garlic, minced**
¼   **cup chopped fresh parsley**
½   **teaspoon dried oregano**
1   **teaspoon dried sweet basil**
¼   **teaspoon fennel seeds**
1   **can (16 ounces) low-sodium tomatoes, undrained**
1   **can (6 ounces) low-sodium tomato paste**
1½   **cups water**
1   **bay leaf**
2   **tablespoons sugar**
¼   **teaspoon pepper**

1. Brown meat, onion, and green pepper. Drain off fat.
2. Add all other ingredients.
3. Cover and simmer about 2 hours, stirring occasionally.

Yield: 6 servings

1 serving contains:

Cal	Prot	Fat	Carb	Sat	Mono	Poly	Chol	Na
190	18	6.2	16	2.3	2.2	0.6	52	49

Exchanges: 1 serving = 2 meats, 1 bread
Recommended for: The Living Heart; Low Calorie; Diabetic; Types I, IIa, IIb, III, IV, and V Diets

Abbreviations: **Cal,** calories; **Prot,** protein; **Carb,** carbohydrate; **Sat,** saturated fat; **Mono,** monounsaturated fat; **Poly,** polyunsaturated fat; **Chol,** cholesterol; **Na,** sodium. Protein, fat, carbohydrate, saturated fat, monounsaturated fat, and polyunsaturated fat are expressed in *grams.* Cholesterol and sodium are expressed in *milligrams.*

Main Dish Meatballs

    1 pound very lean ground beef
    ¼ teaspoon garlic powder
    1 medium onion, finely chopped
    ¼ cup skim milk
    ¼ teaspoon pepper
    ¼ cup wheat germ
    1 teaspoon dry mustard
    1 egg white
    2 low-sodium beef bouillon cubes
 1½ cups plus 1 tablespoon water
    2 teaspoons chopped fresh parsley
    1 tablespoon cornstarch

1. Mix together beef, garlic powder, onion, milk, pepper, wheat germ, dry mustard, and egg white.
2. Form into 12 meatballs and brown on all sides. Drain off fat.
3. Add bouillon cubes, 1½ cups water, and parsley. Cover and cook 20 minutes.
4. Stir cornstarch into 1 tablespoon cold water and add to meatballs to make a gravy.

Yield: 4 servings

1 serving contains:

Cal	Prot	Fat	Carb	Sat	Mono	Poly	Chol	Na
232	28	9.5	7	3.6	3.4	0.9	78	80

Exchanges: 1 serving = 3½ meats, ½ bread
Recommended for: The Living Heart; Diabetic; Types IIa, IIb, III, IV, and V Diets

Applesauce Meat Loaf

 1½ pounds very lean ground beef
    ¾ cup fine, dry low-sodium bread crumbs
    ½ cup applesauce
    ½ cup low-sodium catsup
    1 teaspoon ground sage
    1 teaspoon pepper

1. Preheat oven to 350°F.
2. Combine all ingredients and place in a 9 × 5-inch loaf pan.
3. Bake for 90 minutes.

Yield: 8 servings

1 serving contains:

Cal	Prot	Fat	Carb	Sat	Mono	Poly	Chol	Na
198	19	7.0	14	2.6	2.6	0.5	58	47

Exchanges: 1 serving = 2 meats, 1 bread
Recommended for: The Living Heart; Low Calorie; Types IIa, IIb, III, IV, and V Diets

Lemon Meat Loaf

 1½ pounds very lean ground beef
    1 cup fine, dry low-sodium bread crumbs
    ¼ cup lemon juice
    ¼ cup finely chopped onion
       egg substitute equivalent to 1 egg
    ½ cup low-sodium catsup
    ⅓ cup brown sugar, firmly packed
    1 teaspoon dry mustard
    ¼ teaspoon ground allspice
    ¼ teaspoon ground cloves

1. Preheat oven to 350°F.
2. Combine all ingredients and place in a 9 × 5-inch loaf pan.
3. Bake for 60 minutes.

Yield: 8 servings

1 serving contains:

Cal	Prot	Fat	Carb	Sat	Mono	Poly	Chol	Na
239	21	7.5	21	2.7	2.8	0.8	58	64

Exchanges: 1 serving = 2½ meats, 1 bread, 1 vegetable
Recommended for: The Living Heart; Diabetic; Types IIa, IIb, III, IV, and V Diets

Quick Beef Barbecue

    1 pound very lean ground beef
    1 medium onion, chopped
    1 tablespoon low-sodium prepared mustard
    ½ cup low-sodium catsup
    1 can (6 ounces) low-sodium tomato paste
    ¼ teaspoon ground cloves
    1 tablespoon vinegar
    2 teaspoons sugar
    ½ teaspoon garlic powder
    ½ teaspoon pepper
    ⅛ teaspoon liquid smoke

1. Brown meat and onion. Drain off fat.
2. Add remaining ingredients.
3. Simmer for 15 minutes.

Yield: 4 servings

1 serving contains:

Cal	Prot	Fat	Carb	Sat	Mono	Poly	Chol	Na
279	27	9.2	22	3.5	3.3	0.7	78	72

Exchanges: 1 serving = 3 meats, 1 bread, 1 vegetable
Recommended for: The Living Heart; Diabetic; Types IIa, IIb, III, IV, and V Diets

Chili

1	**pound very lean ground beef**
1½	**cups chopped onion**
1¼	**cups water**
1	**can (6 ounces) low-sodium tomato paste**
4	**teaspoons chili powder**
½	**green pepper, chopped**
1	**bay leaf (optional)**
⅛	**teaspoon dried sweet basil (optional)**

1. Brown meat and onion. Drain off fat.
2. Add remaining ingredients.
3. Cover and simmer 30 minutes, stirring occasionally.

Yield: 4 servings

1 serving contains:

Cal	Prot	Fat	Carb	Sat	Mono	Poly	Chol	Na
249	27	9.0	15	3.5	3.3	0.7	78	72

Exchanges: 1 serving = 3 meats, 1 bread
Recommended for: The Living Heart; Diabetic; Types IIa, IIb, III, IV, and V Diets

Variation:

Chili with Beans: Add 3 cups cooked, unsalted kidney beans. Makes 6 servings.

1 serving contains:

Cal	Prot	Fat	Carb	Sat	Mono	Poly	Chol	Na
281	25	6.5	31	2.4	2.2	0.7	52	52

Exchanges: 1 serving = 2½ meats, 2 breads
Recommended for: The Living Heart; Diabetic; Types IIa, IIb, III, IV, and V Diets

Tamale Pie*

1	**pound very lean ground beef**
2	**medium onions, chopped**
1	**large green pepper, chopped**
2	**cans (6 ounces each) low-sodium tomato paste**
2½	**cups water**
1	**can (8 ounces) low-sodium whole kernel corn, drained**
⅛	**teaspoon garlic powder**
2	**teaspoons sugar**
3	**teaspoons chili powder**
⅛	**teaspoon pepper**
¾	**cup yellow cornmeal**
1	**tablespoon low-sodium corn oil margarine**
1	**cup low-sodium low-fat cheese, cubed**

1. Preheat oven to 375°F.
2. Brown ground beef, onion, and green pepper in a large skillet. Drain off fat. Stir in tomato paste, ½ cup water, corn, garlic, sugar, chili powder, and pepper. Simmer until thick, about 20 minutes.
3. While meat mixture is simmering, stir cornmeal into 2 cups of cold water in saucepan. Cook until thick, stirring constantly. Stir in margarine. Stir cheese into meat mixture and turn into an oiled 9 × 9-inch baking dish.
4. Spoon thickened cornmeal over meat mixture.
5. Bake for 40 minutes.

Yield: 6 servings

1 serving contains:

Cal	Prot	Fat	Carb	Sat	Mono	Poly	Chol	Na
376	27	13.7	36	3.5	4.4	4.4	53	184*

Exchanges: 1 serving = 3 meats, ½ dairy, 2 breads, ½ fat
Recommended for: The Living Heart; Diabetic; Types IIa, IIb, III, and IV Diets

*Limit to 1 serving daily due to sodium content.

Abbreviations: **Cal,** calories; **Prot,** protein; **Carb,** carbohydrate; **Sat,** saturated fat; **Mono,** monounsaturated fat; **Poly,** polyunsaturated fat; **Chol,** cholesterol; **Na,** sodium. Protein, fat, carbohydrate, saturated fat, monounsaturated fat, and polyunsaturated fat are expressed in *grams.* Cholesterol and sodium are expressed in *milligrams.*

Pizza

Dough
1 package active dry yeast
1⅔ cups lukewarm water (95–105°F)
3 tablespoons oil
4 cups flour

Tomato Sauce
1 cup finely chopped onion
3 tablespoons oil
2 cloves garlic, minced
2 cans (16 ounces each) low-sodium tomatoes, undrained, chopped
1 can (6 ounces) low-sodium tomato paste
4 teaspoons dried oregano
2 teaspoons dried sweet basil
2 bay leaves

Topping
8 ounces low-sodium low-fat cheese
½ cup chopped green onion
¼ pound fresh mushrooms, chopped
1 cup chopped green pepper
1 pound very lean ground beef or low-sodium Homemade Sausage (see recipe, this page), browned and drained

1. Dissolve yeast in lukewarm water in a bowl. Add oil and stir in flour. Turn onto lightly floured board and knead until smooth. Place dough in an oiled bowl, turning once to coat the surface.
2. Let rise until double in bulk, about 90 minutes. At this point dough can be punched down, refrigerated for a day or two, or frozen for future use.
3. Punch down and knead again for a few minutes.
4. Divide dough in half and pat into two oiled round 14-inch pizza pans.
5. Add tomato sauce (instructions below) and topping ingredients.
6. Bake in a preheated 400°F oven 20–25 minutes.

Sauce (prepare while dough is rising)
1. Sauté onion in oil until soft and tender. Add garlic and cook 2 minutes more. Add remaining ingredients and simmer uncovered for 60 minutes, stirring occasionally.
2. Remove bay leaf. If a smoother sauce is desired, purée or put mixture through a sieve.

Yield: 2 pizzas (8 servings each)

Note: Half of the dough may be frozen after step 3 and half the sauce if only one pizza is desired.

⅛ pizza contains:

Cal	Prot	Fat	Carb	Sat	Mono	Poly	Chol	Na
281	14	11.0	31	2.0	2.9	5.3	20	100

Exchanges: 1 serving = 2 meats, 2 breads, ½ fat
Recommended for: The Living Heart; Diabetic; Types IIa, IIb, III, and IV Diets

Homemade Sausage

1 pound very lean ground beef
1 teaspoon ground sage
½ teaspoon dried thyme
½ teaspoon garlic powder
1 teaspoon black pepper
1 teaspoon liquid smoke
½ teaspoon crushed red pepper

1. Mix all ingredients together thoroughly and shape into patties.
2. Broil or pan fry. If pan frying, pour off fat as it collects.
3. Drain patties on paper towels.

Yield: 6 servings

Variation:
"Hot" Sausage: Increase crushed red pepper to 1 teaspoon.

1 serving contains:

Cal	Prot	Fat	Carb	Sat	Mono	Poly	Chol	Na
123	16	5.8	0	2.3	2.2	0.3	52	38

Exchanges: 1 serving = 2 meats
Recommended for: The Living Heart; Low Calorie; Diabetic; Types I, IIa, IIb, III, IV, and V Diets

BEEF, LAMB, PORK ENTRÉES

Home-Cooked Beef Stew

1½ pounds lean beef, well trimmed, cut into 1-inch cubes
¼ cup flour
¼ cup oil
2½ cups water
¼ cup chopped fresh parsley
1 clove garlic, minced
2 bay leaves
½ teaspoon dried thyme
¼ teaspoon pepper
4 potatoes, peeled and cubed
5 carrots, cut into 1-inch pieces
3 stalks celery, cut into 1-inch pieces
2 onions, cut into eighths or 6 small white onions, halved

1. Coat beef cubes with flour and brown in oil.
2. Add water and simmer 20 minutes.
3. Chill and skim off fat.
4. Add parsley, garlic, bay leaves, thyme, and pepper.
5. Simmer 60 minutes or until meat is tender. Add more water if needed.
6. Add vegetables and cook 30 minutes more or until vegetables are tender.

Yield: 6 servings

1 serving contains:

Cal	Prot	Fat	Carb	Sat	Mono	Poly	Chol	Na
342	29	15.5	22	3.3	4.1	5.8	78	104

Exchanges: 1 serving = 3 meats, 1 bread, 1 vegetable, 1½ fats
Recommended for: The Living Heart; Diabetic; Types IIa, IIb, III, and IV Diets
For Low Calorie Diets, omit flour and decrease oil to 2 tablespoons. Count as 3 meats, 1 bread, 1 vegetable, ½ fat (286 calories).

Garden Kabobs

½ cup oil
½ cup wine vinegar
½ cup chopped onion
½ teaspoon garlic powder
½ teaspoon pepper
2 pounds lean beef or lamb, well trimmed, cut into 1-inch cubes
10–15 small white onions or 4 yellow onions, quartered
1 green pepper, cut into chunks
¼ pound whole fresh mushrooms
10–15 cherry tomatoes

1. Combine oil, vinegar, onion, garlic powder, and pepper. Pour over meat cubes and marinate several hours or overnight.
2. Remove meat from marinade and alternate with vegetables on skewers. Brush with marinade.
3. Broil 6–8 minutes, turning once, until done.

Yield: 8 servings

1 serving contains:

Cal	Prot	Fat	Carb	Sat	Mono	Poly	Chol	Na
253	27	13.0	6	3.0	3.6	4.3	78	65

Exchanges: 1 serving = 3 meats, 1 vegetable, 1 fat
Recommended for: The Living Heart; Diabetic; Types IIa, IIb, III, and IV Diets

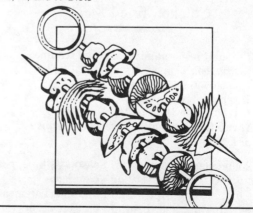

Abbreviations: **Cal,** calories; **Prot,** protein; **Carb,** carbohydrate; **Sat,** saturated fat; **Mono,** monounsaturated fat; **Poly,** polyunsaturated fat; **Chol,** cholesterol; **Na,** sodium. Protein, fat, carbohydrate, saturated fat, monounsaturated fat, and polyunsaturated fat are expressed in *grams.* Cholesterol and sodium are expressed in *milligrams.*

Hungarian Goulash

2 medium onions
2 cloves garlic, minced
2 tablespoons oil
1½ pounds lean beef, well trimmed, cut into 1-inch cubes
⅓ cup chopped green pepper
1 potato, peeled and grated
¼ teaspoon caraway seed
¼ teaspoon crushed red pepper
⅛ teaspoon pepper
1 low-sodium beef bouillon cube
¾ cup water

1. Sauté onion and garlic in oil.
2. Add remaining ingredients and cover.
3. Simmer 3 hours or until meat is tender. Add more water if needed.

Yield: 6 servings

1 serving contains:

Cal	Prot	Fat	Carb	Sat	Mono	Poly	Chol	Na
229	27	10.7	5	2.8	3.0	2.9	78	61

Exchanges: 1 serving = 3 meats, 1 vegetable, ½ fat
Recommended for: The Living Heart; Diabetic; Types IIa, IIb, III, and IV Diets

Chicken Fried Steak

1 pound lean round steak, well trimmed
¼ teaspoon pepper
¼ teaspoon garlic powder
2 egg whites
1 tablespoon skim milk
1 cup fine low-sodium cracker crumbs
3 tablespoons oil

1. Pound steak to tenderize. Season with pepper and garlic. Cut into serving-size pieces.
2. Combine egg whites and skim milk. Dip meat in egg mixture and then into cracker crumbs.
3. Brown coated steak on both sides in oil.
4. Cover and cook over low heat until tender, about 45 minutes.

Yield: 4 servings

1 serving contains:

Cal	Prot	Fat	Carb	Sat	Mono	Poly	Chol	Na
333	29	16.4	16	3.5	4.4	6.2	78	90

Exchanges: 1 serving = 3 meats, 1 bread, 2 fats
Recommended for: The Living Heart; Diabetic; Types IIa, IIb, III, and IV Diets

Burgundy Beef

1 pound lean round steak, well trimmed, sliced into ¼-inch strips
½ teaspoon garlic powder
½ teaspoon pepper
½ teaspoon paprika
2 tablespoons oil
2 tablespoons flour
¼ cup finely chopped onion
¾ cup water
¾ cup burgundy wine
½ cup sliced fresh mushrooms

1. Season steak strips with garlic powder, pepper, and paprika, and brown in oil. Stir in flour.
2. Add remaining ingredients and cover. Simmer until meat is tender, about 45 minutes.

Yield: 4 servings

1 serving contains:

Cal	Prot	Fat	Carb	Sat	Mono	Poly	Chol	Na
251	27	13.0	6	3.1	3.6	4.3	78	59

Exchanges: 1 serving = 3 meats, 1 vegetable, 1 fat
Recommended for: The Living Heart; Diabetic; Types IIa, IIb, III, and IV Diets

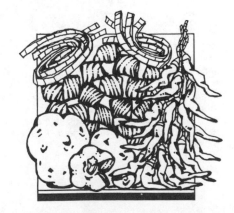

Louisiana Creole Roast

3 pounds lean roast, well trimmed
2 tablespoons oil
½ teaspoon pepper
1 onion, cut into rings
½ cup chopped celery
½ green pepper, cut into rings
2 cans (16 ounces each) low-sodium tomatoes, undrained

1. Brown meat in oil in large pan or Dutch oven.
2. Season with pepper. Add onion rings, celery, and green pepper, stirring until tender.
3. Add tomatoes and cover. Simmer for 1½ to 2 hours until tender or bake in a 325°F oven.
4. Remove fat from drippings and thicken for gravy, if desired.

Yield: 8 servings

1 serving contains:

Cal	Prot	Fat	Carb	Sat	Mono	Poly	Chol	Na
242	26	12.4	6	3.9	4.1	2.7	78	69

Exchanges: 1 serving = 3 meats, 1½ vegetables, ½ fat
Recommended for: The Living Heart; Diabetic; Types IIa, IIb, III, and IV Diets

Curried Lamb

1 pound lean lamb, well-trimmed, cut into 1-inch cubes
1 tablespoon oil
½ cup finely chopped onion
2 teaspoons curry powder
¼ teaspoon pepper
1 teaspoon ground allspice
1 bay leaf
2 teaspoons ground cinnamon
1½ cups water
½ cup raisins

1. Brown meat on all sides in oil.
2. Add remaining ingredients and cook over medium heat 60 minutes or until meat is tender, stirring occasionally.

3. Serve over cooked rice, if desired.

Yield: 4 servings

1 serving contains:

Cal	Prot	Fat	Carb	Sat	Mono	Poly	Chol	Na
277	25	12.2	17	3.9	4.1	2.5	78	64

Exchanges: 1 serving = 3 meats, 1 vegetable, 1 fruit, ½ fat
Recommended for: The Living Heart; Diabetic; Types IIa, IIb, III, and IV Diets
For Low Calorie Diets, omit raisins. Count as 3 meats, 1 vegetable, ½ fat (223 calories).

Barbecued Pork Chops

1 pound lean pork chops, well trimmed
3 slices lemon or 3 tablespoons lemon juice
1 tablespoon brown sugar, firmly packed
⅓ cup low-sodium catsup
¼ cup water

1. Brown chops in skillet without added fat. Drain off fat.
2. Combine remaining ingredients and pour over meat.
3. Cover and simmer 20 minutes. Remove cover and simmer 10 minutes more. Add more water if needed.

Yield: 4 servings

1 serving contains:

Cal	Prot	Fat	Carb	Sat	Mono	Poly	Chol	Na
221	26	8.5	10	2.6	3.5	0.9	75	56

Exchanges: 1 serving = 3 meats, ½ bread
Recommended for: The Living Heart; Low Calorie; Diabetic; Types I, IIa, IIb, III, IV, and V Diets

Abbreviations: **Cal,** calories; **Prot,** protein; **Carb,** carbohydrate; **Sat,** saturated fat; **Mono,** monounsaturated fat; **Poly,** polyunsaturated fat; **Chol,** cholesterol; **Na,** sodium. Protein, fat, carbohydrate, saturated fat, monounsaturated fat, and polyunsaturated fat are expressed in *grams.* Cholesterol and sodium are expressed in *milligrams.*

Glazed Pork Cubes

1   **pound lean pork loin, well trimmed, cut into 1-inch cubes**
1   **tablespoon oil**
3   **tablespoons finely chopped onion**
3   **tablespoons finely chopped green onion**
½   **cup orange juice**
2   **tablespoons lime juice**
2   **tablespoons water**
⅛   **teaspoon dried thyme**
⅛   **teaspoon garlic powder**
¼   **teaspoon pepper**

1. Brown pork cubes in oil.
2. Stir in remaining ingredients and cover.
3. Simmer 30 minutes.
4. Uncover and cook over high heat for 8–10 minutes or until the sauce thickens to a syrupy glaze. Stir frequently.

Yield: 4 servings

1 serving contains:

Cal	Prot	Fat	Carb	Sat	Mono	Poly	Chol	Na
235	26	11.9	6	3.0	4.3	2.8	75	54

Exchanges: 1 serving = 3 meats, 1 vegetable, ½ fat
Recommended for: The Living Heart; Low Calorie; Diabetic; Types IIa, IIb, III, and IV Diets

Pork Skillet Dinner

1½   **pounds lean pork chops, well trimmed**
4   **cups sliced potatoes**
6   **carrots, quartered**
1   **cup sliced onion**
⅔   **cup chopped green pepper**
2   **cans (7¼ ounces each) low-sodium tomato soup**
½   **cup water**

1. Brown pork chops in skillet without added fat. Drain off fat and remove chops from skillet.
2. Layer potatoes, carrots, onions, and green pepper in skillet and place pork chops on top.
3. Combine soup and water, and pour over meat and vegetables.
4. Cover and cook over medium heat 45 minutes or until tender.

Yield: 6 servings

1 serving contains:

Cal	Prot	Fat	Carb	Sat	Mono	Poly	Chol	Na
311	29	8.8	29	2.6	3.5	1.2	75	88

Exchanges: 1 serving = 3 meats, 2 breads
Recommended for: The Living Heart; Diabetic; Types IIa, IIb, III, IV, and V Diets

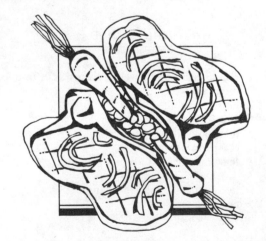

MEATLESS ENTRÉES

Stuffed Onions

6 medium onions, peeled
1 tablespoon low-sodium corn oil margarine, melted
3 tablespoons low-sodium corn oil margarine
¼ cup chopped celery
¼ cup chopped green pepper
¼ teaspoon ground sage
1 clove garlic, minced
⅛ teaspoon pepper
1 tablespoon chopped fresh parsley
1 cup fine, dry low-sodium bread crumbs
¼ cup chopped unsalted walnuts
¼ cup low-sodium low-fat cheese, cubed

1. Preheat oven to 350°F.
2. Cut a thin slice of onion from each end.
3. Pierce each onion from top through center several times with a fork. Place upright, side-by-side (should fit snugly) in a saucepan and cover with water. Cover and simmer 30 minutes or until onions are tender but not soft. Drain.
4. When onions are cool, scoop out centers and set aside.
5. Brush cooked onions with 1 tablespoon melted margarine.
6. Sauté celery, green pepper, and chopped onion centers in remaining margarine until celery is tender. Stir in sage, garlic, pepper, parsley, and bread crumbs.
7. Remove from heat and add nuts and cheese.
8. Spoon mixture into onion cups and bake for 20 minutes.

Yield: 6 servings

1 serving contains:

Cal	Prot	Fat	Carb	Sat	Mono	Poly	Chol	Na
202	5	12.9	18	2.0	4.4	5.5	0	49

Exchanges: 1 serving = ½ meat, 1 bread, 1 vegetable, 2 fats
Recommended for: The Living Heart; Low Calorie; Diabetic; Types IIa, IIb, III, and IV Diets

Stuffed Peppers*

4 green peppers
6 tablespoons chopped onion
2 tablespoons low-sodium corn oil margarine
1 cup long-cooking white rice or brown rice, uncooked
2 cups water
½ teaspoon garlic powder
½ teaspoon pepper
½ teaspoon paprika
1 can (8 ounces) low-sodium tomatoes, undrained
½ teaspoon dried oregano
½ teaspoon dried sweet basil
egg substitute equivalent to 2 eggs
½ of 10-ounce package frozen cut green beans, thawed
½ cup low-sodium low-fat cheese, cubed

1. Preheat oven to 350°F.
2. Cut off top of green peppers. Remove seeds and membrane. Boil in water for 5 minutes and drain.
3. Cook onion in margarine until tender. Add rice, water, garlic powder, pepper, paprika, tomatoes, oregano, and basil. Cover and cook until rice soaks up all of the liquid and is tender.
4. Stir egg substitute, green beans, and cheese into rice mixture.
5. Stuff green peppers and stand upright in a baking dish.
6. Bake for 20 minutes.

Yield: 4 servings

1 serving contains:

Cal	Prot	Fat	Carb	Sat	Mono	Poly	Chol	Na
344	12	10.8	50	1.7	3.8	4.8	1	138*

Exchanges: 1 serving = 1 meat, 3 breads, 1 vegetable, 1½ fats
Recommended for: The Living Heart; Diabetic; Types IIa, IIb, III, and IV Diets

*Limit to 1 serving daily due to sodium content.

Abbreviations: **Cal,** calories; **Prot,** protein; **Carb,** carbohydrate; **Sat,** saturated fat; **Mono,** monounsaturated fat; **Poly,** polyunsaturated fat; **Chol,** cholesterol; **Na,** sodium. Protein, fat, carbohydrate, saturated fat, monounsaturated fat, and polyunsaturated fat are expressed in *grams.* Cholesterol and sodium are expressed in *milligrams.*

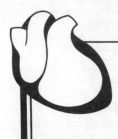

Low-Sodium Vegetables

Green Bean Casserole

1 onion, chopped
½ green pepper, chopped
1 tablespoon oil
1 package (10 ounces) frozen green beans, thawed
1 can (8 ounces) low-sodium tomatoes, drained
⅛ teaspoon crushed red pepper
⅛ teaspoon garlic powder
1 tablespoon low-sodium mayonnaise
¼ cup low-sodium bread crumbs (optional)

1. Preheat oven to 375°F.
2. Sauté onion and green pepper in oil.
3. Add beans, tomatoes, pepper, garlic, and mayonnaise. Stir until heated through.
4. Pour into a baking dish greased with margarine. Sprinkle with bread crumbs and bake 30 minutes.

Yield: 8 servings

1 serving contains:

Cal	Prot	Fat	Carb	Sat	Mono	Poly	Chol	Na
57	1	3.3	6	0.5	0.8	1.8	1	4

Exchanges: 1 serving = 1 vegetable, ½ fat
Recommended for: The Living Heart; Diabetic; Types IIa, IIb, III, and IV Diets

Pinto Beans

1 pound dried pinto beans
4 cups water
4 cans (6 ounces each) low-sodium tomato paste
1 cup chopped onion
½ cup chopped green pepper
8 teaspoons chili powder
½ teaspoon garlic powder
4 teaspoons sugar
1 teaspoon pepper

1. Soak beans in water overnight. Do not drain.
2. Cook beans in water about 60 minutes or until tender.
3. Add remaining ingredients.
4. Simmer 2–3 hours, stirring occasionally.

Yield: 7 cups

½ cup contains:

Cal	Prot	Fat	Carb	Sat	Mono	Poly	Chol	Na
140	8	0.3	28	0.1	0	0.2	0	10

Exchanges: ½ cup = 1 meat, 1 bread, 1 vegetable
Recommended for: The Living Heart; Diabetic; Types I, IIa, IIb, III, IV, and V Diets

Florida Beets*

1 can (16 ounces) low-sodium sliced beets, drained
1 teaspoon grated orange peel
½ cup orange juice concentrate, undiluted
1 tablespoon sugar
1 tablespoon low-sodium corn oil margarine

1. Preheat oven to 350°F.
2. Place beets in a baking dish.
3. Combine all other ingredients and pour over beets.
4. Cover and bake 45 minutes.

Yield: 4 servings

1 serving contains:

Cal	Prot	Fat	Carb	Sat	Mono	Poly	Chol	Na
129	2	3.0	25	0.5	1.2	1.1	0	40*

Exchanges: 1 serving = 1 vegetable, 1½ fruits, 1 fat
Recommended for: The Living Heart; Diabetic; Types IIa, IIb, III, and IV Diets

*Limit to 1 serving daily due to sodium content.

Lemon Broccoli

1 teaspoon sugar
½ teaspoon paprika
¼ teaspoon dry mustard
⅛ teaspoon pepper
1 tablespoon lemon juice
1 tablespoon low-sodium corn oil margarine
1 package (10 ounces) frozen broccoli, cooked without salt, drained

1. Combine all ingredients, except broccoli, in a saucepan until margarine melts.
2. Pour over hot cooked broccoli.

Yield: 4 servings

1 serving contains:

Cal	Prot	Fat	Carb	Sat	Mono	Poly	Chol	Na
49	2	3.1	5	0.5	1.3	1.2	0	11

Exchanges: 1 serving = 1 vegetable, ½ fat
Recommended for: The Living Heart; Diabetic; Types IIa, IIb, III, and IV Diets

Stir-Fried Cabbage

¼ cup chopped onion
1 tablespoon oil
1 pound cabbage, shredded
1 teaspoon sugar
⅛ teaspoon dried tarragon
⅛ teaspoon dried savory
¼ teaspoon pepper

1. Sauté onion in oil.
2. Add cabbage and stir until lightly browned.
3. Add remaining ingredients.
4. Cover and cook until cabbage is tender but not soggy.

Yield: 4 servings

1 serving contains:

Cal	Prot	Fat	Carb	Sat	Mono	Poly	Chol	Na
53	1	3.6	5	0.4	0.8	2.1	0	11

Exchanges: 1 serving = 1 vegetable, ½ fat
Recommended for: The Living Heart; Diabetic; Types IIa, IIb, III, and IV Diets

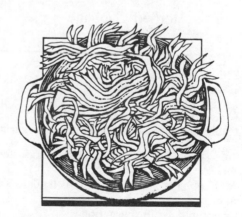

Abbreviations: **Cal,** calories; **Prot,** protein; **Carb,** carbohydrate; **Sat,** saturated fat; **Mono,** monounsaturated fat; **Poly,** polyunsaturated fat; **Chol,** cholesterol; **Na,** sodium. Protein, fat, carbohydrate, saturated fat, monounsaturated fat, and polyunsaturated fat are expressed in *grams.* Cholesterol and sodium are expressed in *milligrams.*

Sweet 'n Sour Red Cabbage

1 **pound red cabbage, cut into 2-inch chunks**
1 **small onion, quartered**
½ **cup water**
⅓ **cup wine vinegar**
3 **tablespoons brown sugar, firmly packed**
¼ **teaspoon pepper**

1. Chop cabbage and onion pieces in a blender.
2. Combine all ingredients in a saucepan. Cover and bring to a boil.
3. Reduce heat and simmer 10–12 minutes, stirring occasionally.

Yield: 4 servings

1 serving contains:

Cal	Prot	Fat	Carb	Sat	Mono	Poly	Chol	Na
64	1	0.2	16	0	0	0.2	0	15

Exchanges: Not applicable for this recipe
Recommended for: The Living Heart and Type IIa Diets

Herbed Cabbage

½ **teaspoon sugar**
¼ **teaspoon dried oregano**
¼ **teaspoon dry mustard**
2 **cups water**
1 **pound cabbage, quartered**
1 **tablespoon low-sodium corn oil margarine**

1. Add sugar, oregano, and mustard to water in a saucepan and bring to a boil.
2. Add cabbage and simmer until tender, 8–10 minutes.
3. Drain and stir in margarine.

Yield: 4 servings

1 serving contains:

Cal	Prot	Fat	Carb	Sat	Mono	Poly	Chol	Na
41	1	3.0	3	0.5	1.2	1.1	0	10

Exchanges: 1 serving = 1 vegetable, ½ fat
Recommended for: The Living Heart; Diabetic; Types IIa, IIb, III, and IV Diets

Glazed Carrots and Raisins

6 **carrots, sliced or julienne cut, partially cooked**
2 **tablespoons low-sodium corn oil margarine**
2 **tablespoons sugar**
½ **cup raisins**
2 **tablespoons lemon juice**

1. Drain carrots when partially cooked.
2. Add remaining ingredients.
3. Cook slowly, stirring constantly, until glazed.

Yield: 6 servings

1 serving contains:

Cal	Prot	Fat	Carb	Sat	Mono	Poly	Chol	Na
110	1	4.0	19	0.7	1.7	1.4	0	29

Exchanges: 1 serving = 1 vegetable, 1 fruit, 1 fat
Recommended for: The Living Heart; Diabetic; Types IIa, IIb, III, and IV Diets

Tangy Buttered Corn

1 **can (16 ounces) low-sodium whole kernel corn**
1 **tablespoon low-sodium prepared mustard**
1 **tablespoon low-sodium corn oil margarine**

1. Heat corn. Drain off some of liquid.
2. Stir in mustard and margarine and heat through.

Yield: 4 servings

1 serving contains:

Cal	Prot	Fat	Carb	Sat	Mono	Poly	Chol	Na
105	2	3.6	15	0.7	1.3	1.3	0	2

Exchanges: 1 serving = 1 bread, ½ fat
Recommended for: The Living Heart; Diabetic; Types IIa, IIb, III, and IV Diets

Ratatouille

4 cloves garlic, minced
4 onions, thinly sliced
3 tablespoons oil
4 green peppers, cut in strips
4 zucchini squash, chopped
1 eggplant, peeled and chopped
6 fresh tomatoes, quartered
½ teaspoon pepper
½ teaspoon dried oregano
½ teaspoon dried sweet basil

1. Sauté garlic and onions in oil.
2. Add green peppers and zucchini. Cook 3–5 minutes.
3. Add remaining ingredients. Cover and cook over low heat about 15 minutes or until vegetables are almost tender. Stir occasionally.
4. Uncover and continue cooking about 10 minutes.

Yield: 16 servings

½ cup contains:

Cal	Prot	Fat	Carb	Sat	Mono	Poly	Chol	Na
54	2	2.8	7	0.3	0.6	1.7	0	7

Exchanges: 1 serving = 1 vegetable, ½ fat
Recommended for: The Living Heart; Low Calorie; Diabetic; Types IIa, IIb, III, and IV Diets

Deluxe Eggplant with Tomatoes

1 eggplant, peeled, cut into ½-inch slices
¼ teaspoon garlic powder
2 tablespoons oil
1 can (16 ounces) low-sodium tomatoes, undrained
1½ tablespoons chopped fresh parsley
½ teaspoon pepper
½ teaspoon dried sweet basil
½ teaspoon dried oregano

1. Sprinkle both sides of eggplant slices with garlic powder and then brown in oil.

2. Add tomatoes and seasonings and heat thoroughly.

Yield: 6 servings

1 serving contains:

Cal	Prot	Fat	Carb	Sat	Mono	Poly	Chol	Na
72	2	4.9	7	0.6	1.1	3.0	0	3

Exchanges: 1 serving = 1 vegetable, 1 fat
Recommended for: The Living Heart; Diabetic; Types IIa, IIb, III, and IV Diets

Baked Okra and Tomatoes

1 pound whole okra, fresh or frozen
1 tablespoon oil
1 onion, chopped
3 tomatoes, chopped
¼ teaspoon pepper
¼ teaspoon garlic powder
¼ cup fine, dry low-sodium bread crumbs (optional)

1. Preheat oven to 400°F.
2. Wash okra and cut off tip ends.
3. Heat oil in saucepan. When hot add okra, onion, tomatoes, pepper, and garlic powder.
4. Cover and simmer until okra is tender, about 15 minutes.
5. Turn into lightly oiled baking dish and top with bread crumbs.
6. Bake for 30 minutes.

Yield: 6 servings

1 serving contains:

Cal	Prot	Fat	Carb	Sat	Mono	Poly	Chol	Na
79	3	2.6	13	0.3	0.6	1.5	0	5

Exchanges: 1 serving = 1 vegetable, ½ bread, ½ fat
Recommended for: The Living Heart; Diabetic; Types IIa, IIb, III, and IV Diets

Abbreviations: **Cal,** calories; **Prot,** protein; **Carb,** carbohydrate; **Sat,** saturated fat; **Mono,** monounsaturated fat; **Poly,** polyunsaturated fat; **Chol,** cholesterol; **Na,** sodium. Protein, fat, carbohydrate, saturated fat, monounsaturated fat, and polyunsaturated fat are expressed in *grams.* Cholesterol and sodium are expressed in *milligrams.*

Honey Glazed Onions

18 white onions about 1½ inches in diameter
¼ cup low-sodium corn oil margarine
2 tablespoons honey
2 teaspoons chopped fresh parsley

1. Preheat oven to 400°F.
2. Blanch onions about 1 minute. Drain. Remove skins and tops. Place onions in a single layer in a small baking dish.
3. Melt margarine in a small saucepan and stir in honey and parsley. Pour over onions.
4. Bake 45 minutes, basting occasionally.

Yield: 6 servings

Note: May bake in microwave oven 15 minutes.

1 serving contains:

Cal	Prot	Fat	Carb	Sat	Mono	Poly	Chol	Na
135	2	7.8	16	1.4	3.3	2.6	0	13

Exchanges: 1 serving = 1 bread, 1½ fats
Recommended for: The Living Heart; Diabetic; Types IIa, IIb, III, and IV Diets

Creamed Potatoes

4 potatoes
1 cup cold skim milk
1 tablespoon cornstarch
2 tablespoons low-sodium corn oil margarine
¼ cup grated onion
¼ teaspoon pepper
¼ cup chopped fresh parsley
paprika

1. Pare, slice, boil, and drain potatoes.
2. Heat cold milk and cornstarch in a saucepan until thickened.
3. Combine all ingredients and heat through.
4. Garnish with paprika.

Yield: 8 servings

1 serving contains:

Cal	Prot	Fat	Carb	Sat	Mono	Poly	Chol	Na
114	3	3.0	19	0.6	1.3	1.0	1	20

Exchanges: 1 serving = 1 bread, 1 fat
Recommended for: The Living Heart; Diabetic; Types IIa, IIb, III, and IV Diets

German Potatoes

¼ cup flour
4 potatoes, peeled and grated
1 onion, grated
egg substitute equivalent to 1 egg
¼ teaspoon pepper
3 tablespoons oil

1. Combine flour, potato, onion, egg substitute, and pepper.
2. Heat oil in skillet. Drop batter from a tablespoon into the hot oil.
3. Fry until golden brown on both sides.

Yield: 12 servings

1 serving contains:

Cal	Prot	Fat	Carb	Sat	Mono	Poly	Chol	Na
96	2	3.8	14	0.5	0.9	2.2	0	12

Exchanges: 1 serving = 1 bread, ½ fat
Recommended for: The Living Heart; Diabetic; Types IIa, IIb, III, and IV Diets

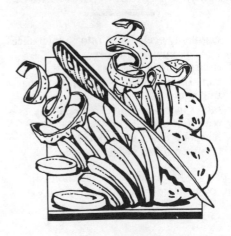

Stuffed Baked Potatoes

4 potatoes, baked
6 tablespoons skim milk
2 tablespoons low-sodium corn oil margarine
¼ cup low-sodium low-fat cheese, shredded
  paprika (optional)
  chopped fresh parsley (optional)

1. Cut potatoes in half lengthwise.
2. Scoop potato out of skin leaving shell intact.
3. Mash potato with milk and margarine. Stir in cheese.
4. Refill potato shells with mixture.
5. Reheat briefly at 350°F, if necessary.
6. Garnish with parsley and paprika, if desired.

Yield: 8 servings

1 serving contains:

Cal	Prot	Fat	Carb	Sat	Mono	Poly	Chol	Na
113	3	3.8	17	0.6	1.4	1.5	0	29

Exchanges: 1 serving = 1 bread, 1 fat
Recommended for: The Living Heart; Diabetic; Types IIa, IIb, III, and IV Diets

Baked Sweet Potatoes

4 medium sweet potatoes, cooked and peeled
½ cup brown sugar, firmly packed
¼ cup low-sodium corn oil margarine
  cinnamon

1. Preheat oven to 375°F.
2. Cut sweet potatoes into ½-inch slices.
3. Layer potatoes, brown sugar, and margarine in a casserole. Sprinkle with cinnamon.
4. Bake, uncovered, for 30 minutes.

Yield: 4 servings

1 serving contains:

Cal	Prot	Fat	Carb	Sat	Mono	Poly	Chol	Na
377	3	12.1	66	2.1	5.0	4.2	0	25

Exchanges: Not applicable for this recipe
Recommended for: The Living Heart and Type IIa Diets

Breaded Stewed Tomatoes

¼ cup finely chopped onion
1 tablespoon low-sodium corn oil margarine
1 can (16 ounces) low-sodium tomatoes, undrained
1 bay leaf
1 whole clove
¼ teaspoon pepper
½ teaspoon ground sage
1 teaspoon sugar
¼ cup fine dry low-sodium bread crumbs
1 tablespoon low-sodium corn oil margarine, melted

1. Sauté onion in margarine in saucepan.
2. Add tomatoes, bay leaf, clove, pepper, sage, and sugar. Cover and cook 10 minutes.
3. Remove bay leaf and clove.
4. Toss bread crumbs in melted margarine.
5. Mix into tomato mixture.

Yield: 4 servings

1 serving contains:

Cal	Prot	Fat	Carb	Sat	Mono	Poly	Chol	Na
127	2	9.1	11	1.6	3.8	3.0	0	6

Exchanges: 1 serving = ½ bread, 2 fats
Recommended for: The Living Heart; Diabetic; Types IIa, IIb, III, and IV Diets

Abbreviations: **Cal,** calories; **Prot,** protein; **Carb,** carbohydrate; **Sat,** saturated fat; **Mono,** monounsaturated fat; **Poly,** polyunsaturated fat; **Chol,** cholesterol; **Na,** sodium. Protein, fat, carbohydrate, saturated fat, monounsaturated fat, and polyunsaturated fat are expressed in *grams.* Cholesterol and sodium are expressed in *milligrams.*

Apple Acorn Squash

2   acorn or winter squash, cut in half
1   cup applesauce
1   tablespoon brown sugar, firmly packed
1   tablespoon low-sodium corn oil margarine
¼   teaspoon ground cinnamon

1. Preheat oven to 350°F.
2. Place squash in baking pan, cut side down. Cover bottom of pan with water.
3. Bake 45 minutes or until squash is tender.
4. Combine remaining ingredients and place in squash cavities.
5. Bake an additional 35 minutes.

Yield: 4 servings

1 serving contains:

Cal	Prot	Fat	Carb	Sat	Mono	Poly	Chol	Na
148	2	3.3	31	0.5	1.2	1.4	0	4

Exchanges: Not applicable for this recipe
Recommended for: The Living Heart and Type IIa Diets

Best-Ever Baked Zucchini

1   pound zucchini squash, unpeeled and sliced
¼   cup sliced green onion
1   tablespoon oil
3   tomatoes, chopped
¼   teaspoon pepper
1   clove garlic, minced
½   green pepper, chopped

1. Preheat oven to 350°F.
2. Sauté zucchini and green onion in oil.
3. Place in casserole and top with remaining ingredients.
4. Cover and bake 30 minutes.

Yield: 6 servings

1 serving contains:

Cal	Prot	Fat	Carb	Sat	Mono	Poly	Chol	Na
43	1	2.4	5	0.3	0.6	1.5	0	4

Exchanges: 1 serving = 1 vegetable, ½ fat
Recommended for: The Living Heart; Low Calorie; Diabetic; Types IIa, IIb, III, and IV Diets

Lemon Zucchini

4–5   zucchini squash, unpeeled, sliced
¾   cup water
2   tablespoons finely chopped onion
⅓   cup chopped fresh parsley
1   tablespoon low-sodium corn oil margarine
¼   teaspoon grated lemon peel
1   tablespoon lemon juice

1. Cook zucchini in water 8–10 minutes or until tender. Drain.
2. While zucchini is cooking, briefly sauté onion and parsley in margarine. Add lemon peel and lemon juice.
3. Heat through and pour over zucchini.

Yield: 4 servings

1 serving contains:

Cal	Prot	Fat	Carb	Sat	Mono	Poly	Chol	Na
36	1	2.9	2	0.5	1.2	1.0	0	1

Exchanges: 1 serving = 1 vegetable, ½ fat
Recommended for: The Living Heart; Low Calorie; Diabetic; Types IIa, IIb, III, and IV Diets

Almond Rice with Curry

3   tablespoons chopped onion
¼   cup thinly sliced celery
1   tablespoon low-sodium corn oil margarine
2   tablespoons slivered unsalted almonds
1   cup long-cooking white rice, uncooked
½   teaspoon curry powder
2   cups hot water

1. Sauté onion and celery in margarine until tender.
2. Add almonds, rice, and curry powder. Cook until lightly browned.
3. Add water and mix well. Heat to boiling and cover.
4. Simmer 15 minutes or until liquid is absorbed and rice is tender.
5. Remove from heat and toss lightly.

Yield: 8 servings

1 serving contains:

Cal	Prot	Fat	Carb	Sat	Mono	Poly	Chol	Na
122	2	2.6	23	0.4	1.3	0.7	0	5

Exchanges: 1 serving = 1½ breads, ½ fat
Recommended for: The Living Heart; Diabetic; Types IIa, IIb, III, and IV Diets

Herbed Rice

1½ **cups water**
 1 **low-sodium chicken bouillon cube**
 ¾ **cup long-cooking white rice, uncooked**
 1 **stalk celery, chopped**
 ¼ **teaspoon dried oregano**
 1 **bay leaf**
1½ **tablespoons chopped fresh parsley**
 1 **teaspoon low-sodium corn oil margarine**

1. Heat water and bouillon cube until cube is dissolved.
2. Add remaining ingredients.
3. Cover and cook until water is absorbed and rice is tender.

Yield: 6 servings

1 serving contains:

Cal	Prot	Fat	Carb	Sat	Mono	Poly	Chol	Na
92	2	0.8	19	0.1	0.4	0.1	0	9

Exchanges: 1 serving = 1½ breads
Recommended for: The Living Heart; Low Calorie; Diabetic; Types IIa, IIb, III, IV, and V Diets

Spanish Rice

 ½ **small onion, finely chopped**
 ¼ **green pepper, chopped**
 1 **cup rice, uncooked**
 2 **tablespoons low-sodium corn oil margarine**
 2 **cups low-sodium tomato juice**
 ½ **teaspoon dried sweet basil**
 ¼ **teaspoon pepper**
 ¼ **teaspoon garlic powder**

1. Sauté onion, green pepper, and rice in margarine until lightly browned.

2. Stir in remaining ingredients.
3. Cover and cook over low heat until rice is tender.

Yield: 8 servings

1 serving contains:

Cal	Prot	Fat	Carb	Sat	Mono	Poly	Chol	Na
124	2	3.0	22	0.5	1.3	1.0	0	4

Exchanges: 1 serving = 1½ breads, ½ fat
Recommended for: The Living Heart; Diabetic; Types IIa, IIb, III, and IV Diets

Sweet Applesauce Dressing

5½ **cups low-sodium bread cubes**
 ½ **cup finely chopped onion**
 1 **cup finely chopped celery**
1½ **cups applesauce**
 ¼ **cup brown sugar, firmly packed**
 1 **teaspoon ground cinnamon**
 ½ **cup low-sodium corn oil margarine, melted**

1. Preheat oven to 350°F.
2. Combine all ingredients thoroughly.
3. Bake on top of well-trimmed pork chops or alone in a baking dish for 75 minutes.

Yield: 10 servings

1 serving contains:

Cal	Prot	Fat	Carb	Sat	Mono	Poly	Chol	Na
226	3	10.3	31	1.9	4.4	3.2	0	21

Exchanges: Not applicable for this recipe
Recommended for: The Living Heart and Type IIa Diets

Abbreviations: **Cal,** calories; **Prot,** protein; **Carb,** carbohydrate; **Sat,** saturated fat; **Mono,** monounsaturated fat; **Poly,** polyunsaturated fat; **Chol,** cholesterol; **Na,** sodium. Protein, fat, carbohydrate, saturated fat, monounsaturated fat, and polyunsaturated fat are expressed in *grams.* Cholesterol and sodium are expressed in *milligrams.*

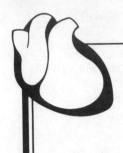

Low-Sodium Salads and Dressings

VEGETABLE SALADS

Marinated Green Bean Salad

2 tablespoons oil
2 tablespoons wine vinegar
2 teaspoons sugar
⅛ teaspoon pepper
1 package (10 ounces) frozen French style green beans, cooked without salt and drained
1 medium onion, cut in thin rings

1. Beat oil, vinegar, sugar, and pepper together with a fork.
2. Toss beans, onion rings, and dressing together.
3. Cover tightly and refrigerate 1–2 hours before serving.

Yield: 4 servings

1 serving contains:

Cal	Prot	Fat	Carb	Sat	Mono	Poly	Chol	Na
94	1	6.9	8	0.9	1.7	4.0	0	4

Exchanges: 1 serving = 1 vegetable, 1½ fats
Recommended for: The Living Heart; Diabetic; Types IIa, IIb, III, and IV Diets

Three Bean Salad

1 can (8 ounces) low-sodium green beans, drained
1 package (10 ounces) frozen wax beans, cooked without salt, drained
1 cup kidney beans, cooked without salt
½ cup chopped green pepper
½ cup chopped onion
½ cup chopped celery
¼ cup vinegar
3 tablespoons oil
½ teaspoon pepper
¼ cup sugar
½ teaspoon celery seed
⅛ teaspoon garlic powder

1. Combine the beans, green pepper, onion, and celery.
2. Combine remaining ingredients. Pour over bean mixture and stir.
3. Refrigerate in covered container for 12 hours before serving, stirring occasionally.
4. Will keep for several days in the refrigerator.

Yield: 10 servings

1 serving contains:

Cal	Prot	Fat	Carb	Sat	Mono	Poly	Chol	Na
91	2	4.2	12	0.5	1.0	2.5	0	9

Exchanges: Not applicable for this recipe
Recommended for: The Living Heart and Type IIa Diets

Beet and Onion Salad

¼ **cup wine vinegar**
1 **teaspoon sugar**
1 **can (16 ounces) low-sodium sliced beets, undrained**
2 **onions, sliced in rings**

1. Combine all ingredients.
2. Allow to marinate at room temperature at least 30 minutes before serving. Stir every 10 minutes.

Yield: 6 servings

1 serving contains:

Cal	Prot	Fat	Carb	Sat	Mono	Poly	Chol	Na
34	1	0.1	8	0	0	0.1	0	29

Exchanges: 1 serving = 1 vegetable
Recommended for: The Living Heart; Low Calorie; Diabetic; Types I, IIa, IIb, III, IV, and V Diets

Cabbage Slaw

⅓ **cup low-sodium mayonnaise**
¼ **cup vinegar**
¼ **cup sugar**
¼ **cup finely chopped green pepper**
2 **tablespoons chopped fresh parsley**
2 **tablespoons finely chopped onion**
3 **cups shredded cabbage**
½ **cup shredded carrots**
¼ **cup thinly sliced radishes**

1. Combine mayonnaise, vinegar, sugar, green pepper, parsley, and onion. Toss with cabbage, carrots, and radishes.
2. Chill before serving.

Yield: 6 servings

1 serving contains:

Cal	Prot	Fat	Carb	Sat	Mono	Poly	Chol	Na
139	1	9.8	13	1.7	2.1	5.0	8	18

Exchanges: 1 serving = 2 vegetables, 2 fats
Recommended for: The Living Heart; Types IIa, IIb, III, and IV Diets

Tossed Salad Deluxe

Dressing
1 **clove garlic, sliced**
2 **tablespoons lemon juice**
½ **teaspoon sugar**
¼ **teaspoon pepper**
½ **teaspoon paprika**
¾ **teaspoon dry mustard**
¼ **cup oil**

1 **head lettuce, shredded**
1 **bunch watercress, torn into small pieces**
½ **avocado, peeled and cut into small pieces**
½ **cup tiny cauliflowerettes**
¼ **cup thin carrot slices**
1 **tomato, cut in wedges**
½ **cup toasted almonds**
1 **tablespoon sesame seeds**

1. Combine dressing ingredients and chill.
2. Place vegetables, almonds, and sesame seeds in salad bowl. Toss with dressing.

Yield: 8 servings

1 serving contains:

Cal	Prot	Fat	Carb	Sat	Mono	Poly	Chol	Na
166	4	14.7	8	1.8	6.2	5.6	0	22

Exchanges: 1 serving = 1½ vegetables, 3 fats
Recommended for: The Living Heart; Diabetic; Types IIa, IIb, III, and IV Diets

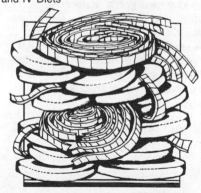

Abbreviations: **Cal,** calories; **Prot,** protein; **Carb,** carbohydrate; **Sat,** saturated fat; **Mono,** monounsaturated fat; **Poly,** polyunsaturated fat; **Chol,** cholesterol; **Na,** sodium. Protein, fat, carbohydrate, saturated fat, monounsaturated fat, and polyunsaturated fat are expressed in *grams.* Cholesterol and sodium are expressed in *milligrams.*

Carrot Raisin Salad

3 cups grated carrots
¾ cup raisins
⅓ cup low-sodium mayonnaise
1 teaspoon sugar
2 tablespoons skim milk
1 tablespoon lemon juice

1. Combine carrots and raisins in large bowl.
2. Mix together remaining ingredients. Toss with carrots and raisins.
3. Chill well before serving.

Yield: 8 servings

1 serving contains:

Cal	Prot	Fat	Carb	Sat	Mono	Poly	Chol	Na
125	1	7.4	16	1.3	1.6	3.8	6	26

Exchanges: 1 serving = 1 fruit, 1 vegetable, 1½ fats
Recommended for: The Living Heart; Diabetic; Types IIa, IIb, III, and IV Diets

Picnic Potato Salad

4 cups boiled potatoes, cubed
½ cup chopped onion
½ cup chopped celery
½ cup chopped green pepper
½ cup grated carrots
1 cucumber, chopped
2 low-sodium pickles, finely chopped
2 teaspoons low-sodium prepared mustard
1 teaspoon garlic powder
½ cup low-sodium mayonnaise
  paprika

1. Combine vegetables, mustard, and garlic powder.
2. Toss lightly with mayonnaise. Sprinkle with paprika.

Yield: 12 servings

½ cup contains:

Cal	Prot	Fat	Carb	Sat	Mono	Poly	Chol	Na
112	2	7.5	10	1.3	1.6	3.8	6	14

Exchanges: ½ cup = 1 bread, 1 fat
Recommended for: The Living Heart; Low Calorie; Diabetic; Types IIa, IIb, III, and IV Diets

Rice Salad

1½ cups cooked unsalted rice
⅓ cup chopped green onion, including tops
¼ cup chopped green pepper
¼ cup chopped red bell pepper
¼ cup chopped celery
¼ cup chopped low-sodium pickle

Dressing
½ cup low-sodium mayonnaise
1 tablespoon vinegar
1½ teaspoons sugar
1½ teaspoons low-sodium prepared mustard
¼ teaspoon pepper

1. Mix rice with vegetables and pickle.
2. In separate bowl, combine dressing ingredients. Toss dressing with rice mixture.
3. Chill at least 2 hours before serving. Garnish with tomato wedges, if desired.

Yield: 6 servings

1 serving contains:

Cal	Prot	Fat	Carb	Sat	Mono	Poly	Chol	Na
200	2	14.9	16	2.6	3.2	7.5	13	12

Exchanges: 1 serving = 1 bread, 3 fats
Recommended for: The Living Heart; Diabetic; Types IIa, IIb, III, and IV Diets

FRUIT SALADS

1 serving contains:

Cal	Prot	Fat	Carb	Sat	Mono	Poly	Chol	Na
79	1	0.1	20	0	0	0.1	0	1

Exchanges: Not applicable for this recipe
Recommended for: The Living Heart; Types I and IIa Diets

Cinnamon Salad

¼ cup cinnamon candies (red-hots)
1½ cups water
1 envelope (1 tablespoon) unflavored gelatin
½ cup applesauce
½ cup chopped celery
½ cup chopped unsalted walnuts

1. Dissolve candies in ½ cup boiling water.
2. Dissolve gelatin in 1 cup hot water.
3. Add candy liquid to dissolved gelatin.
4. Cool in refrigerator until partially set.
5. Add applesauce, celery, and walnuts.
6. Pour into mold and chill.

Yield: 6 servings

1 serving contains:

Cal	Prot	Fat	Carb	Sat	Mono	Poly	Chol	Na
132	3	6.4	18	0.7	1.0	4.2	0	13

Exchanges: Not applicable for this recipe
Recommended for: The Living Heart and Type IIa Diets

Citrus Sparkle Salad

1 cup applesauce
1 envelope (1 tablespoon) unflavored gelatin
1 can (8 ounces) crushed pineapple, packed in own juice, undrained
1 cup clear carbonated beverage

1. Bring applesauce to a boil and add gelatin. Remove from heat.
2. Add remaining ingredients.
3. Pour into mold and chill.

Yield: 6 servings

Lime Sherbet Salad

1 can (15¼ ounces) pineapple chunks, packed in its own juice, drained, reserve liquid
1 envelope (1 tablespoon) unflavored gelatin
1 cup water
1 cup lime sherbet
1 banana, peeled and chopped

1. Add enough water to reserved pineapple juice to equal 1 cup and bring to a boil in saucepan. Remove from heat.
2. Add gelatin and 1 cup water, stirring until gelatin is dissolved.
3. Stir in sherbet until melted. Add banana and pineapple chunks.
4. Pour into mold and chill.

Yield: 6 servings

1 serving contains:

Cal	Prot	Fat	Carb	Sat	Mono	Poly	Chol	Na
121	2	0.8	28	0.4	0.2	0.2	2	16

Exchanges: Not applicable for this recipe
Recommended for: The Living Heart and Type IIa Diets

Variations:

Lemon Sherbet Salad: Substitute pear slices for pineapple and lemon sherbet for lime sherbet (143 calories per serving).
Raspberry Sherbet Salad: Substitute raspberries for pineapple and raspberry sherbet for lime sherbet (147 calories per serving).

Abbreviations: **Cal,** calories; **Prot,** protein; **Carb,** carbohydrate; **Sat,** saturated fat; **Mono,** monounsaturated fat; **Poly,** polyunsaturated fat; **Chol,** cholesterol; **Na,** sodium. Protein, fat, carbohydrate, saturated fat, monounsaturated fat, and polyunsaturated fat are expressed in *grams*. Cholesterol and sodium are expressed in *milligrams*.

Waldorf Fruit Salad

2 cups chopped apple
½ cup chopped celery
⅓ cup chopped unsalted walnuts
⅓ cup low-sodium mayonnaise
1 tablespoon lemon juice

1. Combine all ingredients and toss lightly.
2. Serve on a lettuce leaf, if desired.

Yield: 4 servings

1 serving contains:

Cal	Prot	Fat	Carb	Sat	Mono	Poly	Chol	Na
228	2	20.9	11	3.3	4.1	11.6	13	22

Exchanges: 1 serving = 1 fruit, 4 fats
Recommended for: The Living Heart; Diabetic; Types IIa, IIb, III, and IV Diets

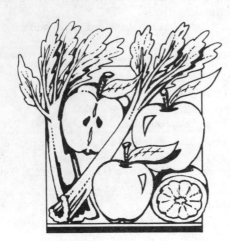

DRESSINGS

Celery Seed Dressing

⅓ cup sugar
1 tablespoon paprika
½ teaspoon dry mustard
½ cup wine or cider vinegar
½ cup oil
1 onion, thinly sliced
1 tablespoon celery seed

1. Place all ingredients in blender for 30 seconds.
2. Store in refrigerator. Shake before serving.

Yield: 1½ cups

1 tablespoon contains:

Cal	Prot	Fat	Carb	Sat	Mono	Poly	Chol	Na
53	0	4.6	3	0.6	1.1	2.7	0	1

Exchanges: 1 tablespoon = 1 fat
Recommended for: The Living Heart and Type IIa Diets

French Dressing

½ **cup oil**
3 **tablespoons vinegar**
2 **tablespoons lemon juice**
1 **teaspoon dry mustard**
1½ **teaspoons paprika**
¼ **teaspoon pepper**
⅛ **teaspoon garlic powder**
⅛ **teaspoon onion powder**
¼ **teaspoon dried sweet basil**

1. Combine all ingredients.
2. Store in covered jar in refrigerator until ready to use. Shake well before using.

Yield: ¾ cup

1 tablespoon contains:

Cal	Prot	Fat	Carb	Sat	Mono	Poly	Chol	Na
82	0	9.1	1	1.2	2.2	5.3	0	0

Exchanges: 1 tablespoon = 2 fats
Recommended for: The Living Heart; Diabetic; Types IIa, IIb, III, and IV Diets

Poppy Seed Dressing

¾ **cup sugar**
1 **teaspoon dry mustard**
⅓ **cup wine vinegar**
¼ **medium onion**
1 **cup oil**
1 **teaspoon poppy seeds**

1. Combine sugar, dry mustard, and vinegar in blender for 10 seconds. Add onion and blend 5 seconds.
2. Add oil slowly, blending constantly, until thick.
3. Pour into storage container. Add poppy seeds.
4. Store in refrigerator. Shake before using.

Yield: 2½ cups

1 tablespoon contains:

Cal	Prot	Fat	Carb	Sat	Mono	Poly	Chol	Na
63	0	5.5	4	0.7	1.4	3.2	0	0

Exchanges: 1 tablespoon = 1 fat
Recommended for: The Living Heart and Type IIa Diets

Italian Dressing

½ **cup oil**
¼ **cup vinegar**
1 **tablespoon lemon juice**
¼ **teaspoon garlic powder**
¼ **teaspoon onion powder**
¼ **teaspoon cayenne pepper**
¼ **teaspoon dry mustard**
1¼ **teaspoons sugar**

1. Combine all ingredients.
2. Store in covered jar in refrigerator until ready to use. Shake well before using.

Yield: ¾ cup

1 tablespoon contains:

Cal	Prot	Fat	Carb	Sat	Mono	Poly	Chol	Na
83	0	9.1	1	1.2	2.2	5.3	0	0

Exchanges: 1 tablespoon = 2 fats
Recommended for: The Living Heart; Diabetic; Types IIa, IIb, III, and IV Diets

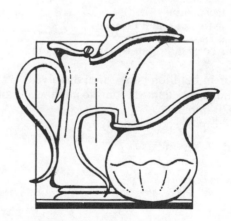

Abbreviations: **Cal,** calories; **Prot,** protein; **Carb,** carbohydrate; **Sat,** saturated fat; **Mono,** monounsaturated fat; **Poly,** polyunsaturated fat; **Chol,** cholesterol; **Na,** sodium. Protein, fat, carbohydrate, saturated fat, monounsaturated fat, and polyunsaturated fat are expressed in *grams.* Cholesterol and sodium are expressed in *milligrams.*

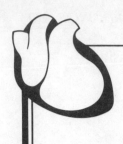

Low-Sodium
Soups, Sauces, Gravies

SOUPS

Cream of Mushroom Soup

1 tablespoon cornstarch
3½ cups water
3 low-sodium chicken bouillon cubes
1 cup finely chopped fresh mushrooms
¾ cup skim milk
½ teaspoon pepper
1 teaspoon onion powder

1. Stir cornstarch into water and heat until boiling.
2. Stir in bouillon cubes until dissolved.
3. Add chopped mushrooms to mixture and simmer 20 minutes.
4. Add milk and seasonings.

Yield: 4 servings

1 serving contains:

Cal	Prot	Fat	Carb	Sat	Mono	Poly	Chol	Na
33	3	0.2	5	0.1	0	0.1	1	28

Exchanges: 1 serving = ½ dairy
Recommended for: The Living Heart; Low Calorie; Diabetic; Types I, IIa, IIb, III, IV, and V Diets

Autumn Vegetable Beef Soup

½ pound very lean ground beef
¾ cup chopped onion
2 cups hot water
¾ cup chopped celery
¾ cup chopped potato
¼ teaspoon pepper
½ bay leaf, crumbled
⅛ teaspoon dried sweet basil
¼ teaspoon chives
⅛ teaspoon garlic powder
⅛ teaspoon dried thyme
1 fresh jalapeño pepper, seeded (optional)
3 fresh tomatoes, chopped
2 carrots, thinly sliced

1. Brown ground beef and onion in large saucepan. Drain off fat.
2. Add remaining ingredients.
3. Bring to a boil. Simmer, covered, for 30 minutes or until vegetables are done.
4. Sprinkle dill as garnish over top.

Yield: 4 servings

1 serving contains:

Cal	Prot	Fat	Carb	Sat	Mono	Poly	Chol	Na
155	15	4.7	14	1.7	1.7	0.5	39	77

Exchanges: 1 serving = 1½ meats, 1 bread
Recommended for: The Living Heart; Low Calorie; Diabetic; Types IIa, IIb, III, IV, and V Diets

Chicken Vegetable Soup

- **1 cup chopped celery**
- **½ cup chopped onion**
- **2 tablespoons low-sodium corn oil margarine**
- **2 cups chopped cooked chicken**
- **1 cup chopped potato**
- **1 cup chopped carrots**
- **⅛ teaspoon pepper**
- **1 teaspoon dried thyme**
- **2 cups low-sodium chicken bouillon**
- **1½ cups water**
- **1 can (8 ounces) low-sodium peas, undrained**

1. Sauté celery and onion in margarine until tender.
2. Add chicken, potato, carrots, pepper, thyme, bouillon, and water.
3. Simmer 20 minutes until potato and carrots are tender.
4. Add peas and heat through.

Yield: 6 servings

1 serving contains:

Cal	Prot	Fat	Carb	Sat	Mono	Poly	Chol	Na
173	16	7.1	11	1.6	2.6	2.1	43	75

Exchanges: 1 serving = 1½ meats, 1 bread, ½ fat
Recommended for: The Living Heart; Low Calorie; Diabetic; Types IIa, IIb, III, and IV Diets

Mulligatawny

- **1 onion, chopped**
- **1 stalk celery, chopped**
- **2 tablespoons low-sodium corn oil margarine**
- **1½ tablespoons flour**
- **1 teaspoon curry powder**
- **3 cups low-sodium chicken bouillon**
- **1 can (8 ounces) tomatoes, undrained**
- **1 carrot, sliced**
- **½ green pepper, chopped**
- **1 apple, peeled, cored, and chopped**
- **1 cup chopped cooked chicken**
- **½ teaspoon pepper**
- **¼ teaspoon dried thyme**
- **½ cup skim milk**

1. Sauté onion and celery in margarine.
2. Blend in flour and curry powder. Stir in bouillon until slightly thickened.
3. Add remaining ingredients except milk and simmer 30 minutes.
4. Add milk and heat through but do not boil.

Yield: 4 servings

1 serving contains:

Cal	Prot	Fat	Carb	Sat	Mono	Poly	Chol	Na
185	13	8.5	15	1.8	3.2	2.6	33	72

Exchanges: 1 serving = 1 meat, 1 bread, 1 fat
Recommended for: The Living Heart; Diabetic; Types IIa, IIb, III, and IV Diets

Hearty Corn Chowder

- **1½ onions, finely chopped**
- **2 tablespoons oil**
- **1 cup hot water**
- **3 potatoes, peeled and chopped**
- **½ teaspoon pepper**
- **1 can (16 ounces) low-sodium corn, drained**
- **2 cups skim milk**

1. Sauté onion in oil.
2. Add water, potatoes, and pepper. Cook until potatoes are tender, about 15 minutes.
3. Mash potatoes slightly.
4. Add corn and milk. Heat until simmering but do not boil.
5. Serve with parsley garnish, if desired.

Yield: 4 servings

1 serving contains:

Cal	Prot	Fat	Carb	Sat	Mono	Poly	Chol	Na
242	8	7.8	35	1.2	1.8	4.5	2	69

Exchanges: 1 serving = 2½ breads, 1½ fats
Recommended for: The Living Heart; Diabetic; Types IIa, IIb, III, and IV Diets

---

Abbreviations: **Cal,** calories; **Prot,** protein; **Carb,** carbohydrate; **Sat,** saturated fat; **Mono,** monounsaturated fat; **Poly,** polyunsaturated fat; **Chol,** cholesterol; **Na,** sodium. Protein, fat, carbohydrate, saturated fat, monounsaturated fat, and polyunsaturated fat are expressed in *grams.* Cholesterol and sodium are expressed in *milligrams.*

Gazpacho

3 tomatoes
1 green pepper
1 onion
1 cucumber, peeled
1½ cups low-sodium tomato juice
2 cloves garlic
½ teaspoon pepper
½ teaspoon dried oregano
½ teaspoon dried sweet basil
1 tablespoon oil

1. Chop ¾ of the vegetables into large chunks.
2. Cut remaining vegetables into small pieces and reserve.
3. Place half of the tomato juice, half of the chunk-sized vegetables, and garlic in blender or food processor, and blend at low speed until finely chopped.
4. Repeat with remaining tomato juice and chunk-sized vegetables.
5. Stir blenderized mixture, small-sized vegetables, pepper, oregano, basil, and oil together.
6. Cover and chill.

Yield: 6 servings

1 serving contains:

Cal	Prot	Fat	Carb	Sat	Mono	Poly	Chol	Na
68	2	2.6	11	0.3	0.6	1.7	0	12

Exchanges: 1 serving = 2 vegetables, ½ fat
Recommended for: The Living Heart; Low Calorie; Diabetic; Types IIa, IIb, III, and IV Diets

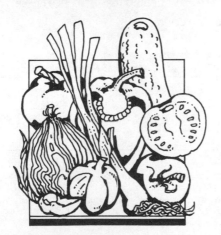

SAUCES AND GRAVIES

Louisiana Creole Sauce

2 tablespoons chopped green onion
2 tablespoons chopped green pepper
¼ cup sliced fresh mushrooms
1 tablespoon oil
½ teaspoon pepper
1 teaspoon dried sweet basil
1 can (16 ounces) low-sodium tomatoes, undrained

1. Sauté onion, green pepper, and mushrooms in oil over low heat 5 minutes.
2. Add remaining ingredients and simmer 20 minutes.
3. Serve with fish, chicken, or beef.

Yield: 2 cups

1 tablespoon contains:

Cal	Prot	Fat	Carb	Sat	Mono	Poly	Chol	Na
7	0	0.5	1	0.1	0.1	0.3	0	1

Exchanges: 1–3 tablespoons = free; ¼ cup = 1 vegetable
Recommended for: The Living Heart; Low Calorie; Diabetic; Types IIa, IIb, III, IV, and V Diets

Tartar Sauce

1 cup low-sodium mayonnaise
3 tablespoons finely chopped low-sodium pickles
1 tablespoon finely chopped onion
2 teaspoons chopped fresh parsley

1. Combine all ingredients.
2. Chill well before serving.

Yield: 1 cup

1 tablespoon contains:

Cal	Prot	Fat	Carb	Sat	Mono	Poly	Chol	Na
99	0	11.0	0	2.0	2.4	5.5	10	2

Exchanges: 1 tablespoon = 2 fats
Recommended for: The Living Heart; Diabetic; Types IIa, IIb, III, and IV Diets

White Sauce

2 tablespoons low-sodium corn oil margarine
2 tablespoons flour
¼ teaspoon pepper
1 cup skim milk

1. Melt margarine in saucepan. Remove from heat.
2. Stir in flour and pepper to make a smooth paste.
3. Add milk slowly, stirring constantly over medium heat, until thickened.

Yield: 1 cup

Variations:

Mushroom Sauce: Add ½ cup sautéed fresh mushrooms to sauce. Serve with chicken or vegetables.
Curry Sauce: Add ¼–½ teaspoon curry powder with dry ingredients. Serve with chicken, lamb, fish, or rice.
Mustard Sauce: Add 1 tablespoon low-sodium prepared mustard. Serve with beef or vegetables.
Cheese Sauce: Add ¼ cup cubed low-sodium low-fat cheese. Serve with macaroni or vegetables.

1 tablespoon White Sauce contains:

Cal	Prot	Fat	Carb	Sat	Mono	Poly	Chol	Na
22	1	1.5	2	0.3	0.6	0.5	0	8

Exchanges: 1 tablespoon White, Curry, or Mustard Sauce = free; 2 tablespoons = 1 fat; 3 tablespoons Mushroom Sauce = 1 fat (45 calories); 1 tablespoon Cheese Sauce = ½ fat (29 calories)
Recommended for: The Living Heart; Diabetic; Types IIa, IIb, III, and IV Diets

Mushroom Gravy

¼ pound fresh mushrooms, finely chopped
2 tablespoons oil
2 drops butter flavoring
½ teaspoon pepper
2 low-sodium beef bouillon cubes
1 cup plus 2 tablespoons water
1 tablespoon cornstarch
¼ cup white wine (optional)

1. Sauté mushrooms in oil 5 minutes. Remove from heat. Add butter flavoring and pepper and set aside.
2. Dissolve bouillon cubes in 1 cup hot water in a separate pan.
3. Combine cornstarch and 2 tablespoons cold water. Stir into bouillon and simmer until thickened.
4. Add mushrooms and wine, simmering 2–3 minutes longer.

Yield: 1¼ cups

1 tablespoon contains:

Cal	Prot	Fat	Carb	Sat	Mono	Poly	Chol	Na
16	0	1.4	1	0.2	0.3	0.8	0	1

Exchanges: 1 tablespoon = free; 2 tablespoons = ½ fat
Recommended for: The Living Heart; Low Calorie; Diabetic; Types IIa, IIb, III, and IV Diets

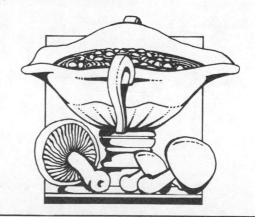

Abbreviations: **Cal,** calories; **Prot,** protein; **Carb,** carbohydrate; **Sat,** saturated fat; **Mono,** monounsaturated fat; **Poly,** polyunsaturated fat; **Chol,** cholesterol; **Na,** sodium. Protein, fat, carbohydrate, saturated fat, monounsaturated fat, and polyunsaturated fat are expressed in *grams.* Cholesterol and sodium are expressed in *milligrams.*

Orange Syrup

1 cup honey
6 tablespoons orange juice concentrate
2 tablespoons low-sodium corn oil margarine

1. Heat all ingredients together until margarine melts.
2. Serve on low-sodium Orange Griddlecakes (see recipe, page 274).

Yield: about 1½ cups

1 tablespoon contains:

Cal	Prot	Fat	Carb	Sat	Mono	Poly	Chol	Na
59	0	1.0	13	0.2	0.4	0.3	0	1

Exchanges: Not applicable for this recipe
Recommended for: The Living Heart and Type IIa Diets

Low-Sodium Breads

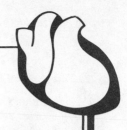

Casserole Cheese Bread*

4½ cups flour
2 packages active dry yeast
3 tablespoons sugar
⅓ cup nonfat dry milk powder
2 tablespoons low-sodium corn oil margarine
1¾ cups hot water (120–130°F)
egg substitute equivalent to 1 egg
1 cup shredded low-sodium low-fat cheese
1 cup dry oatmeal

1. Combine 2 cups flour, yeast, sugar, and milk powder in a large bowl. Add margarine and water. Mix well with electric mixer, about 2 minutes.
2. Add egg substitute, cheese, and ½ cup flour. Mix at high speed for 2 minutes.
3. Stir in oatmeal and remaining flour to make a stiff batter, beating until blended.
4. Cover and let rise in a warm place about 45 minutes.
5. Stir batter down, beating vigorously about 30 seconds.
6. Turn into an oiled casserole.
7. Bake immediately in a preheated 325°F oven 50–55 minutes.

Yield: 1 round loaf (20 slices)

1 slice contains:

Cal	Prot	Fat	Carb	Sat	Mono	Poly	Chol	Na
163	6	3.2	27	0.5	1.0	1.5	0	44*

Exchanges: 1 slice = 2 breads, ½ fat
Recommended for: The Living Heart; Diabetic; Types IIa, IIb, III, and IV Diets

*Limit to 1 slice daily due to sodium content.

Coffee Can Whole Wheat Bread

1 package yeast
½ cup warm water (105–115°F)
3 tablespoons sugar
1 cup skim milk
1 cup whole wheat flour
3 cups flour

1. Dissolve yeast in warm water. Add sugar and stir in milk and both flours.
2. Turn onto lightly floured board and knead 8–10 minutes.
3. Divide dough in half and place each half in an oiled 1-pound coffee can.
4. Oil coffee can lids and cover cans. Let rise until lids pop.
5. Bake in a preheated 350°F oven for 35 minutes.

Yield: 2 small round loaves (10 slices each)

1 slice contains:

Cal	Prot	Fat	Carb	Sat	Mono	Poly	Chol	Na
101	3	0.3	21	0.1	0	0.2	0	7

Exchanges: 1 slice = 1½ breads
Recommended for: The Living Heart; Low Calorie; Diabetic; Types I, IIa, IIb, III, IV, and V Diets

Abbreviations: **Cal,** calories; **Prot,** protein; **Carb,** carbohydrate; **Sat,** saturated fat; **Mono,** monounsaturated fat; **Poly,** polyunsaturated fat; **Chol,** cholesterol; **Na,** sodium. Protein, fat, carbohydrate, saturated fat, monounsaturated fat, and polyunsaturated fat are expressed in *grams*. Cholesterol and sodium are expressed in *milligrams*.

French Bread

2½ cups plus 1 tablespoon water
2 packages active dry yeast
1 tablespoon low-sodium corn oil margarine, melted
7 cups flour
cornmeal
1 egg white

1. Mix 2½ cups warm water (105–115°F) and yeast in mixing bowl until dissolved.
2. Add melted margarine. Stir in 4–5 cups of flour with a spoon.
3. Work in remaining flour until well blended, using hands if necessary. Dough will be sticky.
4. Turn onto lightly floured board and knead 8–10 minutes.
5. Place dough in an oiled bowl, turning once to coat surface. Cover and let rise in a warm place until double, about 1 hour.
6. Divide dough in half. Place one half on a lightly floured board and roll into a rectangle about 10 × 15 inches. Roll up like a jelly roll and tuck in ends.
7. Sprinkle a small amount of cornmeal on an oiled baking sheet.
8. Place roll on sheet, seam side down, and let rise until double, about 30 minutes.
9. Bake in a preheated 375°F oven for 30 minutes.
10. Remove and brush with mixture of egg white and 1 tablespoon water.
11. Bake 10 more minutes.

Yield: 2 loaves (15 slices each)

1 slice contains:

Cal	Prot	Fat	Carb	Sat	Mono	Poly	Chol	Na
111	3	0.7	22	0.1	0.2	0.3	0	3

Exchanges: 1 slice = 1½ breads
Recommended for: The Living Heart; Low Calorie; Diabetic; Types I, IIa, IIb, III, IV, and V Diets

No-Knead Oatmeal Bread

1 package active dry yeast
1 cup water
½ cup dry oatmeal
3 tablespoons low-sodium corn oil margarine
¼ cup honey
3⅛ cups flour
egg substitute equivalent to 1 egg

1. Soften yeast in ¼ cup warm water (105–115°F).
2. Combine ¾ cup boiling water, oatmeal, margarine, and honey in a large bowl. Cool to lukewarm.
3. Stir in 1 cup flour and egg substitute and mix well. Add softened yeast.
4. Stir in remaining flour 1 cup at a time to make a stiff dough.
5. Form into a ball, place in an oiled bowl, turning once to oil top.
6. Cover tightly and refrigerate 2 hours or overnight.
7. Turn onto well-floured board and shape into a loaf. Place in an oiled 9 × 4-inch loaf pan.
8. Cover and let rise in a warm place until double, about 60–90 minutes.
9. Bake in a preheated 375°F oven for 40 minutes.

Yield: 1 loaf (20 slices)

1 slice contains:

Cal	Prot	Fat	Carb	Sat	Mono	Poly	Chol	Na
111	3	2.3	20	0.4	0.9	0.8	0	7

Exchanges: 1 slice = 1 bread, ½ fat
Recommended for: The Living Heart; Low Calorie; Diabetic; Types IIa, IIb, III, and IV Diets

Wheat Bread

4–5 cups unbleached, all-purpose flour
  3 tablespoons sugar
  2 packages active dry yeast
1½ cups water
  ½ cup skim milk
  3 tablespoons low-sodium corn oil margarine
  2 cups whole wheat flour

1. Mix 2 cups all-purpose flour, sugar, and yeast in a large bowl.
2. Heat water, milk, and margarine in a saucepan until hot (120–130°F).
3. Gradually add liquid to dry ingredients. Beat 2 minutes with an electric mixer.
4. Stir in whole wheat flour until well blended.
5. Work in additional all-purpose flour to form a soft dough.
6. Turn onto a lightly floured board and knead 8–10 minutes.
7. Place in an oiled bowl, turning once to oil surface. Cover and let rise in a warm place until double, about 60 minutes.
8. Punch down dough, divide in half, and let rest a few minutes.
9. Shape into two loaves and place in oiled 9 × 5-inch loaf pans.
10. Let rise until double, about 60 minutes.
11. Bake in a preheated 400°F oven 30 minutes.

Yield: 2 loaves (20 slices each)

1 slice contains:

Cal	Prot	Fat	Carb	Sat	Mono	Poly	Chol	Na
90	3	1.2	17	0.2	0.4	0.4	0	2

Exchanges: 1 slice = 1½ breads
Recommended for: The Living Heart; Low Calorie; Diabetic; Types IIa, IIb, III, and IV Diets

Whole Wheat Oatmeal Bread

  1 package active dry yeast
1½ cups warm water (105–115°F)
  3 tablespoons honey
  ½ cup nonfat dry milk powder
2½ cups whole wheat flour
  1 cup enriched, all-purpose flour
  ¼ cup oil
1¼ cups dry oatmeal

1. Dissolve yeast in water.
2. Stir in honey and milk powder.
3. Stir in 1 cup whole wheat flour and 1 cup all-purpose flour until thick batter is formed. Let batter rest 10 minutes.
4. Fold in oil.
5. Stir in additional whole wheat flour and oatmeal.
6. Turn onto lightly floured board and knead 10–15 minutes until dough is smooth.
7. Place in an oiled bowl, turning once to oil surface. Cover and let rise until almost double, about 50 minutes.
8. Punch down, cover, and let rise 40 minutes. (This rising may be omitted, but loaf will be slightly heavier.)
9. Shape into loaf and place in an oiled 9 × 5-inch loaf pan. Let rise until double, about 35 minutes.
10. Bake in a preheated 350°F oven for 60 minutes.

Yield: 1 loaf (20 slices)

1 slice contains:

Cal	Prot	Fat	Carb	Sat	Mono	Poly	Chol	Na
133	4	3.5	22	0.5	0.8	2.0	0	10

Exchanges: 1 slice = 1½ breads, ½ fat
Recommended for: The Living Heart; Diabetic; Types IIa, IIb, III, and IV Diets

Abbreviations: **Cal,** calories; **Prot,** protein; **Carb,** carbohydrate; **Sat,** saturated fat; **Mono,** monounsaturated fat; **Poly,** polyunsaturated fat; **Chol,** cholesterol; **Na,** sodium. Protein, fat, carbohydrate, saturated fat, monounsaturated fat, and polyunsaturated fat are expressed in *grams.* Cholesterol and sodium are expressed in *milligrams.*

Garlic Bread Sticks

3 cups flour
½ teaspoon sugar
2 teaspoons garlic powder
2 packages active dry yeast
1¼ cups plus 1 tablespoon water
1 tablespoon low-sodium corn oil margarine
1 egg white, beaten
½ cup sesame seeds

1. Combine 1 cup flour, sugar, garlic powder, and yeast.
2. Add 1¼ cups warm (105–115°F) water and mix until well combined.
3. Mix in margarine and 1 cup flour.
4. Stir in remaining flour to make a soft dough.
5. Turn onto a lightly floured board and divide into 16 equal portions.
6. Roll each portion into a rope about 18 inches long. Cut each rope into three equal pieces.
7. Place on ungreased baking sheet, cover, and let rise at room temperature about 45 minutes until doubled in size.
8. Combine egg white and 1 tablespoon cold water. Brush over top and sprinkle with seeds.
9. Bake in a preheated 375°F oven 20 minutes.

Yield: 48 sticks

Note: Unbaked bread sticks may be frozen for up to 4 weeks. After rolling the dough into ropes place on a greased baking sheet and cover with plastic wrap and freeze. Transfer to plastic bag when frozen solid. Thaw before proceeding with step 8.

1 bread stick contains:

Cal	Prot	Fat	Carb	Sat	Mono	Poly	Chol	Na
40	1	1.1	6	0.2	0.4	0.4	0	1

Exchanges: 1 bread stick = ½ bread
Recommended for: The Living Heart; Low Calorie; Diabetic; Types IIa, IIb, III, and IV Diets

Sweet Rolls

1 package active dry yeast
¼ cup warm water (105–115°F)
¾ cup skim milk, scalded and cooled
¼ cup sugar
¼ cup oil
3½ cups flour
3 tablespoons low-sodium corn oil margarine
⅓ cup sugar
2 teaspoons ground cinnamon

1. Dissolve yeast in water.
2. Mix in milk, sugar, oil, and half of the flour.
3. Add remaining flour and work into dough. Knead on lightly floured board for 5 minutes.
4. Place in oiled bowl, turning once to oil surface. Cover and let rise until double, about 90 minutes.
5. Punch down and roll into an 18 × 8-inch rectangle.
6. Spread with margarine and sprinkle with sugar and cinnamon.
7. Roll up along wide side to form a roll 18 inches long. Cut into 1-inch slices.
8. Place cut side down on an oiled 9 × 13-inch baking pan or muffin tins.
9. Let rise until double, about 30 minutes.
10. Bake in a preheated 375°F oven 25–30 minutes.

Yield: 18 rolls

1 roll contains:

Cal	Prot	Fat	Carb	Sat	Mono	Poly	Chol	Na
162	3	5.2	26	0.8	1.6	2.5	0	6

Exchanges: Not applicable for this recipe
Recommended for: The Living Heart and Type IIa Diets

Party Surprise Loaf

5½ cups flour
2 packages active dry yeast
⅓ cup sugar
½ cup low-sodium corn oil margarine
1½ cups hot water (120–130°F)
egg substitute equivalent to 2 eggs

1½ cups dry oatmeal
12 dried apricot halves
12 pitted prunes
16 unsalted walnut halves
⅓ cup low-sodium corn oil margarine, melted
¾ cup brown sugar, firmly packed

1. Combine 2 cups flour, yeast, and sugar in a large bowl.
2. Add margarine and water, and mix well with electric mixer.
3. Add egg substitute and 1 cup flour, beating about 1 minute at high speed.
4. Stir in oatmeal and enough of the remaining flour to make a soft dough.
5. Turn onto a lightly floured board and knead 8–10 minutes. Cover with a towel and let rest 20 minutes.
6. Punch dough down and divide into 40 pieces.
7. Shape each piece around 1 apricot, prune, or walnut, and seal.
8. Dip each roll in melted margarine and then roll in brown sugar. Arrange rolls in two layers in an oiled 10-inch tube pan.
9. Cover and let rise in a warm place until nearly doubled, about 45 minutes.
10. Bake in a preheated 350°F oven 45–50 minutes.

Yield: 1 loaf (40 servings)

1 serving contains:

Cal	Prot	Fat	Carb	Sat	Mono	Poly	Chol	Na
150	3	4.9	24	0.9	1.9	1.9	0	8

Exchanges: Not applicable for this recipe
Recommended for: The Living Heart and Type IIa Diets

Garlic Croutons

1 tablespoon low-sodium corn oil margarine
½ teaspoon garlic powder
2 slices low-sodium bread, crusts removed, cut into ½-inch cubes

1. Melt margarine in small skillet.
2. Add garlic powder and bread cubes.
3. Sauté until crisp.

Yield: about 1 cup

Variation:
Add ½ teaspoon herb of your choice.

1 tablespoon contains:

Cal	Prot	Fat	Carb	Sat	Mono	Poly	Chol	Na
16	0	0.9	2	0.2	0.4	3	0	0

Exchanges: 1 tablespoon = free; 2 tablespoons = ½ bread
Recommended for: The Living Heart; Low Calorie; Diabetic; Types IIa, IIb, III, IV, and V Diets

Doughnut Puffs

2 cups flour
¼ cup sugar
1½ tablespoons low-sodium baking powder
1 teaspoon ground nutmeg
¼ cup oil
¾ cup skim milk
2 egg whites
oil
½ cup sugar
1 teaspoon ground cinnamon

1. Mix flour, sugar, baking powder, and nutmeg.
2. Add oil, milk, and egg whites, mixing well with a fork.
3. Drop from a teaspoon into hot oil and fry about 3 minutes or until browned.
4. Drain on paper towels.
5. Mix sugar and cinnamon together and roll warm puffs in sugar mixture.

Yield: 24 puffs

1 puff contains:

Cal	Prot	Fat	Carb	Sat	Mono	Poly	Chol	Na
108	2	4.7	15	0.6	1.1	2.7	0	9

Exchanges: Not applicable for this recipe
Recommended for: The Living Heart and Type IIa Diets

Abbreviations: **Cal,** calories; **Prot,** protein; **Carb,** carbohydrate; **Sat,** saturated fat; **Mono,** monounsaturated fat; **Poly,** polyunsaturated fat; **Chol,** cholesterol; **Na,** sodium. Protein, fat, carbohydrate, saturated fat, monounsaturated fat, and polyunsaturated fat are expressed in *grams.* Cholesterol and sodium are expressed in *milligrams.*

Apple Raisin Coffee Cake

½ cup low-sodium corn oil margarine
1½ cups sugar
  egg substitute equivalent to 2 eggs
1 teaspoon vanilla extract
1½ cups flour
4½ teaspoons low-sodium baking powder
1 teaspoon ground cinnamon
1 teaspoon ground nutmeg
⅛ teaspoon ground cloves
3 apples, cored and finely chopped
½ cup raisins

1. Preheat oven to 350°F.
2. Cream margarine and sugar together.
3. Add egg substitute and vanilla and beat 3–5 minutes.
4. Mix in baking powder, flour, and spices. Stir in apples and raisins.
5. Bake in an oiled and floured 8 × 8-inch pan for 55 minutes.

Yield: 16 servings

1 serving contains:

Cal	Prot	Fat	Carb	Sat	Mono	Poly	Chol	Na
205	2	6.5	36	1.2	2.6	2.3	0	16

Exchanges: Not applicable for this recipe
Recommended for: The Living Heart and Type IIa Diets

Banana Nut Bread

½ cup low-sodium corn oil margarine
½ cup sugar
½ cup honey
  egg substitute equivalent to 2 eggs
1½ cups mashed bananas
1 teaspoon lemon juice
2 cups flour
1½ tablespoons low-sodium baking powder
1 cup chopped unsalted walnuts

1. Preheat oven to 375°F.
2. Cream margarine, sugar, and honey.
3. Add egg substitute and beat 3–5 minutes.

4. Stir in bananas and lemon juice.
5. Blend in flour and baking powder. Add walnuts.
6. Bake in an oiled 9 × 5-inch loaf pan 75 minutes.

Yield: 1 loaf (20 slices)

1 slice contains:

Cal	Prot	Fat	Carb	Sat	Mono	Poly	Chol	Na
188	3	8.9	26	1.3	2.7	4.3	0	12

Exchanges: Not applicable for this recipe
Recommended for: The Living Heart and Type IIa Diets

Pumpkin Bread

3 cups flour
2 cups sugar
1 cup brown sugar, firmly packed
¼ cup low-sodium baking powder
1 teaspoon ground cinnamon
½ teaspoon ground nutmeg
1 cup oil
2 cups cooked pumpkin
⅔ cup water
½ cup chopped unsalted walnuts.

1. Preheat oven to 350°F.
2. Combine dry ingredients.
3. Make a well in the center of the mixture and add oil, pumpkin, and water.
4. Mix well with a spoon. Stir in walnuts.
5. Pour into two oiled and floured 9 × 5-inch loaf pans.
6. Bake 60 minutes.

Yield: 2 loaves (20 slices each)

1 slice contains:

Cal	Prot	Fat	Carb	Sat	Mono	Poly	Chol	Na
157	1	6.5	24	0.8	1.5	3.9	0	2

Exchanges: Not applicable for this recipe
Recommended for: The Living Heart and Type IIa Diets

Squash Bread

1 **cup sugar**
½ **cup brown sugar, firmly packed**
1 **cup mashed cooked winter squash**
½ **cup oil**
 egg substitute equivalent to 2 eggs
¼ **cup water**
2 **cups flour**
1½ **tablespoons low-sodium baking powder**
½ **teaspoon ground nutmeg**
½ **teaspoon ground cinnamon**
¼ **teaspoon ground ginger**
1 **cup raisins**
½ **cup chopped unsalted walnuts**

1. Preheat oven to 350°F.
2. Combine sugars, squash, oil, and egg substitute until well blended.
3. Stir in water. Add dry ingredients and mix well.
4. Stir in raisins and walnuts.
5. Pour into an oiled 9 × 5-inch loaf pan.
6. Bake 70 minutes.

Yield: 1 loaf (20 slices)

1 slice contains:

Cal	Prot	Fat	Carb	Sat	Mono	Poly	Chol	Na
206	3	7.9	33	1.0	1.8	4.8	0	15

Exchanges: Not applicable for this recipe
Recommended for: The Living Heart and Type IIa Diets

Cornbread

1 **cup yellow cornmeal**
1 **cup flour**
3 **tablespoons sugar**
1½ **tablespoons low-sodium baking powder**
¼ **cup oil**
1 **cup skim milk**
 egg substitute equivalent to 2 eggs

1. Preheat oven to 425°F.
2. Combine cornmeal, flour, sugar, and baking powder in a bowl.
3. Stir in oil, milk, and egg substitute only until flour is moistened. Do not overmix.
4. Pour into an oiled 8 × 8-inch pan.
5. Bake 20–25 minutes.

Yield: 16 servings

1 serving contains:

Cal	Prot	Fat	Carb	Sat	Mono	Poly	Chol	Na
114	3	4.1	16	0.6	1.0	2.4	0	22

Exchanges: 1 serving = 1 bread, 1 fat
Recommended for: The Living Heart; Diabetic; Types IIa, IIb, III, and IV Diets

Variation:

Cornmeal Muffins: Line muffin tins with paper liners and fill about ⅔ full. Bake 20 minutes.

Yield: 12 muffins

1 muffin contains:

Cal	Prot	Fat	Carb	Sat	Mono	Poly	Chol	Na
152	4	5.4	22	0.8	1.3	3.1	0	29

Exchanges: 1 muffin = 1½ breads, 1 fat
Recommended for: The Living Heart; Diabetic; Types IIa, IIb, III, and IV Diets

Abbreviations: **Cal,** calories; **Prot,** protein; **Carb,** carbohydrate; **Sat,** saturated fat; **Mono,** monounsaturated fat; **Poly,** polyunsaturated fat; **Chol,** cholesterol; **Na,** sodium. Protein, fat, carbohydrate, saturated fat, monounsaturated fat, and polyunsaturated fat are expressed in *grams.* Cholesterol and sodium are expressed in *milligrams.*

Breakfast Fruit Bars

½ cup low-sodium peanut butter
½ cup oil
⅔ cup honey
egg substitute equivalent to 2 eggs
½ cup skim milk
½ cup raisins
2 bananas, mashed
2 teaspoons vanilla extract
¾ cup whole wheat flour
1 cup flour
½ cup wheat germ
½ cup nonfat dry milk powder
1 tablespoon low-sodium baking powder

1. Preheat oven to 350°F.
2. Mix together peanut butter, oil, honey, egg substitute, milk, raisins, banana, and vanilla.
3. Combine remaining ingredients in a separate bowl and add to wet ingredients ⅓ at a time, stirring well after each addition.
4. Pour into an oiled 8 × 8-inch pan.
5. Bake for 40 minutes.

Yield: 16 servings

1 serving contains:

Cal	Prot	Fat	Carb	Sat	Mono	Poly	Chol	Na
256	7	11.9	33	1.8	3.7	5.7	1	32

Exchanges: Not applicable for this recipe
Recommended for: The Living Heart and Type IIa Diets

Light Muffins

2 cups flour
3 tablespoons sugar
1½ tablespoons low-sodium baking powder
¼ cup oil
1 cup skim milk
1 egg white

1. Preheat oven to 425°F.
2. Combine dry ingredients in a bowl.
3. Combine oil and milk.
4. Add liquid to dry ingredients, stirring only until flour is moistened. Do not overmix.

5. Beat egg white until stiff and fold in.
6. Fill oiled muffin tins ⅔ full.
7. Bake 20 minutes.

Yield: 12 muffins

1 muffin contains:

Cal	Prot	Fat	Carb	Sat	Mono	Poly	Chol	Na
139	3	4.8	21	0.6	1.2	2.8	0	15

Exchanges: 1 muffin = 1½ breads, 1 fat
Recommended for: The Living Heart; Diabetic; Types IIa, IIb, III, and IV Diets

Orange Griddlecakes

1½ cups flour
1 tablespoon low-sodium baking powder
2 tablespoons sugar
egg substitute equivalent to 1 egg
1 cup skim milk
6 tablespoons orange juice concentrate
3 tablespoons oil

1. Combine flour, baking powder, and sugar in a bowl.
2. Mix egg substitute, milk, orange juice concentrate, and oil together in a separate bowl.
3. Add liquid ingredients to dry ingredients, stirring only until blended. Batter will be slightly lumpy.
4. Using about 3 tablespoons batter for each griddlecake, bake on a preheated oiled griddle until browned.
5. Serve with Orange Syrup (see recipe, page 177), if desired.

Yield: 15 3-inch griddlecakes

1 griddlecake contains:

Cal	Prot	Fat	Carb	Sat	Mono	Poly	Chol	Na
99	2	3.1	15	0.4	0.8	1.8	0	16

Exchanges: 1 griddlecake = 1 bread, ½ fat
Recommended for: The Living Heart; Diabetic; Types IIa, IIb, III, and IV Diets

Basic Crêpes

⅔ **cup flour**
  egg substitute equivalent to 2 eggs
¾ **teaspoon grated lemon peel**
4 **teaspoons low-sodium corn oil margarine, melted**
1 **cup skim milk**

1. Combine flour and ½ of egg substitute and beat well at low speed.
2. Add remaining egg substitute and beat 3–5 minutes.
3. Add lemon peel and melted margarine.
4. Gradually stir in enough milk to give the consistency of thin cream.
5. Allow batter to set 2 hours.
6. Brush a 6-inch skillet with oil and heat the skillet.
7. Add ¼ cup batter to pan, tilting the pan so that batter coats the surface evenly. Pour any excess batter back into bowl.
8. Cook the crêpe until lightly brown on bottom, about 1 minute.
9. Turn and brown other side.

Yield: 9 servings

1 crêpe contains:

Cal	Prot	Fat	Carb	Sat	Mono	Poly	Chol	Na
73	3	2.7	9	0.5	1.0	1.1	1	39

Exchange: 1 crêpe = 1 bread
Recommended for: The Living Heart; Low Calorie; Diabetic; Types IIa, IIb, III, and IV Diets

Master Mix

½ **cup low-sodium baking powder**
¼ **cup sugar**
9 **cups flour**
1¼ **cups oil**

1. Sift baking powder and sugar into flour.
2. Sift together twice into a large mixing bowl.
3. Slowly add oil, cutting in with pastry blender until mix is consistency of corn meal.

4. Store in tightly covered container at room temperature or in refrigerator.
5. To measure Master Mix, spoon lightly into cup and level with spatula.
6. Mix will keep 6 weeks.

Yield: 12 cups

1 cup contains:

Cal	Prot	Fat	Carb	Sat	Mono	Poly	Chol	Na
571	10	23.6	79	3.1	5.7	13.8	0	2

Exchanges: Not applicable for this recipe.
This recipe is part of other recipes.

Master Mix Biscuits

⅔ **cup skim milk**
3 **cups low-sodium Master Mix (see recipe, this page)**

1. Preheat oven to 425°F.
2. Add milk all at once to Master Mix, stirring until flour is moistened.
3. Knead 15 times on a lightly floured board.
4. Roll out ½ inch thick and cut with a 2-inch biscuit cutter.
5. Bake 10–12 minutes or until lightly browned.

Yield: 15 biscuits

1 biscuit contains:

Cal	Prot	Fat	Carb	Sat	Mono	Poly	Chol	Na
118	2	4.7	16	0.6	1.1	2.8	0	6

Exchanges: 1 biscuit = 1 bread, 1 fat
Recommended for: The Living Heart; Low Calorie; Diabetic; Types IIa, IIb, III, and IV Diets

Abbreviations: **Cal,** calories; **Prot,** protein; **Carb,** carbohydrate; **Sat,** saturated fat; **Mono,** monounsaturated fat; **Poly,** polyunsaturated fat; **Chol,** cholesterol; **Na,** sodium. Protein, fat, carbohydrate, saturated fat, monounsaturated fat, and polyunsaturated fat are expressed in *grams.* Cholesterol and sodium are expressed in *milligrams.*

Master Mix Drop Biscuits

1 cup skim milk
3 cups low-sodium Master Mix (see recipe, page 275)

1. Preheat oven to 425°F.
2. Add milk all at once to the Master Mix, stirring only until flour is moistened.
3. Drop from a tablespoon onto an oiled baking sheet.
4. Bake 10–12 minutes.

Yield: 15 biscuits

1 biscuit contains:

Cal	Prot	Fat	Carb	Sat	Mono	Poly	Chol	Na
120	3	4.8	17	0.6	1.1	2.8	0	9

Exchanges: 1 biscuit = 1 bread, 1 fat
Recommended for: The Living Heart; Low Calorie; Diabetic; Types IIa, IIb, III, and IV Diets

Master Mix Coffee Cake

½ cup sugar
3 cups low-sodium Master Mix (see recipe, page 275)
¾ cup plus 2 tablespoons skim milk
2 egg whites or egg substitute equivalent to 1 egg

Topping
¼ cup flour
¼ teaspoon ground cinnamon
3 tablespoons brown sugar, firmly packed
¼ cup low-sodium corn oil margarine

1. Preheat oven to 400°F.
2. Add sugar to Master Mix.
3. Combine milk and egg whites or egg substitute.
4. Stir into Master Mix until flour is just moistened.
5. Pour into an oiled 9-inch round pan.

6. Combine topping ingredients and sprinkle over batter.
7. Bake 35 minutes.

Yield: 12 servings

1 serving contains:

Cal	Prot	Fat	Carb	Sat	Mono	Poly	Chol	Na
243	4	10.1	34	1.6	3.2	4.8	0	20

Exchanges: Not applicable for this recipe
Recommended for: The Living Heart and Type IIa Diets

Master Mix Shortcake

2⅓ cups low-sodium Master Mix (see recipe, page 275)
3 tablespoons sugar
3 tablespoons low-sodium corn oil margarine
½ cup skim milk
2 tablespoons sugar

1. Preheat oven to 400°F.
2. Combine Master Mix, 3 tablespoons sugar, margarine, and milk with a fork until a soft dough is formed.
3. Make six round shortcakes on an oiled baking sheet.
4. Bake 15 minutes or until browned.
5. Sprinkle with 2 tablespoons sugar while still warm.

Yield: 6 servings

1 serving contains:

Cal	Prot	Fat	Carb	Sat	Mono	Poly	Chol	Na
320	5	15.0	42	2.3	4.7	7.2	0	12

Exchanges: Not applicable for this recipe
Recommended for: The Living Heart and Type IIa Diets

Crunchy Granola

3 cups dry oatmeal
¼ cup oil
½ cup honey
½ cup brown sugar, firmly packed
1 teaspoon vanilla extract
½ cup sesame seeds
½ cup chopped unsalted walnuts
½ cup toasted wheat germ
½ cup raisins

1. Preheat oven to 350°F.
2. Place oatmeal in a 9 × 13-inch baking pan and toast in oven 10 minutes.
3. Combine oil, honey, brown sugar, and vanilla.
4. Add oil mixture, seeds, and walnuts to toasted oatmeal.
5. Bake 20–30 minutes, stirring every 10 minutes.
6. Cool and add wheat germ and raisins.
7. Store in a covered container in refrigerator.

Yield: 5–6 cups

¼ cup contains:

Cal	Prot	Fat	Carb	Sat	Mono	Poly	Chol	Na
159	3	6.9	23	0.9	1.8	3.7	0	3

Exchanges: Not applicable for this recipe
Recommended for: The Living Heart and Type IIa Diets

Honey Apple Oatmeal

4 teaspoons low-sodium corn oil margarine
3 tablespoons honey
2 teaspoons lemon juice
1½ cups apple slices
3 cups hot cooked oatmeal, cooked without salt

1. Heat margarine, honey, and lemon juice in a skillet.
2. Add apples, stirring until well coated.
3. Cover and simmer 3–4 minutes or until apples are tender.
4. Spoon apple topping onto bowls of hot oatmeal.
5. Serve with skim milk, if desired.

Yield: 6 servings

1 serving contains:

Cal	Prot	Fat	Carb	Sat	Mono	Poly	Chol	Na
135	2	3.9	24	0.7	1.5	1.4	0	2

Exchanges: 1 serving = 1 bread, 1 fruit, ½ fat
Recommended for: The Living Heart; Low Calorie; and Type IIa Diets

Raisin and Spice Oatmeal

2½ cups water
1½ teaspoons ground cinnamon
¼ teaspoon ground nutmeg
⅓ cup raisins
1¼ cups dry quick-cooking oatmeal

1. Bring water, cinnamon, nutmeg, and raisins to a boil.
2. Stir in oatmeal and cook 1 minute, stirring occasionally.
3. Cover pan, remove from heat, and let stand for a few minutes.
4. Serve with skim milk, if desired.

Yield: 6 servings

1 serving contains:

Cal	Prot	Fat	Carb	Sat	Mono	Poly	Chol	Na
90	3	1.3	18	0.2	0.4	0.5	0	3

Exchanges: 1 serving = 1 bread, ½ fruit
Recommended for: The Living Heart; Low Calorie; Diabetic; Types IIa, IIb, III, IV, and V Diets

Abbreviations: **Cal,** calories; **Prot,** protein; **Carb,** carbohydrate; **Sat,** saturated fat; **Mono,** monounsaturated fat; **Poly,** polyunsaturated fat; **Chol,** cholesterol; **Na,** sodium. Protein, fat, carbohydrate, saturated fat, monounsaturated fat, and polyunsaturated fat are expressed in *grams.* Cholesterol and sodium are expressed in *milligrams.*

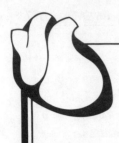

Low-Sodium Desserts

FRUIT-TYPE DESSERTS, PUDDINGS, DESSERT SAUCES

Apple Crisp

    7 apples, peeled, cored, and sliced
    4 teaspoons lemon juice
    1 cup brown sugar, firmly packed
    ½ teaspoon ground cinnamon
    1 cup dry oatmeal
    ½ cup low-sodium corn oil margarine

1. Preheat oven to 400°F.
2. Layer sliced apples in an 8 × 8-inch baking pan.
3. Sprinkle with lemon juice.
4. Combine brown sugar, cinnamon, and oatmeal in a bowl.
5. Cut in margarine. Mixture will look crumbly.
6. Sprinkle mixture over apples.
7. Bake 45 minutes or until topping looks crunchy and apples are tender.

Yield: 16 servings

1 serving contains:

Cal	Prot	Fat	Carb	Sat	Mono	Poly	Chol	Na
148	1	6.3	24	1.1	2.6	2.1	0	5

Exchanges: Not applicable for this recipe
Recommended for: The Living Heart and Type IIa Diets

Apple-Bread Pudding*

    4 slices low-sodium bread
    ¼ cup low-sodium corn oil margarine
    2 apples, peeled, cored, and chopped
       egg substitute equivalent to 2 eggs
    ¼ cup sugar
    1 cup evaporated skim milk, undiluted
    1 cup boiling water
    1 teaspoon vanilla extract
    ¼ cup sugar
    1 teaspoon ground cinnamon

1. Spread bread with margarine and toast in oven.
2. Cut into cubes and place in an 8 × 8-inch baking pan greased with margarine.
3. Add apples.
4. Mix egg substitute, ¼ cup sugar, milk, and water in a separate bowl.
5. Pour mixture over apples and let set 10 minutes.
6. Stir in vanilla.
7. Combine sugar and cinnamon, and sprinkle over the top.
8. Bake in a preheated 350°F oven 40 minutes or until knife inserted in center comes out clean.

Yield: 9 servings

1 serving contains:

Cal	Prot	Fat	Carb	Sat	Mono	Poly	Chol	Na
172	5	6.5	25	1.2	2.6	2.2	1	59*

Exchanges: Not applicable for this recipe
Recommended for: The Living Heart and Type IIa Diets

*Limit to 1 serving daily due to sodium content.

Pineapple Deep-Dish Dessert

5 apples, peeled, cored, and sliced
1 can (8 ounces) crushed pineapple, packed in own juice, undrained
¾ cup brown sugar, firmly packed
3 tablespoons cornstarch
¼ teaspoon ground cinnamon
1 tablespoon low-sodium corn oil margarine

1. Preheat oven to 350°F.
2. Place layers of sliced apples and pineapple in baking dish greased with margarine.
3. Combine sugar, cornstarch, and cinnamon and sprinkle over apples.
4. Dot with margarine.
5. Bake 35–40 minutes.

Yield: 6 servings

Note: May be packaged for freezing before baking, if desired. Bake at 350°F for 60 minutes from frozen state.

1 serving contains:

Cal	Prot	Fat	Carb	Sat	Mono	Poly	Chol	Na
207	0	2.2	49	0.4	0.8	0.9	0	10

Exchanges: Not applicable for this recipe
Recommended for: The Living Heart and Type IIa Diets

Master Mix Quick Peach Cobbler

2 cans (29 ounces each) peach slices, undrained
½ teaspoon almond extract
2⅓ cups low-sodium Master Mix (see recipe, page 275)
3 tablespoons sugar
3 tablespoons low-sodium corn oil margarine, melted
½ cup skim milk
2 tablespoons sugar

1. Preheat oven to 400°F.
2. Heat peaches and almond extract in 9 × 13-inch baking pan in oven 15 minutes.
3. Combine Master Mix, 3 tablespoons sugar, margarine, and milk with a fork until a soft dough is formed.

4. Drop dough from a tablespoon onto hot peaches.
5. Sprinkle with 2 tablespoons sugar.
6. Bake, uncovered, 15–20 minutes or until browned.

Yield: 8 servings

1 serving contains:

Cal	Prot	Fat	Carb	Sat	Mono	Poly	Chol	Na
330	4	11.4	55	1.7	3.5	5.5	0	11

Exchanges: Not applicable for this recipe
Recommended for: The Living Heart and Type IIa Diets

Rhubarb Crisp

2 cups cut fresh or frozen unsweetened rhubarb
½ cup sugar
2 tablespoons flour
⅓ cup brown sugar, firmly packed
3 tablespoons dry oatmeal
¼ cup flour
¼ cup low-sodium corn oil margarine, melted

1. Preheat oven to 325°F.
2. Put rhubarb in baking dish greased with margarine.
3. Mix sugar with 2 tablespoons flour and sprinkle on rhubarb.
4. Combine brown sugar, oatmeal, ¼ cup flour, and melted margarine, and sprinkle over top.
5. Bake 40 minutes.

Yield: 6 servings

1 serving contains:

Cal	Prot	Fat	Carb	Sat	Mono	Poly	Chol	Na
222	1	8.0	37	1.5	3.4	2.5	0	6

Exchanges: Not applicable for this recipe
Recommended for: The Living Heart and Type IIa Diets

Abbreviations: **Cal,** calories; **Prot,** protein; **Carb,** carbohydrate; **Sat,** saturated fat; **Mono,** monounsaturated fat; **Poly,** polyunsaturated fat; **Chol,** cholesterol; **Na,** sodium. Protein, fat, carbohydrate, saturated fat, monounsaturated fat, and polyunsaturated fat are expressed in *grams*. Cholesterol and sodium are expressed in *milligrams*.

Cooked Fruit Compote

½ cup dried apricots, quartered
½ cup dried pitted prunes, quartered
4 cups cold water
1 cinnamon stick
2 lemon slices, ¼-inch thick
2 tablespoons quick-cooking tapioca, uncooked
½ cup sugar
2 tablespoons raisins
½ cup apple slices

1. Soak the dried apricots and prunes in cold water 30 minutes in a saucepan. Do not use aluminum.
2. Add cinnamon stick, lemon slices, tapioca, and sugar.
3. Bring to a boil, cover, and simmer 10 minutes, stirring occasionally.
4. Stir in raisins and apples.
5. Simmer until apples are tender, 5–10 minutes.
6. Pour into a bowl, remove cinnamon stick, and chill.

Yield: 4 servings

1 serving contains:

Cal	Prot	Fat	Carb	Sat	Mono	Poly	Chol	Na
230	1	0.3	60	0	0	0.2	0	8

Exchanges: Not applicable for this recipe
Recommended for: The Living Heart; Types I and IIa Diets

Fruit Poached in Wine

2 cups red or white wine
¾ cup sugar
   sliced peel of ½ fresh lemon
2 tablespoons lemon juice
1 cinnamon stick
4 pieces fresh fruit of choice (pears, peaches, or nectarines), peeled and cored

1. Place wine, sugar, lemon peel, lemon juice, and cinnamon stick in a saucepan. Stir over medium heat until sugar is dissolved and mixture comes to a boil. Reduce heat and simmer 5 minutes.

2. Add fruit and simmer until tender, basting occasionally with juice. Do not allow liquid to boil.
3. Let stand in juice about 20 minutes before serving.
4. Serve with Dessert Topping (see recipe, page 216) or skim milk yogurt, if desired.

Yield: 4 servings

1 serving contains:

Cal	Prot	Fat	Carb	Sat	Mono	Poly	Chol	Na
264	1	0.7	68	0	0	0.7	0	4

Exchanges: Not applicable for this recipe
Recommended for: The Living Heart; Types I and IIa Diets

Layered Fruit Yogurt Pudding

Bottom Layer
1½ tablespoons unflavored gelatin
6 tablespoons cold water
2 cups cranberry juice
¾ cup orange juice
1½ cups sliced bananas
1 can (16 ounces) pineapple chunks, packed in own juice, drained
½ cup chopped unsalted walnuts

Top Layer
1½ teaspoons unflavored gelatin
2 tablespoons cranberry juice
2 tablespoons sugar
1 cup plain skim milk yogurt

Bottom Layer
1. Soften gelatin in cold water.
2. Heat cranberry juice to simmering.
3. Add softened gelatin and stir over low heat until dissolved.
4. Add orange juice.
5. Spread bananas, pineapple chunks, and walnuts in bottom of an 8 × 8-inch baking pan.
6. Pour juice mixture over top and chill until set.

Top Layer
1. Soften gelatin in cranberry juice in small saucepan.
2. Stir over low heat until dissolved.
3. Stir in sugar until dissolved.

4. Blend in yogurt, heating only until combined.
5. Cool to room temperature and spread over bottom layer.
6. Chill several hours.

Yield: 12 servings

1 serving contains:

Cal	Prot	Fat	Carb	Sat	Mono	Poly	Chol	Na
124	3	3.3	22	0.4	0.5	2.2	0	16

Exchanges: Not applicable for this recipe
Recommended for: The Living Heart and Type IIa Diets

Butterscotch Pudding*

½ cup brown sugar, firmly packed
3 tablespoons cornstarch
2 cups skim milk
1 teaspoon vanilla extract
1 tablespoon low-sodium corn oil margarine
¼ teaspoon butter flavoring
10 drops yellow food coloring (optional)
2 drops red food coloring (optional)

1. Combine sugar and cornstarch in saucepan.
2. Gradually add milk, stirring until smooth.
3. Heat to a boil, stirring constantly, and boil 2 minutes. Remove from heat.
4. Stir in vanilla, margarine, butter flavoring, and food colorings.
5. Pour into serving dishes and chill.

Yield: 4 servings

1 serving contains:

Cal	Prot	Fat	Carb	Sat	Mono	Poly	Chol	Na
148	4	3.1	26	0.7	1.3	0.9	2	63*

Exchanges: Not applicable for this recipe
Recommended for: The Living Heart and Type IIa Diets

Variation:

Butterscotch Pie: Make 1½ recipes of pudding and pour into a baked 9-inch low-sodium pie shell of Margarine Pastry *or* Oil Pastry (see recipes, page 290). Top with low-sodium Meringue (see recipe, page 289).

⅛ pie contains:

Cal	Prot	Fat	Carb	Sat	Mono	Poly	Chol	Na
311	6	10.1	50	1.9	4.3	3.2	2	74*

Exchanges: Not applicable for this recipe
Recommended for: The Living Heart and Type IIa Diets

*Limit to 1 serving daily due to sodium content.

Lemon Whip

1 tablespoon (1 envelope) unflavored gelatin
½ cup cold water
¾ cup sugar
¾ cup water
1 teaspoon grated lemon peel
¼ cup lemon juice
2 egg whites

1. Sprinkle gelatin over cold water in small saucepan.
2. Stir over low heat until gelatin dissolves. Remove from heat.
3. Stir in sugar, water, lemon peel, and lemon juice until sugar is dissolved.
4. Chill until soft-set.
5. Turn gelatin mixture into large bowl.
6. Add unbeaten egg whites.
7. Beat at high speed until mixture is fluffy and begins to set, 7–10 minutes.
8. Pour into mold or individual serving dishes and chill.

Yield: 6 servings

1 serving contains:

Cal	Prot	Fat	Carb	Sat	Mono	Poly	Chol	Na
108	2	0	26	0	0	0	0	17

Exchanges: Not applicable for this recipe
Recommended for: The Living Heart; Types I and IIa Diets

Abbreviations: **Cal,** calories; **Prot,** protein; **Carb,** carbohydrate; **Sat,** saturated fat; **Mono,** monounsaturated fat; **Poly,** polyunsaturated fat; **Chol,** cholesterol; **Na,** sodium. Protein, fat, carbohydrate, saturated fat, monounsaturated fat, and polyunsaturated fat are expressed in *grams.* Cholesterol and sodium are expressed in *milligrams.*

Lemon Sauce

1 **cup sugar**
2 **tablespoons cornstarch**
2 **cups water**
2 **tablespoons low-sodium corn oil margarine**
2 **tablespoons lemon juice**
2 **tablespoons grated lemon peel**

1. Mix sugar and cornstarch in saucepan.
2. Stir in water.
3. Bring to a boil and boil 1 minute, stirring constantly. Remove from heat.
4. Stir in margarine and flavorings.
5. Serve over pound cake or other dessert.

Yield: about 2 cups

1 tablespoon contains:

Cal	Prot	Fat	Carb	Sat	Mono	Poly	Chol	Na
32	0	0.7	7	0.1	0.3	0.2	0	0

Exchanges: Not applicable for this recipe
Recommended for: The Living Heart and Type IIa Diets

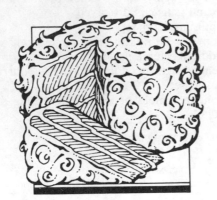

CAKES

Spicy Applesauce Cake

2 **cups sifted flour**
1½ **tablespoons low-sodium baking powder**
1 **teaspoon ground cinnamon**
¼ **teaspoon ground nutmeg**
¼ **teaspoon ground cloves**
1 **cup sugar**
½ **cup oil**
1 **cup applesauce**
1 **teaspoon vanilla extract**
4 **egg whites**
¼ **cup sugar**

1. Preheat oven to 350°F.
2. Sift dry ingredients together.
3. Add oil, applesauce, and vanilla. Mix with electric mixer on low speed 30 seconds, scraping sides of bowl. Beat on high speed 1 minute.
4. In a separate bowl, beat egg whites until frothy. Gradually add ¼ cup sugar while continuing to beat. Beat on high speed to stiff peak stage, 4–5 minutes.
5. Place egg whites in large mixing bowl and pour batter over whites. Fold in gently, 30–35 times.
6. Bake in two oiled and floured 8-inch round pans 25–30 minutes.
7. Cool 5 minutes and remove from pan.

Yield: 24 servings

Variations:

Orange Cake: Omit cinnamon, cloves, and nutmeg. Substitute 1 cup orange juice for applesauce.
Pumpkin Spice Cake: Decrease cinnamon to ½ teaspoon. Increase cloves and nutmeg to ½ teaspoon each. Substitute 1 cup cooked pumpkin and ¼ cup skim milk soured with 1 teaspoon vinegar for the applesauce. Add ½ cup chopped unsalted walnuts in step 8.

1 serving Spicy Applesauce or Orange Cake contains:

Cal	Prot	Fat	Carb	Sat	Mono	Poly	Chol	Na
129	2	4.7	21	0.6	1.1	2.7	0	9

One serving Pumpkin Spice Cake contains 140 calories
Recommended for: The Living Heart and Type IIa Diets

1 serving contains:

Cal	Prot	Fat	Carb	Sat	Mono	Poly	Chol	Na
123	2	4.7	18	0.6	1.1	2.7	0	14

Exchanges: Not applicable for this recipe
Recommended for: The Living Heart and Type IIa Diets

Basic White Cake

   2 cups sifted flour
1½ tablespoons low-sodium baking powder
   1 cup sugar
 ½ cup oil
   1 cup skim milk
   1 teaspoon vanilla extract
 ¼ teaspoon butter flavoring
 ¼ teaspoon almond extract
   4 egg whites
 ¼ cup sugar

1. Preheat oven to 350°F.
2. Sift together flour, baking powder, and 1 cup sugar.
3. Add oil, milk, and flavorings.
4. Mix with electric mixer on low speed 30 seconds, scraping sides of bowl.
5. Beat on high speed 1 minute.
6. In separate bowl, beat egg whites until frothy.
7. Gradually add ¼ cup sugar while continuing to beat.
8. Beat at high speed to stiff peak stage, 4–5 minutes.
9. Place egg whites in large mixing bowl.
10. Pour batter over whites and fold whites gently into batter, 30–35 times.
11. Bake in two oiled and floured 8-inch round pans 25–30 minutes.
12. Cool 5 minutes before removing from pan.

Yield: 24 servings

Variations:

Chocolate Cake: Decrease flour to 1¾ cups. Add ½ cup cocoa powder with dry ingredients.
Lemon Cake: Substitute 2 teaspoons lemon extract and 2 tablespoons grated lemon peel for flavorings.

Quick Snack Cake

2½ cups flour
 ¾ cup sugar
   1 cup brown sugar, firmly packed
   1 teaspoon ground cinnamon
 ¾ cup oil
   1 cup chopped unsalted walnuts
      egg substitute equivalent to 1 egg
1½ tablespoons low-sodium baking powder
   1 cup skim milk

1. Preheat oven to 350°F.
2. Mix flour, sugars, cinnamon, oil, and ½ cup nuts.
3. Set aside 1 cup of above mixture for topping.
4. To remaining mixture, add egg substitute, baking powder, and milk, mixing well.
5. Pour into an oiled 9 × 13-inch pan.
6. Add remaining ½ cup walnuts to the topping mixture and sprinkle over the top of batter.
7. Bake 30 minutes.

Yield: 24 servings

1 serving contains:

Cal	Prot	Fat	Carb	Sat	Mono	Poly	Chol	Na
206	3	10.3	27	1.3	2.2	6.2	0	13

Exchanges: Not applicable for this recipe
Recommended for: The Living Heart and Type IIa Diets

Abbreviations: **Cal,** calories; **Prot,** protein; **Carb,** carbohydrate; **Sat,** saturated fat; **Mono,** monounsaturated fat; **Poly,** polyunsaturated fat; **Chol,** cholesterol; **Na,** sodium. Protein, fat, carbohydrate, saturated fat, monounsaturated fat, and polyunsaturated fat are expressed in *grams.* Cholesterol and sodium are expressed in *milligrams.*

Sheath Cake

½ cup skim milk
1½ teaspoons vinegar
1 cup water
½ cup low-sodium corn oil margarine
6 tablespoons cocoa powder
2 cups flour
2 cups sugar
  egg substitute equivalent to 2 eggs
2 tablespoons low-sodium baking powder
1 teaspoon vanilla extract

Topping
½ cup low-sodium corn oil margarine
6 tablespoons skim milk
6 tablespoons cocoa powder
1 teaspoon vanilla extract
1 box (1 pound) confectioner's sugar
1 cup chopped unsalted pecans or walnuts

1. Preheat oven to 325°F.
2. Mix milk and vinegar together. Set aside to sour.
3. Bring water, margarine, and cocoa to a boil in a saucepan.
4. Mix flour and sugar in a bowl and blend in hot cocoa mixture.
5. Add egg substitute, sour milk, baking powder, and vanilla until well mixed.
6. Bake 50 minutes in a 9 × 13-inch pan lightly greased with margarine.
7. Five minutes before cake is done, melt margarine, milk, cocoa, and vanilla together.
8. Mix in confectioner's sugar and nuts.
9. Spread topping on cake immediately after removing cake from oven.

Yield: 24 servings

1 serving contains:

Cal	Prot	Fat	Carb	Sat	Mono	Poly	Chol	Na
298	3	12.1	48	2.1	5.7	3.6	0	15

Exchanges: Not applicable for this recipe
Recommended for: The Living Heart and Type IIa Diets

Million-Dollar Pound Cake

3 cups sugar
2 cups low-sodium corn oil margarine
  egg substitute equivalent to 6 eggs
½ teaspoon lemon extract
1 teaspoon vanilla extract
1 teaspoon butter flavoring
¼ cup skim milk
4 cups flour

Glaze (optional)
1½ cups confectioner's sugar
¼ cup lemon juice

1. Preheat oven to 325°F.
2. Cream sugar and margarine together.
3. Add egg substitute a small amount at a time, beating well after each addition.
4. Continue beating until batter is very light and fluffy.
5. Add lemon extract, vanilla, butter flavoring, milk, and flour, mixing well.
6. Bake 80 minutes in a bundt pan greased with margarine and floured.
7. Cool in pan 10 minutes before turning out.
8. Combine confectioner's sugar and lemon juice.
9. Pour glaze over warm cake immediately after removing from pan.

Yield: 32 servings

1 serving without glaze contains:

Cal	Prot	Fat	Carb	Sat	Mono	Poly	Chol	Na
244	3	12.4	31	2.3	5.2	4.1	0	23

One serving with glaze contains 266 calories
Recommended for: The Living Heart and Type IIa Diets

Golden Loaf Cake

2 cups flour
1¼ cups sugar
2¼ teaspoons low-sodium baking powder
⅔ cup low-sodium corn oil margarine
2 egg whites
¾ cup skim milk
1 teaspoon vanilla extract
3–4 drops yellow food coloring

1. Preheat oven to 325°F.
2. Mix flour, sugar, and baking powder together in a mixing bowl.
3. Add margarine, egg whites, and ¼ cup milk.
4. Mix with electric mixer 2 minutes at medium speed.
5. Add remaining milk, vanilla, and food coloring and mix 2 minutes more.
6. Pour batter into an oiled and floured 9 × 5-inch loaf pan.
7. Bake 60 minutes or until cake springs back when lightly touched. Cake will have crack on top.
8. Allow to cool before cutting. Good with low-sodium Lemon Sauce (see recipe, page 282).

Yield: 14 servings

1 serving contains:

Cal	Prot	Fat	Carb	Sat	Mono	Poly	Chol	Na
220	3	9.0	32	1.7	3.8	2.9	0	16

Exchanges: Not applicable for this recipe
Recommended for: The Living Heart and Type IIa Diets

COOKIES AND BARS

Old-Fashioned Oatmeal Cookies

½ cup low-sodium corn oil margarine
½ cup brown sugar, firmly packed
¼ cup sugar
2 egg whites, slightly beaten or egg substitute equivalent to 1 egg
1 teaspoon vanilla extract
1 cup flour
1 tablespoon low-sodium baking powder
1 cup dry oatmeal
½ cup chopped unsalted pecans
½ cup raisins

1. Preheat oven to 375°F.
2. Cream margarine and sugars until fluffy.
3. Add egg whites or egg substitute and vanilla and mix well.
4. Blend in flour and baking powder.
5. Add oatmeal, nuts, and raisins.
6. Drop from a teaspoon onto a lightly oiled baking sheet.
7. Bake 10–12 minutes.

Yield: 48 two-inch cookies

1 cookie contains:

Cal	Prot	Fat	Carb	Sat	Mono	Poly	Chol	Na
59	1	2.9	8	0.5	1.4	0.9	0	4

Exchanges: Not applicable for this recipe
Recommended for: The Living Heart and Type IIa Diets

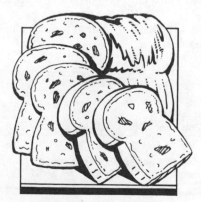

Abbreviations: **Cal,** calories; **Prot,** protein; **Carb,** carbohydrate; **Sat,** saturated fat; **Mono,** monounsaturated fat; **Poly,** polyunsaturated fat; **Chol,** cholesterol; **Na,** sodium. Protein, fat, carbohydrate, saturated fat, monounsaturated fat, and polyunsaturated fat are expressed in *grams.* Cholesterol and sodium are expressed in *milligrams.*

Banana Oatmeal Cookies

1½ cups flour
 1 cup sugar
 1 tablespoon low-sodium baking powder
 ¼ teaspoon ground nutmeg
 ¾ teaspoon ground cinnamon
 ¾ cup low-sodium corn oil margarine
      egg substitute equivalent to 1 egg
 1 cup mashed banana
1¾ cups dry oatmeal
 ½ cup chopped unsalted walnuts

1. Preheat oven to 400°F.
2. Sift flour, sugar, baking powder, nutmeg, and cinnamon into a large mixing bowl.
3. Add margarine, egg substitute, and banana, beating well.
4. Mix in oatmeal and walnuts until thoroughly blended.
5. Drop from a teaspoon onto an ungreased baking sheet.
6. Bake 12–15 minutes or until cookies are done. Remove from sheet immediately.

Yield: 54 cookies

Variation:

Banana Raisin Oatmeal Cookies: Add ½ cup raisins with nuts.

1 cookie without raisins contains:

Cal	Prot	Fat	Carb	Sat	Mono	Poly	Chol	Na
71	1	3.6	9	0.6	1.3	1.4	0	3

One cookie with raisins contains 78 calories
Recommended for: The Living Heart and Type IIa Diets

Lemon Doodle Cookies

 ⅔ cup low-sodium corn oil margarine
 ½ cup brown sugar, firmly packed
 ½ teaspoon lemon extract
 ⅔ cup flour
1½ cups oatmeal
      sugar

1. Preheat oven to 325°F.
2. Cream margarine and brown sugar.
3. Add lemon extract, flour, and oatmeal, and mix well.
4. Form dough into small balls (walnut size) and place on an oiled baking sheet.
5. Flatten balls with bottom of glass dipped in sugar.
6. Bake 13–15 minutes.

Yield: 36 1½-inch cookies

1 cookie contains:

Cal	Prot	Fat	Carb	Sat	Mono	Poly	Chol	Na
67	1	3.7	8	0.7	1.6	1.2	0	1

Exchanges: Not applicable for this recipe
Recommended for: The Living Heart and Type IIa Diets

Peanut Butter Cookies

 1 cup low-sodium corn oil margarine
 1 cup sugar
 1 cup brown sugar, firmly packed
 5 tablespoons evaporated skim milk, undiluted
 1 teaspoon vanilla extract
 1 cup low-sodium peanut butter
 2 cups flour
 1 tablespoon low-sodium baking powder

1. Preheat oven to 350°F.
2. Thoroughly cream margarine, sugars, milk, and vanilla.
3. Stir in peanut butter.
4. Stir in flour and baking powder.
5. Drop from a teaspoon onto an ungreased baking sheet.
6. Press with back of floured fork to make criss-cross pattern.
7. Bake 15 minutes.

Yield: 72 two-inch cookies

1 cookie contains:

Cal	Prot	Fat	Carb	Sat	Mono	Poly	Chol	Na
80	2	4.4	9	0.8	1.9	1.3	0	3

Exchanges: Not applicable for this recipe
Recommended for: The Living Heart and Type IIa Diets

Walnut Crispies

3 egg whites
1 teaspoon vanilla extract
1 cup sugar
2 cups chopped unsalted walnuts

1. Preheat oven to 350°F.
2. Beat egg whites until stiff.
3. Add vanilla.
4. Gradually add sugar while continuing to beat.
5. Fold in nuts.
6. Drop from a teaspoon onto an oiled cookie sheet.
7. Bake 2–3 minutes.
8. Turn off oven. Remove cookies after 1 hour.

Yield: 72 cookies

1 cookie contains:

Cal	Prot	Fat	Carb	Sat	Mono	Poly	Chol	Na
33	1	2.1	3	0.2	0.3	1.4	0	2

Exchanges: Not applicable for this recipe
Recommended for: The Living Heart and Type IIa Diets

Brownies

1¼ cups low-sodium corn oil margarine
⅔ cup cocoa powder
2 cups sugar
egg substitute equivalent to 4 eggs
2 teaspoons vanilla extract
1½ cups flour
1 cup chopped unsalted walnuts
confectioner's sugar (optional)

1. Preheat oven to 350°F.
2. Heat margarine and cocoa in saucepan until margarine is melted.
3. Place in bowl with sugar and mix well.
4. Add egg substitute gradually, beating very well after each addition.
5. Add vanilla, flour, and nuts, and mix thoroughly.
6. Spread in 9 × 13-inch baking pan greased with margarine.
7. Bake 35 minutes. Do not overbake.

8. Cool before cutting. May sprinkle with confectioner's sugar if desired.

Yield: 24 brownies

1 brownie contains:

Cal	Prot	Fat	Carb	Sat	Mono	Poly	Chol	Na
227	3	13.9	25	2.5	5.0	5.5	0	20

Exchanges: Not applicable for this recipe
Recommended for: The Living Heart and Type IIa Diets

Black Raspberry Bars

¾ cup low-sodium corn oil margarine
1 cup brown sugar, firmly packed
1¾ cups flour
1 tablespoon low-sodium baking powder
1½ cups dry oatmeal
1 can (16 ounces) black raspberries, drained

1. Preheat oven to 400°F.
2. Cream margarine and sugar.
3. Mix in flour and baking powder until well blended.
4. Stir in oatmeal.
5. Press half of the mixture into a 9 × 13-inch baking pan greased with margarine.
6. Spread raspberries over mixture.
7. Sprinkle with remaining oatmeal mixture.
8. Bake 25 minutes.
9. Cool 5 minutes before cutting into bars.

Yield: 24 servings

1 bar contains:

Cal	Prot	Fat	Carb	Sat	Mono	Poly	Chol	Na
159	2	6.3	25	1.1	2.6	2.0	0	4

Exchanges: Not applicable for this recipe
Recommended for: The Living Heart and Type IIa Diets

Abbreviations: **Cal,** calories; **Prot,** protein; **Carb,** carbohydrate; **Sat,** saturated fat; **Mono,** monounsaturated fat; **Poly,** polyunsaturated fat; **Chol,** cholesterol; **Na,** sodium. Protein, fat, carbohydrate, saturated fat, monounsaturated fat, and polyunsaturated fat are expressed in *grams*. Cholesterol and sodium are expressed in *milligrams*.

PIES AND TOPPINGS

Honey Apple Pie

1   unbaked low-sodium 9-inch pie shell of Margarine Pastry *or* Oil Pastry (see recipes, page 290)
6–7   apples, peeled, cored, and sliced
½   cup honey
¼   cup low-sodium corn oil margarine
1   cup whole wheat flour
1   teaspoon ground cinnamon
⅓   cup sugar

1. Preheat oven to 375°F.
2. Place apples in unbaked pie shell and drizzle with honey.
3. Combine margarine, flour, cinnamon, and sugar, and sprinkle over apples.
4. Bake 35 minutes.

Yield: 8 servings

1 serving contains:

Cal	Prot	Fat	Carb	Sat	Mono	Poly	Chol	Na
370	4	14.1	61	2.6	5.8	4.7	0	5

Exchanges: Not applicable for this recipe
Recommended for: The Living Heart and Type IIa Diets

Cherry Nut Pie

1   cup sugar
2½   tablespoons cornstarch
⅓   cup light corn syrup
1   teaspoon grated lemon peel
¾   cup water
1   can (16 ounces) water-packed cherries, drained, reserve liquid
½   cup chopped unsalted walnuts
1   tablespoon low-sodium corn oil margarine
1   unbaked low-sodium 9-inch pie shell and pastry for lattice top of Margarine Pastry *or* Oil Pastry (see recipes, page 290)

1. Preheat oven to 425°F.
2. Mix sugar, cornstarch, corn syrup, lemon peel, water, and reserved cherry juice in a saucepan.
3. Bring to a boil, add cherries, and boil 5 minutes. Remove from heat.
4. Add nuts and margarine.
5. When cooled to lukewarm, pour into pie shell and criss-cross pastry on top to form lattice design.
6. Bake 20 minutes.
7. Reduce temperature to 375°F and bake an additional 20 minutes.

Yield: 8 servings

1 serving contains:

Cal	Prot	Fat	Carb	Sat	Mono	Poly	Chol	Na
483	5	22.1	69	3.7	8.1	8.7	0	13

Exchanges: Not applicable for this recipe
Recommended for: The Living Heart and Type IIa Diets

Lemon Meringue Pie

1½   cups sugar
6   tablespoons cornstarch
2   cups water
4   drops yellow food coloring
¼   cup low-sodium corn oil margarine
¼   cup lemon juice
1   tablespoon grated lemon peel
1   baked low-sodium 9-inch pie shell of Margarine Pastry *or* Oil Pastry (see recipes, page 290)
    low-sodium Meringue for 9-inch pie (see recipe, page 289)

1. Preheat oven to 400°F.
2. Stir together sugar, cornstarch, water, and food coloring in saucepan until smooth.
3. Cook over medium heat, stirring until thickened. Continue to cook 1 minute, then remove from heat.
4. Add margarine, lemon juice, and lemon peel.
5. Pour into baked pie shell.
6. Spread Meringue on pie, sealing edges.
7. Bake 8–10 minutes.

Yield: 8 servings

1 serving contains:

Cal	Prot	Fat	Carb	Sat	Mono	Poly	Chol	Na
385	3	13.5	65	2.5	5.8	4.3	0	21

Exchanges: Not applicable for this recipe
Recommended for: The Living Heart and Type IIa Diets

Pumpkin Pie*

egg substitute equivalent to 2 eggs
2 cups cooked pumpkin
¾ cup sugar
1 teaspoon ground cinnamon
½ teaspoon ground ginger
¼ teaspoon ground cloves
1 can (13 ounces) evaporated skim milk, undiluted
1 unbaked low-sodium 9-inch pie shell of Margarine Pastry *or* Oil Pastry (see recipes, page 290)

1. Preheat oven to 425°F.
2. Beat egg substitute 5 minutes.
3. Mix in pumpkin, sugar, spices, and milk.
4. Pour into pie shell.
5. Bake 15 minutes.
6. Reduce temperature to 350°F and continue baking 45–50 minutes or until knife inserted in center comes out clean.

Yield: 8 servings

1 serving contains:

Cal	Prot	Fat	Carb	Sat	Mono	Poly	Chol	Na
276	8	9.0	42	1.6	3.6	3.2	2	91*

Exchanges: Not applicable for this recipe
Recommended for: The Living Heart and Type IIa Diets

*Limit to 1 serving daily due to sodium content.

Meringue

3 egg whites
½ teaspoon vanilla extract
6 tablespoons sugar

1. Preheat oven to 350°F.
2. Beat egg whites with vanilla until soft peaks form.
3. Gradually add sugar while continuing to beat until stiff and glossy.
4. Spread meringue on pie filling, sealing against pastry.
5. Bake 12–15 minutes or until peaks are golden brown.

Yield: meringue for one 9-inch pie

⅛ recipe for 9-inch pie contains:

Cal	Prot	Fat	Carb	Sat	Mono	Poly	Chol	Na
42	1	0	9	0	0	0	0	19

Exchanges: Not applicable for this recipe
Recommended for: The Living Heart and Type IIa Diets

Note: For meringue for 8-inch pie, use 2 egg whites and decrease sugar to 4 tablespoons.

⅛ recipe for 8-inch pie contains:

Cal	Prot	Fat	Carb	Sat	Mono	Poly	Chol	Na
28	1	0	6	0	0	0	0	13

Exchanges: Not applicable for this recipe
Recommended for: The Living Heart and Type IIa Diets

Abbreviations: **Cal,** calories; **Prot,** protein; **Carb,** carbohydrate; **Sat,** saturated fat; **Mono,** monounsaturated fat; **Poly,** polyunsaturated fat; **Chol,** cholesterol; **Na,** sodium. Protein, fat, carbohydrate, saturated fat, monounsaturated fat, and polyunsaturated fat are expressed in *grams.* Cholesterol and sodium are expressed in *milligrams.*

Margarine Pastry

⅓ **cup low-sodium corn oil margarine**
1 **cup flour**
2–3 **tablespoons water**

1. Cut margarine into flour until coarse meal texture is obtained.
2. Sprinkle water over flour, mixing gradually with a fork.
3. Form into ball and chill 10 minutes.
4. Roll out from center to edge until about ⅛-inch thick.
5. Fit into 9-inch pie pan and flute edges.
6. If baked shell is needed, bake in a preheated 425°F oven 12–15 minutes.

Yield: one 9-inch pie shell

Note: Double recipe for two-crust pie or pie with lattice top.

⅛ *of single crust recipe contains:*

Cal	Prot	Fat	Carb	Sat	Mono	Poly	Chol	Na
124	2	7.8	12	1.4	3.3	2.5	0	1

Exchanges: ⅛ of single crust recipe = 1 bread, 1½ fats
Recommended for: The Living Heart; Low Calorie; Diabetic; Types IIa, IIb, III, and IV Diets

Oil Pastry

1 **cup flour**
¼ **cup oil**
2 **tablespoons cold water**

1. Blend oil into flour with a fork.
2. Sprinkle water over mixture, mixing well.
3. Shape into ball and chill.
4. Roll out between two pieces of waxed paper.
5. Remove top layer of waxed paper and invert dough into pie pan.
6. Peel off other sheet of waxed paper and flute edges of crust.
7. If baked shell is needed, bake in a preheated 450°F oven 10–12 minutes.

Yield: one 9-inch pie shell

Note: Double recipe for two-crust pie or pie with lattice top.

⅛ *of single crust recipe contains:*

Cal	Prot	Fat	Carb	Sat	Mono	Poly	Chol	Na
117	2	7.0	12	0.9	1.7	4.1	0	0

Exchanges: ⅛ of single crust recipe = 1 bread, 1 fat
Recommended for: The Living Heart; Low Calorie; Diabetic; Types IIa, IIb, III, and IV Diets

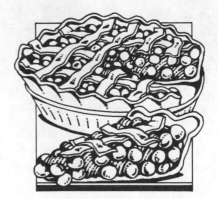

Managing Your Diet

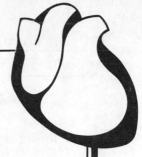

The Living Heart Diet: Menus

Living Heart Diet Menus

The following menus have been designed for *The Living Heart Diet* and may be used by individuals on the Type IIa Diet. A week (7 days) of sample menus is given with the nutrient analysis for each day, including calories, protein, fat, carbohydrate, calcium, phosphorus, iron, sodium, potassium, vitamin A, thiamin, riboflavin, niacin, ascorbic acid, saturated fat, monounsaturated fat, polyunsaturated fat, and cholesterol. For each day's menu, the percent of calories from protein, carbohydrate, and fat is shown, along with the percent of calories from polyunsaturated, saturated, and monunsaturated fat, as well as the P/S ratio. The sodium value for each menu does not include the use of any salt other than that listed in each recipe.

The asterisks indicate recipes that may be found in this book. Amounts are abbreviated as follows: g = grams; mg = milligrams; IU = international units.

The Living Heart Diet Menu: Day 1

Breakfast
  Broiled pink grapefruit half
  *Crunchy Granola (½ cup) over
  Skim milk yogurt (1 cup)
  Whole wheat toast (1 slice) with
  Tub margarine (1 teaspoon)
  Coffee

Lunch
  *Hearty Corn Chowder (¼ recipe)
  *Honey Wheat Loaf (2 slices) with
  Tub margarine (2 teaspoons)
  Carrot sticks (½ carrot) and green pepper
    rings (½ pepper)
  Skim milk (1 cup)

Dinner
  *Tangy Italian Mushrooms (½ cup)
  *Chicken Cacciatore (1 serving) with
  Spaghetti (1 cup)
  Broccoli spears with
  Tub margarine (½ teaspoon)
  *Garlic Bread Sticks (4) with
  Tub margarine (1½ teaspoons)
  Iced tea

Caloric and Nutritional Values

Calories	2,067.00
Protein	96.09 g
Fat	66.37 g
Carbohydrate	291.23 g
Calcium	1,359.00 mg
Phosphorus	2,066.00 mg
Iron	16.57 mg
Sodium	3,609.00 mg
Potassium	4,641.00 mg
Vitamin A	17,162.00 IU
Thiamin	2.18 mg
Riboflavin	2.83 mg
Niacin	21.13 mg
Ascorbic acid	404.00 mg
Saturated fat	11.42 g
Monounsaturated fat	18.31 g
Polyunsaturated fat	32.76 g
Cholesterol	89.00 mg

Percent as calories	
Protein	18%
Carbohydrate	56%
Fat	28%
Polyunsaturated	14%
Saturated	5%
Monounsaturated	8%
P/S ratio	2.86

The Living Heart Diet Menu: Day 2

Breakfast
  Breakfast Puff (1 serving) with
  Blueberries (canned in syrup, 1 cup)
  Sautéed ham slice (1 ounce)
  Skim milk (1 cup)
  Coffee

Lunch
  Autumn Vegetable Beef Soup (1 serving)
  Saltine crackers (10) with
  Pimento Cheese Spread (¼ cup)
  Cherry Nut Pie (1 slice)
  Skim milk (1 cup)

Dinner
  Pastry Cheese Puffs (2)
  Burgundy Flank Steak (1 serving)
  Eggplant with Tomatoes (1 serving)
  Tossed salad (1 cup) with
  Creamy Buttermilk Dressing (1 tablespoon)
  Hard roll (1) with
  Tub margarine (1 teaspoon)
  Fresh Fruit Kabob (1)
  Iced tea

Caloric and Nutritional Values

Calories	2,137.00
Protein	102.67 g
Fat	81.22 g
Carbohydrate	257.11 g
Calcium	1,154.00 mg
Phosphorus	1,884.00 mg
Iron	16.47 mg
Sodium	4,448.00 mg
Potassium	3,446.00 mg
Vitamin A	10,534.00 IU
Thiamin	1.25 mg
Riboflavin	1.96 mg
Niacin	17.17 mg
Ascorbic acid	136.00 mg
Saturated fat	19.14 g
Monounsaturated fat	25.36 g
Polyunsaturated fat	32.92 g
Cholesterol	179.00 mg

Percent as calories

Protein	19%
Carbohydrate	48%
Fat	34%
Polyunsaturated	14%
Saturated	8%
Monounsaturated	11%
P/S ratio	1.71

The Living Heart Diet Menu: Day 3

Breakfast

Pineapple juice (1 cup)
Scrambled egg substitute (¼ cup)
*Homemade Sausage (2 ounces)
Whole wheat toast (2 slices) with
Tub margarine (1 teaspoon)
Skim milk (1 cup)
Coffee

Lunch

*Ratatouille (2 cups)
*Casserole Cheese Bread (2 slices) with
Tub margarine (1 teaspoon)
Fresh granny apple (1)
Skim milk (1 cup)

Dinner

*Stuffed Fish Rolls (¼ recipe)
*Glazed Carrots and Raisins (1 serving)
*Cottage Cheese Stuffed Baked Potato (1)
*Light Muffins (1) with
Tub margarine (1½ teaspoons)
*Rhubarb Crisp (1 serving)
Iced Tea

Caloric and Nutritional Values

Calories	1,991.00
Protein	93.43 g
Fat	63.17 g
Carbohydrate	270.88 g
Calcium	1,185.50 mg
Phosphorus	1,613.10 mg
Iron	15.62 mg
Sodium	4,366.00 mg
Potassium	4,359.00 mg
Vitamin A	14,030.00 IU
Thiamin	1.59 mg
Riboflavin	2.24 mg
Niacin	17.32 mg
Ascorbic acid	265.00 mg
Saturated fat	12.85 g
Monounsaturated fat	19.50 g
Polyunsaturated fat	28.50 g
Cholesterol	135.00 mg

Percent as calories

Protein	18%
Carbohydrate	54%
Fat	28%
Polyunsaturated	13%
Saturated	6%
Monounsaturated	9%
P/S ratio	2.22

The Living Heart Diet Menu: Day 4

Breakfast
*Honey Apple Oatmeal (1 cup)
Cinnamon toast (1 slice) with
Tub margarine (1 teaspoon)
Low-fat cottage cheese (1 cup)
Coffee

Lunch
*Chili with Beans (1 serving)
*Toasted Tortilla Chips (12)
*Cool Cuke Salad (1 serving)
Fresh peach (1)
Skim milk (1 cup)

Dinner
*Stuffed Onions (2)
French style green beans (½ cup) with
Tub margarine (½ teaspoon)
*Cinnamon Salad (1 serving)
*Quick Bran Bread (2 slices) with
Tub margarine (1 teaspoon)
Iced tea

Caloric and Nutritional Values

Calories	2,048.00
Protein	99.22 g
Fat	67.84 g
Carbohydrate	267.05 g
Calcium	1,127.00 mg
Phosphorus	1,677.00 mg
Iron	17.27 mg
Sodium	4,876.00 mg
Potassium	2,987.00 mg
Vitamin A	5,974.00 IU
Thiamin	1.09 mg
Riboflavin	1.74 mg
Niacin	11.95 mg
Ascorbic acid	78.00 mg
Saturated fat	15.22 g
Monounsaturated fat	20.73 g
Polyunsaturated fat	27.53 g
Cholesterol	80.00 mg
Percent as calories	
Protein	19%
Carbohydrate	52%
Fat	29%
Polyunsaturated	12%
Saturated	7%
Monounsaturated	9%
P/S ratio	1.80

The Living Heart Diet Menu: Day 5

Breakfast

> *Orange juice (1 cup)*
> *English muffin (1 whole)*
> *Tub margarine (2 teaspoons)*
> *Skim milk (1 cup)*
> *Coffee*

Lunch

> **Clam Mushroom Bisque (1 serving)*
> **Whole Wheat Rusks (2) with*
> *Tub margarine (1 teaspoon)*
> **Cinnamon Salad (1 serving)*
> *Low-fat cheese (2 ounces)*
> *Iced tea*

Dinner

> **Guacamole Dip (2 tablespoons)*
> **Toasted Tortilla Chips (6)*
> **Easy Enchiladas (1)*
> **Mexican Marinated Salad (1 serving)*
> *Pinto beans (1 cup)*
> *Fresh pineapple (1 cup)*
> *Iced tea*

Caloric and Nutritional Values

Calories	1,964.00
Protein	94.40 g
Fat	62.23 g
Carbohydrate	268.03 g
Calcium	1,259.00 mg
Phosphorus	2,238.60 mg
Iron	20.41 mg
Sodium	3,391.00 mg
Potassium	5,776.00 mg
Vitamin A	18,712.00 IU
Thiamin	1.51 mg
Riboflavin	1.93 mg
Niacin	15.05 mg
Ascorbic acid	924.20 mg
Saturated fat	14.89 g
Monounsaturated fat	18.43 g
Polyunsaturated fat	22.45 g
Cholesterol	137.00 mg

Percent as calories	
Protein	19%
Carbohydrate	54%
Fat	27%
Polyunsaturated	11%
Saturated	7%
Monounsaturated	9%
P/S ratio	1.51

The Living Heart Diet Menu: Day 6

Breakfast
*Orange Griddlecakes (2) with
Tub margarine (2 teaspoons) and
*Orange Syrup (2 tablespoons)
Soy-based bacon substitute (2 slices)
Skim milk (1 cup)
Coffee

Lunch
*Luncheon Tuna Salad (1 serving)
*Whole Wheat Oatmeal Bread (2 slices)
Lettuce wedge with
*Zesty French Dressing (1½ tablespoons)
Fresh strawberries (1 cup)
Skim milk (1 cup)

Dinner
*Oriental Soup (1 cup)
*Chinese Style Vegetable Dinner (1 serving)
Brown rice (1 cup)
Hard rolls (2)
Tub margarine (1 teaspoon)
*Fresh Fruit Ice (1 serving)

Caloric and Nutritional Values

Calories	2,113.00
Protein	76.50 g
Fat	56.45 g
Carbohydrate	333.70 g
Calcium	1,050.10 mg
Phosphorus	1,452.60 mg
Iron	19.77 mg
Sodium	4,861.00 mg
Potassium	3,445.00 mg
Vitamin A	4,862.00 IU
Thiamin	1.75 mg
Riboflavin	1.88 mg
Niacin	20.54 mg
Ascorbic acid	269.60 mg
Saturated fat	10.91 g
Monounsaturated fat	16.19 g
Polyunsaturated fat	26.17 g
Cholesterol	48.00 mg

Percent as calories

Protein	14%
Carbohydrate	63%
Fat	23%
Polyunsaturated	11%
Saturated	5%
Monounsaturated	7%
P/S ratio	2.39

The Living Heart Diet Menu: Day 7

Breakfast
  *Date Bran Muffins (2)
  Breakfast cut broiled pork chop (1 ounce)
  Banana (1) and orange (1) slices
  Skim milk (1 cup)
  Coffee

Lunch
  *New England Baked Soybeans (1 cup)
  *Jalapeño Cornbread (1 slice) with
  Tub margarine (1 teaspoon)
  *Caraway Slaw (1 serving)
  Fresh apple (1)
  Skim milk (1 cup)

Dinner
  *Home-Cooked Beef Stew (1 serving)
  Tossed salad (1 cup) with
  *Celery Seed Dressing (1 tablespoon)
  *Biscuits (2) with
  Tub margarine (1 teaspoon)
  *Baked Custard (1 serving)
  Iced tea

Caloric and Nutritional Values

Calories	2,053.00
Protein	101.38 g
Fat	79.37 g
Carbohydrate	251.72 g
Calcium	1,495.00 mg
Phosphorus	1,891.00 mg
Iron	19.37 mg
Sodium	3,377.00 mg
Potassium	4,889.00 mg
Vitamin A	14,094.00 IU
Thiamin	2.06 mg
Riboflavin	2.75 mg
Niacin	17.86 mg
Ascorbic acid	150.00 mg
Saturated fat	16.45 g
Monounsaturated fat	23.65 g
Polyunsaturated fat	35.78 g
Cholesterol	117.00 mg

Percent as calories

Protein	19%
Carbohydrate	49%
Fat	34%
Polyunsaturated	16%
Saturated	7%
Monounsaturated	11%
P/S ratio	2.17

Low-Calorie Menus

The following sample menus each contain approximately 1,500 calories. They have been formulated as examples of how to incorporate recipes in the book into exchanges. The calorie level can be adjusted upward or downward according to the calorie level prescribed by your physician. Those of you who need to control your calories and/or carbohydrate intake and are following a diet for diabetics or a low-calorie, Type IIb, Type III, Type IV, or Type V diet will find these menus helpful. A week (7 days) of sample menus is given with the nutrient analysis for each day, including calories, protein, fat, carbohydrate, calcium, phosphorus, iron, sodium, potassium, vitamin A, thiamin, riboflavin, niacin, ascorbic acid, saturated fat, monounsaturated fat, polyunsaturated fat, and cholesterol. For each day's menu, the percent of calories from protein, carbohydrate, and fat is shown, along with the percent from polyunsaturated, saturated, and monounsaturated fat and the P/S ratio. The sodium value for each menu does not include the use of any salt other than that listed in each recipe.

The asterisks indicate recipes that may be found in this book. Amounts are abbreviated as follows: g = grams; mg = milligrams; IU = international units.

301

The Low-Calorie Menu: Day 1

Breakfast	Exchanges
Broiled pink grapefruit half	1 fruit
*Raisin and Spice Oatmeal (½ cup) with	1 bread, ½ fruit
Tub margarine (1½ teaspoons)	1½ fats
Skim milk (1 cup)	1 dairy
Coffee	

Lunch

*Old-Fashioned Mushroom Soup (1 serving)	1 bread, ½ fat
*Monk's Bread (1 slice) with	1 bread, ½ fat
Tub margarine (1 teaspoon)	1 fat
Carrot sticks (½ carrot) and green pepper rings (½ pepper)	2 vegetables
Low-fat cottage cheese (1 cup) with	3 meats[1]
Pineapple rings (2)	1 fruit
Skim milk (1 cup)	1 dairy

Dinner

*Tangy Italian Mushrooms (⅓ cup)	1 vegetable
*Chicken Cacciatore (1 serving) with	3 meats, 1 bread, 1 fat
Spaghetti (½ cup)	1 bread
Broccoli spears (1) with	1 vegetable
Tub margarine (½ teaspoon)	½ fat
*Garlic Bread Sticks (2) with	1 bread
Tub margarine (2 teaspoons)	2 fats
Fresh strawberries (1⅛ cups)	1½ fruits
Iced tea	

Total Exchanges

6 meats, 2 dairies, 6 bread and cereals, 7 fats, 4 fruits, 4 vegetables

Caloric and Nutritional Values

Calories	1.605.00
Protein	103.16 g
Fat	49.46 g
Carbohydrate	193.50 g
Calcium	1,138.00 mg
Phosphorus	1,666.00 mg
Iron	13.89 mg
Sodium	3,766.00 mg
Potassium	4,284.00 mg
Vitamin A	17,833.00 IU
Thiamin	1.50 mg
Riboflavin	2.84 mg
Niacin	20.26 mg
Ascorbic acid	486.00 mg
Saturated fat	10.89 g
Monounsaturated fat	14.76 g
Polyunsaturated fat	21.11 g
Cholesterol	105.00 mg

Percent as calories	
Protein	25%
Carbohydrate	48%
Fat	27%
Polyunsaturated	12%
Saturated	6%
Monounsaturated	9%
P/S ratio	1.93

---

[1]This is an example of counting a dairy product as a meat exchange when eating a meatless meal.

The Low-Calorie Menu: Day 2

Breakfast
	Exchanges
Breakfast Puff (1 serving)	1 meat, 1 bread, 2 fats
Blueberries (diet pack, ¾ cup)	1½ fruits
Very thin sliced ham (½ ounce)	½ meat
Skim milk (1 cup)	1 dairy
Coffee	

Lunch
Autumn Vegetable Beef Soup (1 serving)	1½ meats, 1 bread
Saltine crackers (12) with	2 breads
Tub margarine (2 teaspoons)	2 fats
Tomato slices (2 tomatoes)	2 vegetables
Fresh pear (1)	1 fruit
Skim milk (1 cup)	1 dairy

Dinner
Herbed Tomato Starter (1 serving)	free
Burgundy Flank Steak (1 serving)	3 meats
Tangy Buttered Corn (⅓ cup)	1 bread
Tossed salad (2 cups) with	2 vegetables
Creamy Buttermilk Dressing (2 tablespoons)	1 fat
Hard roll (1) with	1 bread
Tub margarine (2 teaspoons)	2 fats
Fresh Fruit Kabob (1 serving)	1½ fruits
Iced tea	

Total Exchanges
6 meats, 2 dairies, 6 bread and cereals, 7 fats, 4 fruits, 4 vegetables

Caloric and Nutritional Values
Calories	1,497.18
Protein	83.86 g
Fat	49.19 g
Carbohydrate	184.77 g
Calcium	912.01 mg
Phosphorus	1,291.94 mg
Iron	15.30 mg
Sodium	3,426.10 mg
Potassium	3,793.22 mg
Vitamin A	11,892.38 IU
Thiamin	1.05 mg
Riboflavin	1.93 mg
Niacin	17.02 mg
Ascorbic acid	185.44 mg
Saturated fat	12.14 g
Monounsaturated fat	17.04 g
Polyunsaturated fat	18.64 g
Cholesterol	133.95 mg

Percent as calories
Protein	22%
Carbohydrate	49%
Fat	29%
Polyunsaturated	11%
Saturated	8%
Monounsaturated	10%
P/S ratio	1.53

The Low-Calorie Menu: Day 3

Breakfast	Exchanges
Apple juice (⅓ cup)	1 fruit
*Cheesy Scrambled Eggs (1)	2 meats, ½ dairy, 1½ fats
*Homemade Sausage (1½ ounces)	1½ meats
Whole wheat toast (1½ slices) with	1½ breads
Tub margarine (1 teaspoon)	1 fat
Skim milk (1 cup)	1 dairy
Coffee	

Lunch	
*Ratatouille (1½ cups)	3 vegetables, 1½ fats
*Monk's Bread (2 slices) with	2 breads, 1 fat
Tub margarine (1 teaspoon)	1 fat
Fresh granny apple (1)	1 fruit
Skim milk (½ cup)	½ dairy

Dinner	
*Stuffed Fish Rolls (¼ recipe)	2½ meats
*Fluffy Stuffed Baked Potato (1)	1½ breads
*Glazed Carrots (1 serving)	1 vegetable, 1 fruit
*Yeast Biscuits (1) with	1 bread, ½ fat
Tub margarine (½ teaspoon)	½ fat
*Full-of-Berries Gelatin (1 serving)	1 fruit
Iced tea	

Total Exchanges

6 meats, 2 dairies, 6 bread and cereals, 7 fats, 4 fruits, 4 vegetables

Caloric and Nutritional Values

Calories	1,562.00
Protein	89.98 g
Fat	50.90 g
Carbohydrate	192.61 g
Calcium	1,090.00 mg
Phosphorus	1,908.00 mg
Iron	12.97 mg
Sodium	4,671.00 mg
Potassium	3,685.00 mg
Vitamin A	17,041.00 IU
Thiamin	1.29 mg
Riboflavin	1.87 mg
Niacin	15.02 mg
Ascorbic acid	256.00 mg
Saturated fat	11.66 g
Monounsaturated fat	15.63 g
Polyunsaturated fat	21.66 g
Cholesterol	136.00 mg

Percent as calories	
Protein	23%
Carbohydrate	49%
Fat	29%
Polyunsaturated	13%
Saturated	6%
Monounsaturated	10%
P/S ratio	1.85

The Low-Calorie Menu: Day 4

Breakfast

	Exchanges
Honey Apple Oatmeal (1 cup)	2 breads, 2 fruits, 1 fat
Cinnamon toast (1 slice) with	1 bread
Tub margarine (1 teaspoon)	1 fat
Low-fat cottage cheese (¾ cup)	2½ meats
Coffee	

Lunch

Better Broiled Burger (1 serving) on	3 meats, 1 vegetable
Hamburger bun (½) with	1 bread
Mayonnaise (2 teaspoons)	1 fat
Cool Cuke Salad (1 serving)	1 vegetable
Fresh peach	1 fruit
Skim milk (1 cup)	1 dairy

Dinner

Stuffed Onion (1)	½ meat, 1 bread, 1 vegetable, 2 fats
French style green beans (½ cup) with	1 vegetable
Tub margarine (½ teaspoon)	½ fat
Molded Fruit Salad (1 serving)	1 fruit
Quick Bran Bread (1 slice) with	1 bread, ½ fat
Tub margarine (1 teaspoon)	1 fat
Skim milk (1 cup)	1 dairy

Total Exchanges

6 meats, 2 dairies, 6 bread and cereals, 7 fats, 4 fruits, 4 vegetables

Caloric and Nutritional Values

Calories	1,471.00
Protein	86.91 g
Fat	50.89 g
Carbohydrate	170.37 g
Calcium	1,067.00 mg
Phosphorus	1,389.00 mg
Iron	11.47 mg
Sodium	3,571.00 mg
Potassium	2,526.00 mg
Vitamin A	4,960.00 IU
Thiamin	.90 mg
Riboflavin	1.73 mg
Niacin	10.05 mg
Ascorbic acid	71.00 mg
Saturated fat	13.51 g
Monounsaturated fat	17.11 g
Polyunsaturated fat	18.12 g
Cholesterol	105.00 mg

Percent as calories

Protein	23%
Carbohydrate	46%
Fat	31%
Polyunsaturated	11%
Saturated	9%
Monounsaturated	11%
P/S ratio	1.34

The Low-Calorie Menu: Day 5

Breakfast

	Exchanges
Breakfast Steak (1½ ounces)	1½ meats
English muffin (1) with	2 breads
Tub margarine (2 teaspoons)	2 fats
Tomato slices (1 tomato)	1 vegetable
Skim milk (1 cup)	1 dairy
Coffee	

Lunch

*Clam-Mushroom Bisque (1 serving)	1 meat, 1 dairy, 1 fat
*Whole Wheat Rusks (5) with	2½ breads
Tub margarine (2 teaspoons)	2 fats
*Mexican Slaw Salad (1 serving)	1 vegetable
Fresh plums (2)	2 fruits

Dinner

*Hearty Cheese Fondue (¼ cup) with	1 meat
Fresh cauliflowerettes (½ cup)	1 vegetable
*Zippy Broiled Fillets (1 serving)	2½ meats
*Herbed Rice (1 serving)	1½ breads
Asparagus spears (4) with	1 vegetable
Tub margarine (1 teaspoon)	1 fat
*Baked Apple (1)	2 fruits, 1 fat
Iced tea	

Total Exchanges

6 meats, 2 dairies, 6 bread and cereals, 7 fats, 4 fruits, 4 vegetables

Caloric and Nutritional Values

Calories	1,516.00
Protein	90.50 g
Fat	52.80 g
Carbohydrate	174.90 g
Calcium	941.70 mg
Phosphorus	1,660.20 mg
Iron	15.13 mg
Sodium	2,901.00 mg
Potassium	2,657.00 mg
Vitamin A	4,645.00 IU
Thiamin	1.38 mg
Riboflavin	1.75 mg
Niacin	16.31 mg
Ascorbic acid	117.20 mg
Saturated fat	12.20 g
Monounsaturated fat	17.60 g
Polyunsaturated fat	21.30 g
Cholesterol	185.00 mg

Percent as calories	
Protein	24%
Carbohydrate	46%
Fat	31%
Polyunsaturated	13%
Saturated	7%
Monounsaturated	11%
P/S ratio	1.75

The Low-Calorie Menu: Day 6

Breakfast

	Exchanges
Orange juice (½ cup)	1 fruit
*Bacon Biscuits (2) with	2 breads, 1 fat
Tub margarine (2 teaspoons)	2 fats
Skim milk yogurt (1 cup)	1 dairy
Coffee	

Lunch

*Fat-Free Fried Chicken (1 serving)	3 meats
*Savory Green Beans (1 serving)	1 vegetable
*Whole Wheat Oatmeal Bread (1 slice) with	1½ breads, ½ fat
Tub margarine (1½ teaspoon)	1½ fats
Fresh strawberries (¾ cup)	1 fruit
Skim milk (1 cup)	1 dairy

Dinner

*Oriental Soup (1 serving)	1 vegetable
*Beef Sukiyaki (1 serving)	3 meats, 2 vegetables
Brown rice (¾ cup)	1½ breads
Hard roll (1) with	1 bread
Tub margarine (2 teaspoons)	2 fats
*Fresh Fruit Ice (1 serving)	2 fruits
Iced tea	

Total Exchanges
6 meats, 2 dairies, 6 bread and cereals, 7 fats, 4 fruits, 4 vegetables

Caloric and Nutritional Values

Calories	1,658.00
Protein	95.71 g
Fat	45.56 g
Carbohydrate	214.66 g
Calcium	1,097.50 mg
Phosphorus	1,473.80 mg
Iron	15.18 mg
Sodium	4,834.00 mg
Potassium	4,027.00 mg
Vitamin A	5,297.00 IU
Thiamin	1.95 mg
Riboflavin	2.19 mg
Niacin	23.48 mg
Ascorbic acid	503.00 mg
Saturated fat	12.17 g
Monounsaturated fat	15.98 g
Polyunsaturated fat	20.30 g
Cholesterol	126.00 mg

Percent as calories	
Protein	23%
Carbohydrate	52%
Fat	25%
Polyunsaturated	11%
Saturated	6%
Monounsaturated	8%
P/S ratio	1.67

The Low-Calorie Menu: Day 7

Breakfast	Exchanges
*Date Bran Muffin (1)	1 bread, 1 fat
Breakfast-cut broiled pork chop (1 ounce)	1 meat
Banana (½ banana) and orange (1 orange) slices	2 fruits
Skim milk (1 cup)	1 dairy
Coffee	

Lunch

*New England Baked Soybeans (1 cup)	2 meats, 2 breads, 2 fats
*Cornbread (1 slice) with	1 bread, 1 fat
Tub margarine (1 teaspoon)	1 fat
*Caraway Slaw (1 serving)	1½ vegetables
Fresh apple (1)	1 fruit
Skim milk (1 cup)	1 dairy

Dinner

*Home-Cooked Beef Stew (1 serving)	3 meats, 1 bread, 1 vegetable, ½ fat
Tossed salad (1½ cups) with	1½ vegetables
*Herbed French Dressing (2 tablespoons)	free
*Biscuit (1) with	1 bread
Tub margarine (1½ teaspoons)	1½ fats
Fresh cantaloupe (¼)	1 fruit
Iced tea	

Total Exchanges

6 meats, 2 dairies, 6 bread and cereals, 7 fats, 4 fruits, 4 vegetables

Caloric and Nutritional Values

Calories	1,647.00
Protein	88.13 g
Fat	62.00 g
Carbohydrate	198.22 g
Calcium	1,223.00 mg
Phosphorus	1,498.00 mg
Iron	16.96 mg
Sodium	2,631.00 mg
Potassium	4,578.00 mg
Vitamin A	17,032.00 IU
Thiamin	1.73 mg
Riboflavin	2.08 mg
Niacin	15.47 mg
Ascorbic acid	182.00 mg
Saturated fat	13.52 g
Monounsaturated fat	18.86 g
Polyunsaturated fat	26.75 g
Cholesterol	112.00 mg

Percent as calories	
Protein	21%
Carbohydrate	48%
Fat	33%
Polyunsaturated	15%
Saturated	7%
Monounsaturated	10%
P/S ratio	1.97

Low-Sodium Menus

A week (7 days) of sample low-sodium menus is given on the following pages. The total amount of sodium in each day's menu is between 500 and 600 milligrams. This is a very low-sodium content, and the diet should be used only by those who have been told by their physician to follow such a low-sodium diet. Others who need a higher, yet still restricted, sodium diet can add regular margarine to the menus. Each tablespoon of regular soft tub margarine contains 140 milligrams of sodium. Regular bread can also be added to the menus to increase the sodium content; 1 slice of whole wheat bread adds 132 milligrams of sodium. A dietitian will be able to assist you in making other modifications to achieve your prescribed sodium level.

Below each menu is given the nutrient analysis for each day, including: calories, protein, fat, carbohydrate, calcium, phosphorus, iron, sodium, potassium, vitamin A, thiamin, riboflavin, niacin, ascorbic acid, saturated fat, monounsaturated fat, polyunsaturated fat, and cholesterol. For each day's menu, the percent of calories from protein, carbohydrate, and fat is shown along with the percent of calories from polyunsaturated, saturated, and monounsaturated fat, as well as the P/S ratio.

The asterisks indicate recipes that may be found in this book. Amounts are abbreviated as follows: g = grams; mg = milligrams; IU = international units.

The Low-Sodium Menu: Day 1

Breakfast
Pineapple-grapefruit juice (½ cup)
*Raisin and Spice Oatmeal (1 cup)
*Coffee Can Whole Wheat Bread (1 slice) with
Low-sodium corn oil margarine (1 teaspoon)
Skim milk (1 cup)
Coffee

Lunch
*Chicken Curry Sandwiches (1 sandwich)
*Picnic Potato Salad (½ cup)
Carrot sticks (1 carrot)
Skim milk (1 cup)

Dinner
*Spaghetti Sauce (1 serving) with
Spaghetti (1 cup)
Tossed salad (1 cup) with
*Italian Dressing (1 tablespoon)
*Garlic Bread Sticks (4) with
Low-sodium corn oil margarine (2 teaspoons)
*Fruit Poached in Wine (1 serving)
Iced tea

Caloric and Nutritional Values

Calories	2,087.00
Protein	85.93 g
Fat	65.62 g
Carbohydrate	298.09 g
Calcium	937.00 mg
Phosphorus	1,399.00 mg
Iron	16.65 mg
Sodium	492.00 mg
Potassium	3,637.00 mg
Vitamin A	12,845.00 IU
Thiamin	1.54 mg
Riboflavin	1.93 mg
Niacin	17.77 mg
Ascorbic acid	147.00 mg
Saturated fat	13.22 g
Monounsaturated fat	18.91 g
Polyunsaturated fat	28.11 g
Cholesterol	138.00 mg

Percent as calories	
Protein	16%
Carbohydrate	57%
Fat	28%
Polyunsaturated	12%
Saturated	6%
Monounsaturated	8%
P/S ratio	2.12

The Low-Sodium Menu: Day 2

Breakfast
 Orange juice (½ cup)
 *Homemade Sausage (2 ounces)
 *Master Mix Biscuits (2)
 *Mushroom Gravy (¼ cup)
 Skim milk
 Coffee

Lunch
 *Okay Deviled Eggs (½ egg)
 *Mulligatawny soup (1 serving)
 *Light Muffins (1) with
 Low-sodium corn oil margarine (1 teaspoon)
 Fresh pear (1)
 Skim milk (1 cup)

Dinner
 *Burgundy Beef (1 serving)
 *Creamed Potatoes (1 serving)
 Broccoli spear (1) with
 Low-sodium corn oil margarine (½ teaspoon)
 *Whole Wheat Oatmeal Bread (2 slices) with
 Low-sodium corn oil margarine (1 teaspoon)
 *Cooked Fruit Compote (1 serving)
 Iced tea

Caloric and Nutritional Values

Calories	2,077.00
Protein	102.64 g
Fat	70.28 g
Carbohydrate	267.10 g
Calcium	1,211.00 mg
Phosphorus	1,886.00 mg
Iron	15.73 mg
Sodium	581.00 mg
Potassium	4,836.00 mg
Vitamin A	8,209.00 IU
Thiamin	1.33 mg
Riboflavin	2.19 mg
Niacin	20.59 mg
Ascorbic acid	154.00 mg
Saturated fat	15.13 g
Monounsaturated fat	22.12 g
Polyunsaturated fat	29.32 g
Cholesterol	174.00 mg

Percent as calories	
Protein	19%
Carbohydrate	51%
Fat	30%
Polyunsaturated	13%
Saturated	7%
Monounsaturated	10%
P/S ratio	1.93

The Low-Sodium Menu: Day 3

Breakfast
  Grapefruit sections (1 cup)
  *Honey Apple Oatmeal (1 cup)
  Low-sodium toast (1 slice) with
  Low-sodium corn oil margarine (1 teaspoon)
  Skim milk (1 cup)
  Coffee

Lunch
  *Quick Beef Barbecue (1 serving)
  *Cornbread (2 slices)
  Green pepper rings (½ pepper)
  *Lemon Whip (1 serving)
  Skim milk (1 cup)

Dinner
  *Gazpacho (1 serving)
  *Fancy Parisian Fillets (1 serving)
  *Stuffed Baked Potato (1)
  *Lemon Zucchini (1 serving)
  *Coffee Can Whole Wheat Bread (2 slices) with
    Low-sodium corn oil margarine (1 teaspoon)
  *Waldorf Fruit Salad (1 serving)
  Iced tea

Caloric and Nutritional Values

Calories	2,094.00
Protein	98.95 g
Fat	69.19 g
Carbohydrate	279.62 g
Calcium	1,111.00 mg
Phosphorus	1,747.00 mg
Iron	16.79 mg
Sodium	572.00 mg
Potassium	4,576.00 mg
Vitamin A	7,067.00 IU
Thiamin	1.63 mg
Riboflavin	1.99 mg
Niacin	19.24 mg
Ascorbic acid	308.00 mg
Saturated fat	14.37 g
Monounsaturated fat	20.96 g
Polyunsaturated fat	29.16 g
Cholesterol	168.00 mg

Percent as calories	
Protein	18%
Carbohydrate	53%
Fat	29%
Polyunsaturated	13%
Saturated	6%
Monounsaturated	9%
P/S ratio	2.02

The Low-Sodium Menu: Day 4

Breakfast
*Cooked Fruit Compote (1 serving)
*Banana Nut Bread (1 slice) with
  Low-sodium corn oil margarine (1 teaspoon)
  Skim milk yogurt (1 cup)
  Coffee

Lunch
*Chili with Beans (1 serving)
  Low-sodium crackers (10)
  Low-sodium low-fat cheese (1 ounce)
  Tossed salad (1 cup) with
*Italian Dressing (2 tablespoons)
  Iced tea

Dinner
*Hearty Chicken Stew with Dumplings (1 serving)
*Lemon Broccoli (1 serving)
*Citrus Sparkle Salad (1 serving)
*Sheath Cake (1 slice)
  Iced tea

Caloric and Nutritional Values

Calories	2,076.00
Protein	86.19 g
Fat	64.35 g
Carbohydrate	301.49 g
Calcium	1,195.00 mg
Phosphorus	1,717.00 mg
Iron	15.44 mg
Sodium	592.00 mg
Potassium	3,922.00 mg
Vitamin A	7,781.00 IU
Thiamin	.92 mg
Riboflavin	1.64 mg
Niacin	14.31 mg
Ascorbic acid	127.00 mg
Saturated fat	11.96 g
Monounsaturated fat	20.87 g
Polyunsaturated fat	27.05 g
Cholesterol	110.00 mg

Percent as calories	
Protein	16%
Carbohydrate	58%
Fat	27%
Polyunsaturated	12%
Saturated	5%
Monounsaturated	9%
P/S ratio	2.26

The Low-Sodium Menu: Day 5

Breakfast
Light Muffin (1)
Homemade Sausage (2 ounces)
Sliced tomato (1 tomato)
Skim milk (1 cup)
Coffee

Lunch
Autumn Vegetable Beef Soup (1 serving)
French Bread (2 slices) with
Low-sodium corn oil margarine (2 teaspoons)
Skim milk yogurt (1 cup)
Canned peach slices (1 cup)
Iced tea

Dinner
Barbecued Pork Chops (1)
Spanish Rice (2 servings)
French style green beans (½ cup) with
Low-sodium corn oil margarine (½ teaspoon)
Wheat Bread (2 slices) with
Low-sodium corn oil margarine (2 teaspoons)
Fresh Fruit Kabobs (2)
Iced tea

Caloric and Nutritional Values

Calories	2,109.00
Protein	104.61 g
Fat	59.25 g
Carbohydrate	295.06 g
Calcium	1,073.00 mg
Phosphorus	1,536.00 mg
Iron	20.36 mg
Sodium	547.00 mg
Potassium	4,165.00 mg
Vitamin A	11,310.00 IU
Thiamin	2.09 mg
Riboflavin	2.29 mg
Niacin	24.04 mg
Ascorbic acid	187.00 mg
Saturated fat	14.22 g
Monounsaturated fat	21.76 g
Polyunsaturated fat	18.77 g
Cholesterol	174.00 mg

Percent as calories	
Protein	19%
Carbohydrate	56%
Fat	25%
Polyunsaturated	8%
Saturated	6%
Monounsaturated	10%
P/S ratio	1.32

The Low-Sodium Menu: Day 6

Breakfast
Broiled grapefruit half
*Light Muffins (2) with
Low-sodium corn oil margarine (1 teaspoon)
Skim milk yogurt (1 cup)
Coffee

Lunch
*Tuna Macaroni Casserole (1 serving)
Lettuce wedge with
*Celery Seed Dressing (1 tablespoon)
*Whole Wheat Oatmeal Bread (2 slices) with
Low-sodium corn oil margarine (1 teaspoon)
*Peanut Butter Cookies (3)
Iced tea

Dinner
*Gazpacho (1 serving)
*Veal Scallopini (1 serving)
Rice (1 cup)
Asparagus spears (4) with
Low-sodium corn oil margarine (½ teaspoon)
*Raspberry Sherbet Salad (1 serving)
Iced tea

Caloric and Nutritional Values

Calories	2,061.00
Protein	90.75 g
Fat	66.29 g
Carbohydrate	280.95 g
Calcium	1,097.00 mg
Phosphorus	1,669.07 mg
Iron	15.02 mg
Sodium	488.00 mg
Potassium	3,510.00 mg
Vitamin A	4,096.00 IU
Thiamin	1.44 mg
Riboflavin	2.01 mg
Niacin	25.46 mg
Ascorbic acid	172.00 mg
Saturated fat	12.59 g
Monounsaturated fat	22.03 g
Polyunsaturated fat	28.21 g
Cholesterol	114.00 mg

Percent as calories	
Protein	17%
Carbohydrate	54%
Fat	29%
Polyunsaturated	12%
Saturated	5%
Monounsaturated	10%
P/S ratio	2.24

The Low-Sodium Menu: Day 7

Breakfast
*Crunchy Granola (¼ cup)
Skim milk yogurt (1 cup)
Fresh strawberries (1 cup)
Coffee

Lunch
*Chicken and Rice Salad (1 serving)
*Casserole Cheese Bread (1 slice) with
Low-sodium corn oil margarine (1 teaspoon)
Fresh zucchini strips (½ cup)
Skim milk (1 cup)

Dinner
*Stuffed Pepper (1)
*Florida Beets (1 serving)
Lettuce wedge with
*French Dressing (1 tablespoon)
*French Bread (2 slices) with
Low-sodium corn oil margarine (1 teaspoon)
*Honey Apple Pie (1 slice)
Iced tea

Caloric and Nutritional Values

Calories	2,102.00
Protein	70.76 g
Fat	72.98 g
Carbohydrate	299.49 g
Calcium	1,140.00 mg
Phosphorus	1,407.00 mg
Iron	14.90 mg
Sodium	617.00 mg
Potassium	3,306.00 mg
Vitamin A	5,250.00 IU
Thiamin	1.75 mg
Riboflavin	2.14 mg
Niacin	15.08 mg
Ascorbic acid	377.00 mg
Saturated fat	12.49 g
Monounsaturated fat	22.48 g
Polyunsaturated fat	32.76 g
Cholesterol	56.00 mg

Percent as calories	
Protein	13%
Carbohydrate	56%
Fat	31%
Polyunsaturated	14%
Saturated	6%
Monounsaturated	10%
P/S ratio	2.62

The Living Heart Diet: Food Guides

MEAT, FISH, AND POULTRY GUIDE

The Living Heart Diet: Select only lean, well-trimmed cuts of meat. Limit to no more than 6 ounces daily.

The Low-Calorie Living Heart Diet: Limit amount to exchanges specified for desired calorie level on page 32. Remove bone and skin before weighing each cooked portion of meat, fish, or poultry.

1 ounce meat, fish, or poultry = 1 meat exchange

¼ cup flaked, cubed, or chopped meat = 1 ounce = 1 meat exchange

Each exchange (1 ounce) has approximately: 59 calories, 8 grams protein, and 3 grams fat.

Yes[a]	No
Beef ("Choice" or "Good" graded meat)	**Beef** (all "Prime" graded meat)
Lean and well trimmed	Beef bacon
Chipped or dried	Beef sausage
Chuck—arm, eye, blade (pot roast or steak)	Brisket
Flank steak—plain, cubed, or rolled	Chili meat
Ground beef—chuck or round	Corned beef (except lean corned beef round)
Light-weight beef	Hamburger meat
Loin—porterhouse, T-bone, sirloin, tenderloin (steak or roast)	Pastrami
	Plate ribs—short or spare
Round—bottom, heel, rump, tip, or top (roast or steak)	Rib eye—steak or standing rib roast
Veal	**Veal**
All well-trimmed cuts	Breast riblets

[a]See page 320 to estimate the number of ounces per average serving.

Yes	No

Pork—fresh, lean and well trimmed
  Leg (fresh ham)
  Loin—rib or chop
  Pork cubed steak
  Ribs—center or shank
	Pork—fresh
	  Boston (roast or steak)
	  Ground pork
	  Loin back ribs
	  Shoulder arm picnic (roast or steak)
	  Shoulder blade
	  Spareribs

Pork—smoked (cured), lean, and well trimmed
  Canadian bacon
  Ham—center slices, rump, or shank
  Loin—rib or chop
	Pork—smoked (cured)
	  Bacon
	  Canned deviled ham
	  Ham—country, dry cure
	  Neckbones
	  Pickled pigs' feet
	  Pork hock
	  Pork jowl
	  Pork shoulder picnic or roll
	  Salt pork
	  Sausage—all kinds

Lamb
  Leg—roast, center whole shank, sirloin (roast or chops)
  Loin—chop or roast
  Rib—chop or roast
  Shank
  Shoulder—chop or roast
	Lamb
	  Ground lamb
	  Mutton

Fish and shellfish
  All freshwater and saltwater fish
  Anchovy fillet—8 thin
  Clams—2 medium = 1 ounce
  Crabs—¼ cup = 1 ounce
  Lobster—¼ cup = 1 ounce
  Octopus—1 ounce
  Oysters—3 to 4 medium = 1 ounce
  Salmon and mackerel (drain the oil) ¼ cup = 1 ounce
  Sardines—number may vary by size; 1 ounce (approximately 3 = 1 ounce)
  Scallops—3 to 4 medium = 1 ounce
  Shrimp—4 medium or 2 large = 1 ounce (limit to 3 ounces per month)
  Squid—1 ounce
  Tuna—(drain the oil or use water pack) ¼ cup = 1 ounce
	Fish and shellfish
	  Caviar
	  Crayfish
	  Eel
	  Shrimp—more than 3 ounces per month
	  Frozen breaded fish products
	  Fish roe, including caviar

Yes	No

Poultry (no skin)
  Chicken—thigh and drumstick = 3 ounces;
    ½ breast = 3 ounces
  Chicken, canned, deboned, or whole
  Rock Cornish hen—½ hen = 4 ounces
  Turkey
	Poultry
	  Poultry skin
	  Duck
	  Goose

Game—lean and well trimmed
  Alligator
  Armadillo
  Dove
  Frog
  Goat
  Pheasant
  Quail
  Rabbit
  Squirrel
  Turtle
  Venison
	Game
	  Opossum
	  Raccoon
	  Venison sausage

Luncheon meat
  Thinly sliced lean beef, chicken, turkey, or
    ham
  Turkey ham
  Turkey pastrami
	Luncheon meat—all varieties of fresh or canned
	  Bologna
	  Bratwurst
	  Frankfurters, beef, pork, and poultry
	  Headcheese
	  Liverwurst
	  Salami

Organ meats
  Beef tripe
  Liver (beef, pork, lamb)—limit to 3 ounces per
    month
	Organ meats
	  Brains
	  Chicken liver
	  Chitterlings
	  Gizzard
	  Heart
	  Kidney
	  Liver (beef, pork, lamb)—more than 3 ounces
	    per month
	  Pork maw
	  Sweetbreads

Soybean products—limit to no more than 1
    serving per day on The Low-Calorie Living
    Heart Diet—unlimited on The Living Heart
    Diet
  Soybean meat substitutes which have no
    saturated fat added
  Soybean meat extenders (textured vegetable
    protein)
	Soybean products
	  Textured vegetable protein added to *fatty*
	    ground meat (meat containing greater than
	    10% fat)

	Miscellaneous
	  Commercially fried meat, fish, or poultry
	  Meats canned or frozen in gravy or sauce

Meat Substitutes

The following foods may be substituted in the quantities listed for 1 ounce of meat:

Cottage cheese:
　½ cup dry curd = 1 meat exchange
　⅓ cup low-fat = 1 meat exchange
　¼ cup regular = 1 meat exchange

2 ounces low-fat cheese (1 to 8% butterfat) = 1 meat exchange

1 ounce vegetable oil cheese[a] = 1 meat exchange

½ cup cooked dried peas or beans[b] = 1 meat exchange

2 tablespoons peanut butter[c] = 1 meat exchange

---

[a]In addition to being 1 meat exchange, this food must also be counted as 1 fat exchange.
[b]In addition to being 1 meat exchange, this food must also be counted as 1 bread exchange.
[c]In addition to being 1 meat exchange, this food must also be counted as 2 fat exchanges.

Estimating Portion Size of Meat, Fish, and Poultry (Cooked Weights)

	Number of ounces per average serving
Fish, 1 piece (3 × 2½ × ½″)	3
Chicken, ½ large breast	3
Chicken leg (drumstick plus thigh)	3
Cornish hen, ½ of whole (no skin)	3
Ground meat, 1 pound lean, divided into 4 equal portions, 1 patty cooked	3
Roast beef, 1 lean slice (3 × 3 × ¾″)	3
Ham, 1 lean slice (3 × 3 × ¾″)	3
Pork chop, 1 medium (½″ thick)	2
Chopped meat, fish, or poultry (¼ cup)	1
Scallops, approximately 10 medium	3
Oysters, approximately 10 medium	3
Shrimp, 12 medium—*limit to once a month*	3
Liver, pork or calf, 1 slice (3 × 2¼ × ⅜″)—*limit to once a month*	3

EGG GUIDE

The Living Heart Diet and The Low-Calorie Living Heart Diet recommend no more than 2 egg yolks per week, including those used in cooking. As it is difficult to count egg yolks used in cooking—BE CAREFUL! Egg substitutes without cholesterol may be used if additional eggs are desired. Egg whites may be used as desired, without counting calories. In many recipes 1 whole egg may be replaced by 2 egg whites.

1 whole egg = 79 calories
1 egg white = 16 calories

The calories in egg substitutes vary according to brand.

Yes	No
Egg yolks (2 per week) including those used in cooking	Egg yolks—no more than the 2 allowed per week
Egg whites—free	
	Cakes, batters, sauces, rolls, and other foods containing egg yolks
	Commercial cookies, cakes, mixes, and other commercial foods containing egg yolks
	Custards containing egg yolks (unless figured into weekly allowance)
Egg substitutes—cholesterol-free (1 egg equivalent = 1 ounce meat on The Low-Calorie Living Heart Diet)	Egg substitutes that are not cholesterol-free
	Eggnog and other beverages containing egg yolks

DAIRY PRODUCTS GUIDE

The table on pages 42 to 43 specifies the number of cups of milk needed daily by each age group.

The Living Heart Diet: Skim milk dairy products can be used freely. Low-fat dairy products and those containing moderate amounts of fat are allowed; the number of servings should be limited according to the desired calorie plan on page 32.

The Low-Calorie Living Heart Diet: The amount listed is equal to 1 exchange. Limit amount to exchange specified for desired calorie level on page 32. Each exchange contains approximately 80 calories, 12 grams carbohydrate, 8 grams protein, and 1 gram fat or less.

Yes	No
Milk	**High-Fat Dairy Products**
Skim or fluid nonfat milk—1 cup	American, Cheddar, Swiss, and other cheeses containing 9% butterfat or more
Low-fat milk (1% butterfat)—1 cup[a]	Butter
Buttermilk (made from skim milk)—1 cup	Chocolate milk
Buttermilk (made from low-fat milk)—1 cup[b]	Condensed milk
Buttermilk, powdered—⅓ cup powder *or* 1 cup reconstituted	Cream cheese
Nonfat dry milk—⅓ cup powder *or* 1 cup reconstituted	Evaporated milk
Low-fat milk (1½ to 2% butterfat)—1 cup[b]	Half and half
Low-fat dry milk—1 cup[b]	Ice cream
Evaporated skim milk—½ cup undiluted *or* 1 cup diluted	Mellorine
Evaporated low-fat milk—½ cup undiluted *or* 1 cup diluted[b]	Sour cream
Dairy vegetable blend—½ cup[b]	Yogurt made from whole milk
Whole milk—½ cup[b]	Whipping cream
Cheese	
Imitation cheese made from skim milk (1% butterfat)—2 ounces	
Hand cheese, made from skim milk—2 ounces	
Imitation cheese, made with skim milk and polyunsaturated oil—1 ounce	
Sap Sago skim milk cheese—2 ounces	
Cottage cheese, dry curd—½ cup	
Cottage cheese, low-fat—½ cup[a]	
Cottage cheese, creamed—½ cup[b]	
Cheese, 4–8% butterfat—2 ounces	
Yogurt	
Yogurt, plain, skim milk—¾ cup	
Yogurt, plain, low-fat—1 cup[b]	
Desserts	
Frozen yogurt[c]—¼ cup[d]	
Fruited yogurt, low-fat[c]—½ cup[d]	
Ice milk[c]—½ cup[a]	

[a]In addition to being 1 dairy exchange, this food must also be counted as ½ fat exchange.
[b]In addition to being 1 dairy exchange, this food must also be counted as 1 fat exchange.
[c]High sugar content; not recommended for diabetics.
[d]In addition to being 1 dairy exchange, this food must also be counted as 1 fruit exchange.

Dairy Substitutes

The Living Heart Diet: Most dairy substitutes should not be used on The Living Heart Diet because they contain either coconut oil, palm kernel oil, or hydrogenated fat. If the product lists a polyunsaturated oil as an ingredient, however, it may be included and can be substituted for 1 exchange of bread.

The Low-Calorie Living Heart Diet: 1 serving = 1½ ounces of allowed dairy substitute = 1 bread exchange

Yes	No
If product lists a recommended oil as ingredient, it may be included when properly exchanged from the daily food plan.	Imitation sour creams—tub, powdered, or canned
1½ ounces = 1 bread exchange	Imitation whipped toppings—tub, powdered, aerosol, or frozen
	Imitation coffee creamers—liquid, powdered or frozen
	Filled milk
	Imitation milk

BREAD AND CEREAL GUIDE

The Living Heart Diet: 4 servings daily or more as desired.

The Low-Calorie Living Heart Diet: Limit number of exchanges according to specific calorie level on page 32.

Any one of the following is a serving in the amount listed.

1 serving = 1 bread exchange

Each exchange contains approximately 68 calories, 15 grams carbohydrate, and 2 grams protein.

Yes	No
All whole-grain and enriched bread products including:	**Bread products**
Bagels (except those made with egg or cheese) (3″ diameter)—½	Bagels made with eggs or cheese
Biscuits*a* (2″ diameter)—1	Butter rolls
Breads—1 slice	Cheese breads
French	Canned biscuits
Italian	Commercial doughnuts, muffins, sweet rolls, waffles, and pancakes
Oatmeal	Croissants
Pumpernickel	Egg breads
Raisin (no icing)	
Rye	
Sour dough	
Whole wheat	
White	
Bread crumbs—3 tablespoons	
Cornbread*a* (2 × 2 × 1″)—1 piece or ¹⁄₁₆ of 9″ pan	
Corn muffin*a* (2″ diameter)—1	
English muffin (4″ diameter)—½	
Hamburger bun—½	
Hot dog bun—½	
Muffins*a*—1	
Pancakes*a* (5 × ½″)—1	
Pita bread—½ small pocket	
Roll, plain—1	
Roll, French—1 small or ½ large	
Hard roll—1	
Tortillas, (6″ diameter) soft	
Corn—1	
Flour*a*—1	
Waffles*a* (5 × ½″)—1	

*a*Prepared with recommended ingredients. Count also as 1 fat exchange on The Low-Calorie Diet.

Yes	No
Cereal products Dry cereals which do not contain coconut or palm oil—1 ounce (see nutrition label on package for serving size) Barley, cooked—½ cup Bran, shredded or bud type—⅓ cup Bran flakes—½ cup Flake or puff type—¾ cup Hot cereal—½ cup Grits, cooked—½ cup Rice, cooked—½ cup Wheat germ—3 tablespoons	**Cereals** Cereals containing coconut or coconut oil Presweetened cereals
Pastas (cooked) Lasagna—½ cup Macaroni—½ cup Noodles, lasagna or spinach—½ cup Spaghetti—½ cup	**Pastas** Egg noodles Chow mein noodles

Crackers and snacks
Animal crackers—6
Bread sticks (5 × ½″)—4
Graham crackers (2½″ square)—2
Matzo (4 × 6″)—½
Melba toast (3½ × 1½ × ⅛″)—4
Oyster crackers—20
Pretzels
    Large three-ring (2½″ across)—4
    Small three-ring (1½″ across)—12
    Rods (8″)—1
    Sticks (3⅛ × ⅛″)—25
Rye crackers (wafers) (3½ × 2″)—3
Saltines (2″ square)—6
Soda crackers (2½″ square)—4
	Crackers
	Corn chips
	Potato chips
	Tortilla chips
	Other commercial crackers

Other Foods to Be Counted as Bread Exchanges

Although the following foods are not bread, they contain an approximately equivalent amount of carbohydrate. Any one of the following foods, in the amount listed, can be substituted for 1 exchange from the Bread Group.

Yes	No
Desserts	**Desserts**
Angel food cake (3 × 1 × ½″)—1 slice	Cheesecake pastries
Fruit ice—¼ cup	Commercial cakes, pies, cookies, fried pies,
Gelatin (regular)—⅓ cup	and cupcakes
Frozen yogurt—⅓ cup	Commercial mixtures containing dried eggs,
Ice milk—⅓ cup	whole milk, coconut, coconut oil, and/or
Sherbet—¼ cup	hydrogenated shortening
	Commercial sweet rolls
	Ice cream
	Mellorine
Starchy vegetables (cooked)	
Acorn squash—½ cup	
Baked beans, canned or homemade (no pork)— ¼ cup	
Corn—⅓ cup or ½ large corn-on-the-cob	
Dried beans, peas, lentils, chick peas, garbanzos, soybeans, or lima beans—½ cup	
Green peas—½ cup	
Hominy—½ cup	
Parsnips—⅔ cup	
Popcorn (popped in oil), no fat added after popping—2 cups[a]	
Popcorn (air-popped), no fat added after popping—3 cups	
Potato, white[b]—1 small or ½ cup mashed	
Pumpkin (without milk, eggs or sugar)—¾ cup	
Sweet potatoes or yams—¼ cup mashed[b]	
Winter squash, acorn or butternut—½ cup	

[a]In addition to being 1 bread exchange, this food must also be counted as 1 fat exchange.

[b]Without added fat in preparation. If desired, use recommended ingredients and remember to count added fat into your daily allowance.

Soups

Certain soups (e.g., fat-free broth, bouillon, and consommé) may be included in the diet *freely* because they contain a negligible amount of calories. Those that are higher in calories (listed below) can be substituted for 1 exchange of bread or bread and meat.

Vegetable soup: count soups made from starchy vegetables (e.g., corn, peas, beans, potatoes) as ½ cup = 1 bread exchange.

Beef stew: count ounces of meat as meat exchanges and ½ cup starchy vegetables as 1 bread exchange.

Mixed vegetable or tomato soup: 1 cup = 1 bread exchange.

Alcohol

Any one of the following in the amount listed is 1 exchange and may be substituted for 1 exchange from the Bread and Cereal Guide. Such substitutions should be *limited to 2 exchanges per day.* The allowance should not be accumulated.

1 ounce bourbon, gin, rum, Scotch, tequila, vodka, whiskey = 1 bread exchange

1½ ounces dessert or sweet wine = 1 bread exchange

2½ ounces dry table wine = 1 bread exchange

5 ounces regular beer = 1 bread exchange

8 ounces light beer (96 calories per 12 ounces) = 1 bread exchange (check label for calorie and carbohydrate content)

Miscellaneous

Any of the following foods may be counted as 1 bread exchange:

Bread crumbs—3 tablespoons
Catsup—¼ cup
Chili sauce—¼ cup
Cocoa—5 tablespoons
Cornmeal—2 tablespoons
Cornstarch—2 tablespoons
Flour—2½ tablespoons
Tapioca—2 tablespoons
Tomato paste—6 tablespoons
Tomato sauce—1 cup

FAT GUIDE

The Living Heart Diet: Margarine, oil, salad dressings, nuts, and seeds should be limited according to the desired calorie plan on page 32.

The Low-Calorie Living Heart Diet: Use the number of exchanges specified on desired calorie level on page 32. Any one of the following is a serving or exchange in the amount listed.

Each exchange contains approximately: 45 calories, and 4 grams fat.

Yes	No
Margarine—1 teaspoon Tub margarine listing liquid safflower oil, sunflower oil, or liquid corn oil as the first ingredient	**Margarine** Any tub margarine not listing either safflower, sunflower, or corn oil as the first ingredient Diet margarine Squeeze margarine
Oil—1 teaspoon Recommended oils: Safflower oil Sunflower oil Corn oil Other oils for occasional use: Cottonseed oil (or blends of soybean and cottonseed oils) Olive oil[a] Peanut oil[a] Sesame oil Soybean oil	**Saturated vegetable oils and shortening** Coconut oil Palm kernel oil Palm oil Partially hydrogenated vegetable oils Solid shortening
Salad dressings—2 teaspoons Commercial dry package mixes containing recommended ingredients French dressing, commercial Italian dressing, commercial Mayonnaise, commercial or homemade Mayonnaise type dressing, commercial Russian dressing, commercial Thousand Island dressing, commercial Homemade dressings with recommended ingredients	**Salad dressings** Blue cheese dressing Green goddess dressing Roquefort dressing Salad dressings made with sour cream or cheese
Nuts Almonds 7 whole Brazil nuts 2 Chestnuts 5 small Filberts 5 Hazelnuts 5 Hickory 7 small Mixed nuts 4–6	**Nuts** Cashew Macadamia Pistachio

[a]REMEMBER: Monounsaturated or neutral fats do not affect cholesterol levels, but they do have the same number of calories per unit as saturated and polyunsaturated fats.

Yes		No
Peanuts		
Spanish	20 whole	
Virginia	10 whole	
Pecans	6 halves	
Soynuts, toasted	3 tablespoons	
Walnuts (high in polyunsaturated fat)	5 halves	

Seeds
Pumpkin—1 tablespoon
Sesame—1 tablespoon
Sunflower—1 tablespoon

Foods containing monounsaturated fat—May be used occasionally	**Foods containing saturated fats**
Avocado (4″ diameter)—⅛	Bacon
Olives—5 small	Butter
Peanut butter—2 teaspoons	Chocolate
	Coconut
	Cream sauces
	Gravy made from meat drippings
	Ham hocks
	Lard
	Meat drippings
	Meat fat
	Salt pork

Hidden Fat

It is often difficult to detect the amount of fat in certain foods, especially when eating away from home. Even though these fats may not be visible, they do add extra calories. The following guidelines will help you count those "hidden fats." These figures also apply when the food is cooked in or contains a fat that may not be recommended in The Living Heart Diets.

How Much Fat?

Meats, fish, poultry
Pan-fried   ½ teaspoon (2 grams) fat per ounce of meat

Breaded and fried   1 teaspoon (4 grams) fat per ounce of meat

Basted   ½ teaspoon (2 grams) fat per ounce of meat

Marinated   Disregard fat if meat is not basted during cooking; count ½ teaspoon (4 grams) fat per ounce of meat if basted with marinade during cooking.

Vegetables
Stir-fried   ½ teaspoon (2 grams) fat per ½ cup portion

Seasoned with margarine, oil, or other fat   ½ teaspoon (2 grams) fat per ½ cup portion

Breaded and fried   1 teaspoon (4 grams) fat per ½ cup portion

French fries   1 teaspoon (4 grams) fat per 10 French fries

Eggs

Fried	1 teaspoon (4 grams) fat per egg
Scrambled	Absorbs all fat used in cooking

Example: If 1 teaspoon margarine is used when cooking the eggs, count 1 teaspoon (4 grams) fat.

Salads

Potato or macaroni salad	1 tablespoon (12 grams) fat per ½ cup salad
Slaw type or fruit salad	4 teaspoons (16 grams) fat per ½ cup salad
Meat or egg salad	4 teaspoons (16 grams) fat per ½ cup salad

Sauces

Gravy (homemade)	1 teaspoon (4 grams) fat per 2 tablespoons gravy
White sauce (homemade)	1 teaspoon (4 grams) fat per 2 tablespoons white sauce
Tartar sauce	1 teaspoon (4 grams) fat per 2 teaspoons tartar sauce

Miscellaneous

The following foods are high in saturated fat and are *not* recommended on The Living Heart Diet. However, they often cannot be avoided when eating away from home. If they are included in various foods, they should be counted accordingly. The following amounts are equal to approximately 1 fat exchange:

Food	Amount = 1 fat exchange (45 calories)
Bacon	1 slice
Butter	1 teaspoon
Cream cheese	1 tablespoon
Coffee cream (light)	2 tablespoons
Cream (heavy), whipped	1 tablespoon
Half and half	3 tablespoons
Sour cream	2 tablespoons
Imitation coffee creamer	2 tablespoons (liquid)
	1 tablespoon (powder)
Imitation sour cream	2 tablespoons
Imitation whipped topping	5 tablespoons (aerosol)
	3 tablespoons (frozen or powdered)
Commercial dips	2 tablespoons
Coconut (unsweetened, dried, shredded, flaked)	2 tablespoons

FRUIT GUIDE

Each day select at least one serving of fruit that is high in vitamin C. Good sources are indicated with a (C).

The Living Heart Diet: All fruits are allowed.

The Low-Calorie Living Heart Diet: Fruits may be fresh, frozen, or canned *without* sugar. Each of the following is an exchange in the amount listed.

Each exchange contains approximately: 40 calories, 10 grams carbohydrate.

Yes	No
Apple (2″ diameter)—1	Commercial fruit pie fillings
Apple juice (frozen or canned)—⅓ cup	Commercial fruit whips
Applesauce, unsweetened—½ cup	Fruits in sugar syrup
Apricots, fresh—2 medium	
Apricots, dried—4 halves	
Avocado—See *Fat Guide*, pages 328–330	
Banana—½ small	
Blackberries—½ cup	
Blueberries—½ cup	
(C) Cantaloupe (6″ diameter)—¼	
Cherries—10 large	
Cider—⅓ cup	
Cranberries—free, if no sugar added	
Cranberry juice cocktail	
Low calorie—¾ cup	
Regular—¼ cup	
Cranberry sauce—2 tablespoons	
Dates—2	
Dewberries—½ cup	
Figs, fresh—1 medium	
Figs, dried—1	
Fruit cocktail, unsweetened—½	
(C) Grapefruit—½	
(C) Grapefruit juice (fresh, frozen, canned)—½ cup	
Grapes, Tokay—12	
Grapes, green seedless—18	
Grape juice—¼ cup	
Honeydew melon (7″ diameter)—⅛	
Kumquats—4 medium	
Mandarin orange sections—½ cup	
(C) Mango—½ small	
Mixed fruit (canned), unsweetened—½ cup	
Nectar—¼ cup	
Nectarine—½ large or 1 small	
(C) Orange (2½″ diameter)—1	
(C) Orange juice—½ cup	
(C) Papaya—⅓ medium or ¾ cup	
Peach—1 medium	
Pear—1 small	
Persimmon—1 medium	

Yes	No
Pineapple, unsweetened	
Chunk—½ cup	
Slices—2 small	
Juice—⅓ cup	
Plums—2 medium	
Prunes, dried—2 medium	
Prune juice—¼ cup	
Raisins—2 tablespoons	
Raspberries—½ cup	
(C) Strawberries—¾ cup	
(C) Tangerine—1 medium	
(C) Tangerine juice—½ cup	
(C) Tomato juice—up to 1 cup free	
Vegetable juice cocktail—up to 1 cup free	
Watermelon—1 cup	

VEGETABLE GUIDE

The Living Heart Diet: Nonstarchy vegetables (listed below) are low in calories. However, for the diabetic it is important to account for all sources of carbohydrate and protein; therefore, each ½ cup of cooked or raw vegetables is 1 exchange. For persons trying to lose weight, it is usually not necessary to account for these calories; therefore the nonstarchy vegetables can be consumed freely. On page 334 there is a list of vegetables which everyone can use without counting. They have negligible calories. Remember, starchy vegetables (e.g., potatoes and corn) are listed in the Bread and Cereal Guide on page 326. Good sources of vitamin A are indicated with an (A).

Each exchange contains approximately 28 calories, 5 grams carbohydrate, and 2 grams protein.

Yes	No
½ CUP = 1 EXCHANGE	Commercially fried vegetables, e.g., fried
Artichoke	potatoes, French fries, onion rings, okra,
Asparagus	eggplant
Avocado—See *Fat Guide*, pages 328 to 330	Commercial vegetables, frozen or canned,
Bamboo shoots	packaged in a sauce or butter
Bean sprouts	Dried beans or peas seasoned with bacon fat, salt
Beans, green and wax	pork, or ham hocks
Beets	Frozen French fries and fried onion rings
(A) Broccoli	
Brussels sprouts	
Cabbage	
(A) Carrots	
Cauliflower	
Celery	
Cucumbers	
Eggplant	
Ginger root	
(A) Greens	

Beet	Kale
Chard	Mustard
Collard	Spinach
Dandelion	Turnip

Kohlrabi
Leeks
Mushrooms
Okra
Onions
Peas—See *Bread and Cereal Guide*, pages 324 to 327
Pepper, green and red
Pimento
Pumpkin—See *Bread and Cereal Guide*, pages 324 to 327
Rhubarb, unsweetened
Rutabaga
Sauerkraut
Shallots
Spinach

Yes	No

Sprouts (alfalfa and bean)
Summer squash (zucchini and yellow)
Tomatoes
Tomato juice
Turnips
Vegetable juice
Water chestnuts
Winter squash—See *Bread and Cereal Guide*,
   pages 324 to 327
Zucchini

Free Vegetables
The following raw vegetables have negligible
  calories and may be used as desired:
(A) Chicory
   Chinese cabbage
   Endive
(A) Escarole
   Lettuce
   Parsley
   Pickles
   Radishes
(A) Watercress

MISCELLANEOUS FOOD GUIDE

Some foods, such as those listed below, are low enough in calories that it is not necessary to consider the calories in them. Spices and herbs add flavor without adding calories. Many beverages (e.g., coffee, tea, and diet carbonated drinks) can add variety to the diet.

Yes: The Low-Calorie Living Heart Diet	**Yes: The Living Heart Diet**
These foods are very low in calories and may be eaten *freely*. Bitters Bouillon (fat-free) Broth (fat-free) Club soda Cocoa (limit 1 tablespoon free) Coffee, black Consommé (fat-free) Cranberries (unsweetened) Decaffeinated coffee Diet salad dressing (limit 1 tablespoon per meal) Diet gelatin Diet soft drinks[a] Dietetic jelly, jam, preserves, syrup[a] Flavoring essence (maple, butter, vanilla, etc.) Gelatin, unflavored Horseradish Hot sauce Lemon Lime Liquid smoke Mustard Picante sauce Pickles (unsweetened) Rennet tablets Rhubarb (unsweetened) Soy sauce Spices and herbs Sugar-free carbonated beverages Sugar substitute[a] Sugarless gum Tea, no sugar Vinegar Worcestershire sauce	These foods are high in calories and may lead to a weight gain and/or an elevation in triglycerides; however, they are low in fat and can be *used in moderation*. Alcoholic beverages—beer, wine, whiskey (recommended limit of no more than 2 exchanges daily)—see *Bread and Cereal Guide*, pages 324 to 327 Candy, hard sugar type Carbonated beverages Fruit-flavored drinks, punches, or ades Fruit whips Gelatin, flavored (sweetened) Honey Jelly, jam, marmalade, preserves, molasses Popsicles Punches and fruit-flavored drinks Sherbet Sugar Syrup The following foods are high in calories and contain fat. They can be calculated into the diet if recommended ingredients (e.g., skim milk, egg substitute, egg white, oil, margarine, or cocoa) are used. Candy, homemade Cakes Cookies Pastries Pies Puddings

[a]Subject to current warnings about saccharin.

Appendix

TABLE 1. *Desirable weights for men and women, 25 years and older*

MEN						WOMEN			
Height		Small frame	Medium frame	Large frame		Height		Small frame	Medium frame	Large frame
Feet	Inches					Feet	Inches			
5	2	128–134	131–141	138–150		4	10	102–111	109–121	118–131
5	3	130–136	133–143	140–153		4	11	103–113	111–123	120–134
5	4	132–138	135–145	142–156		5	0	104–115	113–126	122–137
5	5	134–140	137–148	144–160		5	1	106–118	115–129	125–140
5	6	136–142	139–151	146–164		5	2	108–121	118–132	128–143
5	7	138–145	142–154	149–168		5	3	111–124	121–135	131–147
5	8	140–148	145–157	152–172		5	4	114–127	124–138	134–151
5	9	142–151	148–160	155–176		5	5	117–130	127–141	137–155
5	10	144–154	151–163	158–180		5	6	120–133	130–144	140–159
5	11	146–157	154–166	161–184		5	7	123–136	133–147	143–163
6	0	149–160	157–170	164–188		5	8	126–139	136–150	146–167
6	1	152–164	160–174	168–192		5	9	129–142	139–153	149–170
6	2	155–168	164–178	172–197		5	10	132–145	142–156	152–173
6	3	158–172	167–182	176–202		5	11	135–148	145–159	155–176
6	4	162–176	171–187	181–207		6	0	138–151	148–162	158–179

Prepared by Metropolitan Life Insurance Co.; data derived primarily from Build and Blood Pressure Study, 1979, Society of Actuaries and Association of Life Insurance Medical Directors of America, 1980.
Weights are given in pounds, according to height and frame, in indoor clothing.

TABLE 2. Nutrient analysis of common foods

Food	Unit	Weight (g)	Cal	CHO (g)	Prot (g)	Fat (g)	Sat fat (g)	Mono fat (g)	Poly fat (g)	Chol (mg)	Na (mg)
Almonds: dried, shelled, slivered (not packed)	1 tbsp	7	43	1.4	1.3	3.9	0.3	2.7	0.7	0	tr
Anchovy: 1–4" flat	1 whole	4	5	0.0	0.8	0.3	0.1	0.1	0.1	5	32
Angel food cake: see *Cake*											
Apple: raw with skin	1 whole	150	80	20.0	0.3	0.8	0	0	0.8	0	1
Apple: raw, pared, ¼" slices or diced pieces	1 cup	110	59	15.5	0.2	0.3	0	0	0.3	0	1
Apple butter	1 tbsp	18	33	8.2	0.1	0.1	0	0	0.1	0	tr
Apple juice: canned or bottled	1 cup	248	117	29.5	0.2	0	0	0	0.0	0	2
Applesauce: canned, sweetened	1 cup	255	232	60.7	0.5	0.3	0	0	0.3	0	5
Apricots: raw	3 whole	114	55	13.7	1.1	0.2	0	0	0.2	0	1
Apricot nectar: canned or bottled	1 cup	251	143	36.6	0.8	0.3	0	0	0.3	0	tr
Artichoke: frozen, cooked, bud or globe	1 whole	300	52	11.9	3.4	0.2	0	0	0.2	0	36
Asparagus: canned spears, ½" diameter	4 spears	80	17	2.7	1.9	0.3	0	0	0.3	0	189
Asparagus: canned, cut spears, low sodium	1 cup	235	47	7.3	6.1	0.7	0	0	0.7	0	7
Avocado: California, raw, 3⅛" diameter	1 whole	284	369	12.9	4.7	36.7	7.3	16.5	4.8	0	9
Avocado: California, raw, puréed, mashed, or sieved (unpeeled)	1 tbsp	14	25	0.9	0.3	2.4	0.5	1.1	0.3	0	1
Bacon: Canadian, cooked, 3⅜ × 3/16"	1 oz	28	78	0.1	7.7	5.0	1.7	1.9	0.4	25	726
Bacon: cooked (approximately 20 slices/lb raw)	2 slices	15	86	.5	3.8	7.8	2.7	3.4	0.8	11	153
Bacon bits: with coconut oil	1 tsp	3	15	0.9	1.3	0.6	0.6	0.1	0	0	115
Bacon bits: with soy oil	1 tsp	3	14	0.9	1.4	0.6	0.1	0.2	0.2	0	115
Bagel: water	1 whole	73	212	41.1	7.9	1.3	0.2	0.2	0.3	0	120
Baking powder: double acting	1 tsp	3	3	0.7	0	0	0	0	0	0	290
Baking powder: low sodium	1 tsp	4	7	1.8	0	0	0	0	0	0	tr
Baking soda	¼ tsp	4	0	0	0	0	0	0	0	0	345
Banana: raw, medium	1 whole	175	101	26.4	1.3	0.2	0.1	0	0.2	0	1
Barbecue sauce: commercial (corn oil)	1 tbsp	16	14	1.3	0.2	1.1	0.1	0.3	0.6	0	127
Beans: garbanzos or chickpeas	1 cup	185	248	42.1	14.1	3.3	1.0	0.3	2.0	0	18
Beans: pork and beans in tomato sauce, canned	1 cup	255	311	48.5	15.6	6.6	2.4	2.8	0.6	6	1,181
Beans: kidney	1 cup	185	218	39.6	14.4	0.9	0.3	0.1	0.6	0	6
Beans: lentils	1 cup	200	212	38.6	15.6	0	0	0	0	0	4
Beans: lima, frozen, cooked	1 cup	170	168	32.5	10.2	0.2	0	0	0.1	0	172
Beans: lima, canned	1 cup	170	163	31.1	9.2	0.5	0.2	0	0.3	0	401
Beans: lima, canned, low sodium	1 cup	170	162	30.1	9.9	0.5	0.1	0	0.2	0	7
Beans: pinto, calico, red Mexican	1 cup	185	218	39.6	14.4	0.9	0.3	0.1	0.6	0	6
Beans: mung, sprouts, cooked and drained	1 cup	125	35	6.5	4.0	0.3	0	0	0.3	0	5

This information is current as of this printing. Check the manufacturer's label for updated analysis.

A dash (—) indicates that data are not available. Trace (tr) indicates that a very small amount of the constituent is present.

Abbreviations used in this table are: tbsp = tablespoon; tsp = teaspoon; oz = ounce; lb = pound; gm = gram; mg = milligrams; " = inches; Cal = calories; CHO = carbohydrate; Prot = protein; Sat fat = saturated fat; Mono fat = monounsaturated fat; Poly fat = polyunsaturated fat; Chol = cholesterol; Na = Sodium.

Food	Measure	gm	Cal	CHO	Prot	Fat	Sat fat	Mono fat	Poly fat	Chol	Na
Beans: mung, sprouts, uncooked	1 cup	105	37	6.9	4.0	0.2	0	0	0	0	5
Beans: green, snap, fresh, frozen, cooked	1 cup	130	34	7.8	2.1	0.1	0	0	0.1	0	3
Beans: green, snap, canned	1 cup	135	32	7.0	1.9	0.3	0	0	0	0	319
Beans: green, snap, canned, low sodium	1 cup	135	30	6.5	2.0	0.1	0.1	0	0.1	0	3
Beans: white, Great Northern, navy, cooked	1 cup	180	212	38.2	14.0	1.1	0.3	0.1	0.7	0	13
Beans: yellow or wax, frozen, cooked	1 cup	125	28	5.8	1.8	0.3	0	0	0.3	0	4
Beans: yellow or wax, canned	1 cup	135	32	7.0	1.9	0.4	0	0	0.4	0	319
Beans: yellow or wax, canned, low sodium	1 cup	135	28	6.3	1.6	0.1	0	0	0.1	0	3
Beef: dried, chipped, uncooked	1 oz	28	58	0	9.7	1.8	0.8	0.8	0	26	1,219
Beef: <6% fat; flank, round, Pike's Peak (lean only)	1 oz	28	53	0	8.9	1.7	0.9	0.8	0.1	26	19
Beef: 10% fat; chuck, filet mignon, New York strip, porterhouse, T-bone, tenderloin, ground round, choice grade (lean only)	1 oz	28	61	0	8.5	2.7	1.3	1.1	0.1	26	19
Beef: 15% fat; club, rib eye roast, choice grade (lean only)	1 oz	28	74	0	8.1	4.4	2.2	2.0	0.2	27	18
Beef: 20% fat; ground chuck	1 oz	28	82	0	7.7	5.5	2.9	2.6	0.2	27	16
Beef: 25% fat; ground beef (hamburger), chuck, steak, pot roast (lean and fat)	1 oz	28	93	0	7.4	6.8	3.4	3.1	0.3	27	16
Beef: >30% fat; brisket, rib eye steak, standing rib roast, spareribs (lean and fat)	1 oz	28	110	0	6.5	9.1	4.8	4.4	0.3	27	15
Beef: corned	1 oz	28	110	0	6.5	9.1	4.4	4.4	0.3	27	264
Beef: tongue: medium-fat, cooked, 3 × 2 × 1/8"	1 slice	20	49	0.1	4.3	3.3	1.8	2.0	0.1	18	12
Beef: kidney, cooked, 1/2 × 1/2 × 1/4"	1 oz	140	353	1.1	46.2	16.8	6.6	2.5	2.7	1,126	354
Beef: liver	1 oz	28	40	1.5	5.7	1.1	0.4	0.2	0.2	86	39
Beef: tallow: suet	1 tbsp	14	120	0	0.2	13.2	6.8	5.9	0.6	11	0
Beer: regular	12 oz	360	151	13.7	1.1	0	0	0	0	0	25
Beets: red, canned, diced, sliced, or whole	1 cup	170	63	15.0	1.7	0.2	0	0	0.2	0	401
Beets: red, canned, diced, sliced, or whole, low sodium	1 cup	170	63	14.8	1.5	0.2	0	0	0.2	0	78
Biscuit: made with shortening	1 whole	28	103	12.8	2.1	4.8	—	—	—	—	175
Blackberries: raw (also boysenberries, dewberries)	1 cup	144	84	18.6	1.7	1.3	0.3	0.3	0.7	0	1
Bologna: 1 slice	1 oz	28	86	0.3	3.4	8.3	3.4	4.0	0.3	52	287

This information is current as of this printing. Check the manufacturer's label for updated analysis.

A dash (—) indicates that data are not available. Trace (tr) indicates that a very small amount of the constituent is present.

Abbreviations used in this table are: tbsp = tablespoon; tsp = teaspoon; oz = ounce; lb = pound; gm = gram; mg = milligrams; " = inches; Cal = calories; CHO = carbohydrate; Prot = protein; Sat fat = saturated fat; Mono fat = monounsaturated fat; Poly fat = polyunsaturated fat; Chol = cholesterol; Na = Sodium.

TABLE 2. (continued)

Food	Unit	Weight (g)	Cal	CHO (g)	Prot (g)	Fat (g)	Sat fat (g)	Mono fat (g)	Poly fat (g)	Chol (mg)	Na (mg)
Bouillon cube: all kinds (1 tsp instant bouillon)	1 cube	4	5	0.2	0.8	0.1	0.1	0	0	0	960
Braunschweiger (liver sausage)	1 oz	28	90	0.7	4.2	9.2	3.1	4.4	1.2	—	287
Bread: cracked wheat	1 slice	25	66	13.0	2.2	0.6	0.1	0.2	0.2	0	132
Bread: English muffin	1 whole	57	133	25.5	4.4	1.4	0.4	0.6	0.4	0	263
Bread: French, enriched; 2½ × 2 × ½"	1 slice	15	44	8.3	1.4	0.5	0.1	0.2	0.1	0	87
Bread: pita, pocket	1 large	52	145	30.0	5.0	1.0	0.3	0.4	0.2	0	86
Bread: pumpernickel (dark rye)	1 slice	32	79	17.0	2.9	0.4	0.1	0.2	0.1	0	182
Bread: raisin	1 slice	25	66	13.4	1.7	0.7	0.1	0.3	0.1	0	91
Bread: rye (light)	1 slice	25	61	13.0	2.3	0.3	0.1	0.2	0.1	0	139
Bread: white, enriched	1 slice	25	68	12.6	2.2	0.8	0.2	0.2	0.2	0	127
Bread: whole wheat, firm crumb	1 slice	25	61	11.9	2.6	0.8	0.1	0.4	0.2	0	132
Bread: white, low sodium	1 slice	28	76	14.1	2.4	0.9	0.2	0.3	0.2	0	3
Broccoli: medium stalk, fresh, cooked, and drained	1 stalk	180	47	8.1	5.6	0.5	0	0	0.5	0	18
Brussels sprouts: frozen, cooked, and drained	1 cup	155	51	10.1	5.0	0.3	0	0	0.3	0	22
Butter: 1 pat	1 tsp	5	36	0	0	4.1	2.5	1.2	0.2	12	49
Buttermilk: made from skim milk	1 cup	245	88	12.5	8.8	0.2	0.1	0.1	0	2	319
Buttermilk: made from low-fat milk	1 cup	245	99	11.7	8.1	2.2	1.3	0.6	0.1	9	257
Cabbage: common or Chinese; shredded, cooked, and drained	1 cup	145	29	6.2	1.6	0.3	0	0	0.3	0	20
Cabbage: common or Chinese varieties, raw, shredded	1 cup	90	22	4.9	1.2	0.2	0	0	0.2	0	18
Cake: angel food, 1/12 of 10" tube cake	1 slice	60	161	36.1	4.3	0.1	0.1	0	0.1	0	170
Cake: coffee cake (mix), 2⅝ × 2¾ × 1¼"	1 slice	72	232	37.7	4.5	6.9	2.0	3.2	1.3	35	310
Cake: cream cheese, without crust or topping	1 slice	85	368	25.7	7.6	26.8	6.0	6.0	1.0	163	173
Cake: devil's food (frozen), 1/6 of 7½" cake	1 slice	85	323	47.3	3.7	15.0	7.7	5.4	0.7	37	357
Cake: devil's food cupcake with icing (mix), 2½" diameter	1 whole	35	119	20.4	1.5	4.3	1.8	2.1	0.4	17	92
Cake: gingerbread (mix), 2¾ × 2¾ × 1⅛"	1 slice	63	174	32.2	2.0	4.3	1.1	2.1	1.0	0.6	192
Cake: marble with white icing (mix), 1/12 of layer cake	1 slice	87	288	53.9	3.8	7.6	4.8	2.1	0.7	40	225
Cake: yellow with chocolate icing (mix), 1/12 of layer cake	1 slice	92	310	53.0	3.8	10.4	4.6	5.5	0.9	44	209

This information is current as of this printing. Check the manufacturer's label for updated analysis.

A dash (—) indicates that data are not available. Trace (tr) indicates that a very small amount of the constituent is present.

Abbreviations used in this table are: tbsp = tablespoon; tsp = teaspoon; oz = ounce; lb = pound; gm = gram; mg = milligrams; " = inches; Cal = calories; CHO = carbohydrate; Prot = protein; Sat fat = saturated fat; Mono fat = monounsaturated fat; Poly fat = polyunsaturated fat; Chol = cholesterol; Na = Sodium.

Food	Serving	Weight (gm)	Cal	CHO (gm)	Prot (gm)	Fat (gm)	Sat fat (gm)	Mono fat (gm)	Poly fat (gm)	Chol (mg)	Na (mg)
Candy; candy corn, approximately 72 pieces	1/4 cup	50	182	44.8	0	1.0	0.3	0.5	0.2	0	106
Candy[a]: chocolate, bittersweet	1 oz	28	135	13.3	2.2	11.3	6.3	4.2	0.2	5	1
Candy[a]: chocolate, sweet	1 oz	28	150	16.4	1.2	10.0	5.6	3.7	0.2	5	9
Candy: chocolate covered mint, 1 3/8 × 3/8"	1 small	11	45	8.9	0.2	1.2	0.4	0.7	0.1	0.6	20
Candy: chocolate covered raisins	1 cup	190	808	134.0	10.3	32.5	18.1	11.8	0.7	19	122
Candy: chocolate covered vanilla cream	1 piece	13	56	9.1	0.5	2.2	0.8	1.0	0.1	2	24
Candy: fudge, plain, 1 cubic inch	1 piece	21	84	15.8	0.6	2.6	0.9	1.2	0.4	1	44
Candy: gum drops, 1 large or 8 small	1 large	10	34	8.7	0	0.1	0	0	0.1	0	4
Candy: jellybeans	10 pieces	28	104	26.4	0	0.1	0	0	0.5	0	3
Candy: M & M® type	1/4 cup	49	230	35.8	2.6	9.7	5.4	3.5	0.2	3	36
Candy: peanut brittle, 2 1/2 × 2 1/2 × 1/3" piece	1 oz	28	119	23.0	1.6	2.9	0.6	1.3	0.9	0	9
Candy: chocolate-flavored roll (Tootsie Roll®) 1 × 1/2"	1 piece	7	28	5.8	0.2	0.6	0.2	0.3	0.1	1	14
Candy bar[a]: chocolate coated almonds, or peanut bar (Mr. Goodbar®)	1 oz	28	161	11.2	3.5	12.4	2.1	8.2	1.6	—	17
Candy bar[a]: chocolate coated with coconut center (Mound®)	1 oz	28	124	20.4	0.8	5.0	2.9	1.9	0	3	56
Candy bar[a]: fudge, peanut, caramel (O'Henry®, Snicker®, Rally®, Baby Ruth®)	1 oz	28	130	16.6	2.7	6.5	1.8	3.5	1.0	3	36
Candy bar[a]: Hershey Krackel® or Nestlés Crunch®	1 oz	28	144	15.0	2.3	8.3	4.4	3.1	0.6	3	35
Candy bar[a]: milk chocolate bar or 7 chocolate kisses	1 oz	28	147	16.1	2.2	9.2	5.1	3.3	0.2	5	27
Cantaloupe: 5" diameter	1 whole	91	159	39.8	3.7	0.5	0	0	0.5	0	64
Cantaloupe: cubed or diced, approximately 20/cup	1 cup	160	48	12.0	1.1	0.2	0	0	0.2	0	19
Carbonated beverage: Coca-Cola®, Mr. Pibb®	12 oz	369	144	37.2	0	0	0	0	0	0	30
Carbonated beverage: ginger ale	12 oz	366	108	28.8	0	0	0	0	0	0	—
Carbonated beverage: Sprite®	12 oz	366	143	36.0	0	0	0	0	0	0	63
Carbonated beverage: Sprite® without sugar	12 oz	366	5	0	0	0	0	0	0	0	63
Carbonated beverage: Mr. Pibb® without sugar	12 oz	366	2	0.4	0	0	0	0	0	0	56

[a]The weight of candy bars often changes. The analysis here is given for 1 ounce and can be calculated for the total unit (1 piece of candy).

This information is current as of this printing. Check the manufacturer's label for updated analysis.
A dash (—) indicates that data are not available. Trace (tr) indicates that a very small amount of the constituent is present.
Abbreviations used in this table are: tbsp = tablespoon; tsp = teaspoon; oz = ounce; lb = pound; gm = gram; mg = milligrams; " = inches; Cal = calories; CHO = carbohydrate; Prot = protein; Sat fat = saturated fat; Mono fat = monounsaturated fat; Poly fat = polyunsaturated fat; Chol = cholesterol; Na = Sodium.

TABLE 2. (continued)

Food	Unit	Weight (g)	Cal	CHO (g)	Prot (g)	Fat (g)	Sat fat (g)	Mono fat (g)	Poly fat (g)	Chol (mg)	Na (mg)
Carbonated beverage: Fresca®	12 oz	366	3	0	0	0	0	0	0	0	86
Carbonated beverage: Tab®	12 oz	366	1	0.1	0	0	0	0	0	0	45
Carrot: raw, approximately 1⅛ × 7½"	1 whole	81	30	7.0	0.8	0.1	0	0	0.1	0	34
Carrots: fresh, cooked, sliced	1 cup	155	48	11.0	1.4	0.3	0	0	0.3	0	51
Carrots: canned solids, sliced	1 cup	155	47	10.4	1.2	0.5	0	0	0.5	0	366
Carrots: canned solids, sliced, low sodium	1 cup	155	39	8.7	1.2	0.2	0	0	0.2	0	60
Cashew: roasted in oil, unsalted (14 large, 18 medium, or 26 small)	1 oz	28	159	8.3	4.9	12.8	2.6	7.3	2.1	0	4
Catfish: freshwater, raw	1 oz	28	29	0	5.0	1.0	0.2	0.3	0.3	—	17
Cauliflower: frozen, cooked, approximately 7 flowerettes	1 cup	180	32	5.9	3.4	0.4	0	0	0.4	0	18
Caviar: sturgeon, granular	1 tbsp	16	42	0.5	4.3	2.4	0.6	0.7	1.0	48	352
Celery: green, raw, 8 × 1½" stalk	1 stalk	40	7	1.6	0.4	0	0	0	0	0	50
Cereal: bran, unprocessed, 1.17 cup	1 oz	28	91	12.3	3.9	0.4	0.2	0.2	0.7	0	2
Cereal: bran buds	1 cup	60	144	44.6	7.6	1.8	0.3	0.3	1.1	0	493
Cereal: 40% bran flakes	1 cup	35	106	28.2	3.6	0.6	0.1	0.1	0.3	0	207
Cereal: Cheerios® or puffed oats	1 cup	25	99	18.8	3.0	1.4	0.3	0.5	0.6	0	317
Cereal: corn flakes	1 cup	25	97	21.3	2.0	0.1	0	0	0.1	0	251
Cereal: corn grits, enriched, cooked without salt	1 cup	245	125	27.0	2.9	0.2	0	0	0.1	0	2
Cereal: cream of rice, cooked without salt	1 cup	245	123	27.4	2.0	0	0	0	0	0	2
Cereal: cream of wheat, cooked without salt	1 cup	240	180	40.6	5.3	1.0	0.2	0.1	0.5	0	2
Cereal: farina, enriched, regular, cooked without salt	1 cup	245	103	21.3	3.2	0.5	0.1	0	0.2	0	4
Cereal: farina, enriched, quick-cooking, cooked with salt	1 cup	245	105	21.8	3.2	0.5	0.1	0	0.2	0	466
Cereal: farina, enriched, instant-cooking, cooked without salt	1 cup	245	135	27.9	4.2	0.5	0.1	0	0.2	0	13
Cereal: granola, without coconut or other saturated fat	¼ cup	28	139	16.9	2.9	6.7	5.1	0	0.6	0	30
Cereal: granola, cooked (¼ cup dry = ½ cup cooked)	½ cup	120	100	21.0	3.0	1.0	0.2	0.4	0.4	0	30
Cereal: Grape-Nuts®	1 cup	110	430	92.8	11.0	0.7	0	0	0.7	0	814
Cereal: oatmeal, cooked without salt	1 cup	240	132	23.3	4.8	2.4	0.4	0.8	1.0	0	2

This information is current as of this printing. Check the manufacturer's label for updated analysis.

A dash (—) indicates that data are not available. Trace (tr) indicates that a very small amount of the constituent is present.

Abbreviations used in this table are: tbsp = tablespoon; tsp = teaspoon; oz = ounce; lb = pound; gm = gram; mg = milligrams; " = inches; Cal = calories; CHO = carbohydrate; Prot = protein; Sat fat = saturated fat; Mono fat = monounsaturated fat; Poly fat = polyunsaturated fat; Chol = cholesterol; Na = Sodium.

Food	Portion	Wt (g)	Cal	CHO	Prot	Fat	Sat fat	Mono fat	Poly fat	Chol	Na
Cereal: puffed rice	1 cup	15	60	13.4	0.9	0.1	0	0	0.1	0	0
Cereal: puffed wheat	1 cup	15	54	11.8	2.3	0.2	0.1	0.1	0.2	0	1
Cereal: raisin bran	1 cup	50	144	39.7	4.2	0.7	0	0	0.4	0	212
Cereal: Rice Krispies®	1 cup	30	117	26.3	1.8	0.1	0	0	0.1	0	283
Cereal: Spoon Size Shredded Wheat®, approximately 50 biscuits per cup	1 cup	50	180	40.0	5.0	1.3	0.2	0.2	0.7	0	2
Cereal: Shredded Wheat® biscuit, 3¾ × 2¼ × 1"	1 whole	25	90	20.0	2.5	0.6	0.1	0.1	0.3	0	1
Cereal: sugar-coated corn flakes	1 cup	40	154	36.5	1.8	0.1	0	0	0.1	0	267
Cereal: Wheat Chex®	⅓ cup	28	110	23.0	2.0	1.0	0.9	0.1	0.1	0	198
Cereal: wheat germ	1 tbsp	6	23	3.0	1.8	0.7	0.1	0.1	0.4	0	1
Cereal: Wheaties® or Total®	1 cup	30	104	24.2	3.1	0.7	0.1	0.1	0.4	0	310
Cheese: American	1 oz	28	106	0.5	6.3	8.9	5.6	2.5	0.3	27	406
Cheese: blue	1 oz	28	100	0.7	6.1	8.2	5.3	2.2	0.2	21	396
Cheese: brick	1 oz	28	105	0.8	6.6	8.4	5.3	2.4	0.2	27	159
Cheese: brie	1 oz	28	95	0.1	5.9	7.9	—	—	—	28	178
Cheese: camembert	1 oz	28	85	0.1	5.6	6.9	4.3	2.0	0.2	20	239
Cheese: cheddar	1 oz	28	114	0.4	7.1	9.4	6.0	2.7	0.3	30	176
Cheese: colby	1 oz	28	112	0.4	6.7	9.1	5.7	2.6	0.3	27	171
Cheese: cottage, creamed (4% fat)	¼ cup	53	54	1.4	6.6	2.4	1.5	0.7	0.1	8	212
Cheese: cottage, low fat (2% fat)	¼ cup	57	51	2.1	7.8	1.1	0.7	0.3	0	5	230
Cheese: cottage, dry curd	¼ cup	36	31	0.7	6.3	0.2	0.1	0	0	3	5
Cheese: cream cheese, 2 tbsp	1 oz	28	99	0.8	2.1	9.9	6.2	2.8	0.4	31	84
Cheese: edam	1 oz	28	101	0.4	7.1	7.9	5.0	2.3	0.2	25	274
Cheese: feta	1 oz	28	75	1.2	4.0	6.0	4.2	1.3	0.2	25	316
Cheese: gouda	1 oz	28	101	0.6	7.1	7.8	5.0	2.2	0.2	32	232
Cheese: gruyere	1 oz	28	117	0.1	8.5	9.2	5.4	2.9	0.5	31	95
Cheese: monterey	1 oz	28	106	0.2	6.9	8.6	—	—	—	—	152
Cheese: mozzarella, part-skim, low-moisture	1 oz	28	79	0.9	7.8	4.9	3.1	1.4	0.1	15	150
Cheese: mozzarella, whole milk	1 oz	28	80	0.6	5.5	6.1	3.7	1.9	0.2	22	106
Cheese: muenster	1 oz	28	104	0.3	6.6	8.5	5.4	2.5	0.2	27	178
Cheese: neufchatel	1 oz	28	74	0.8	2.8	6.6	4.2	1.9	0.2	22	113
Cheese: parmesan, grated	1 tbsp	5	23	0.2	2.1	1.5	1.0	0.4	0	4	93
Cheese: provolone	1 oz	28	100	0.6	7.3	7.6	4.8	2.1	0.2	20	248
Cheese: ricotta, whole milk (13% fat)	¼ cup	62	108	1.9	7.0	8.1	5.2	2.3	0.2	32	52

This information is current as of this printing. Check the manufacturer's label for updated analysis.

A dash (—) indicates that data are not available. Trace (tr) indicates that a very small amount of the constituent is present.

Abbreviations used in this table are: tbsp = tablespoon; tsp = teaspoon; oz = ounce; lb = pound; gm = gram; mg = milligrams; " = inches; Cal = calories; CHO = carbohydrate; Prot = protein; Sat fat = saturated fat; Mono fat = monounsaturated fat; Poly fat = polyunsaturated fat; Chol = cholesterol; Na = Sodium.

TABLE 2. *(continued)*

Food	Unit	Weight (g)	Cal	CHO (g)	Prot (g)	Fat (g)	Sat fat (g)	Mono fat (g)	Poly fat (g)	Chol (mg)	Na (mg)
Cheese: ricotta, part skim milk (8% fat)	¼ cup	62	86	3.2	7.1	4.9	3.1	1.4	0.2	19	77
Cheese: romano	1 oz	28	110	1.0	9.0	7.6	—	—	—	29	340
Cheese: roquefort	1 oz	28	105	0.6	6.1	8.7	5.5	2.4	0.4	26	513
Cheese: Swiss	1 oz	28	95	0.6	7.0	7.1	4.6	2.0	0.2	24	388
Cheese: Velveeta® (cheese spread)	1 oz	28	82	2.5	4.7	6.0	3.8	1.8	0.2	16	381
Cheese: 1% butterfat (Countdown®)	1 oz	28	40	3.6	6.6	0.3	0.2	0.1	0	1	409
Cheese: 4–8% butterfat, processed (Breeze®, Chef's Delight®, Country Club®, Mellow Age®, Tasty®, Lite-Line®, low-fat DI-ET®)	1 oz	28	50	2.8	5.8	1.7	1.1	0.5	0	10	428
Cheese: 5% butterfat, natural (St. Otho)	1 oz	28	49	3.1	9.1	1.1	0.8	0.3	0	10	—
Cheese: 19–32% polyunsaturated fat (Golden® Image®, Cheez-ola®, Dorman®, Nutrend®, Scandic®, Unique®)	1 oz	28	98	1.1	6.2	7.5	1.5	1.4	4.1	4	330
Cheese: 23% polyunsaturated fat, low sodium (Cheez-ola®)	1 oz	28	90	0.6	6.8	6.3	0.8	1.5	3.6	1	156
Cherries: raw, sweet, unpitted	10 whole	75	47	11.7	0.9	0.2	0	0	0.2	0	1
Cherries: canned, sweet, syrup-packed, pitted	1 cup	257	208	52.7	2.3	0.5	0	0	0.5	0	3
Chicken: gizzard, all classes, cooked, chopped	1 cup	145	215	1.0	39.2	4.8	1.4	1.8	1.2	283	83
Chicken: light meat, no skin	1 oz	28	51	0	9.2	1.4	0.4	0.7	0.3	22	18
Chicken: dark meat, no skin	1 oz	28	52	0	8.3	1.8	0.5	0.6	0.4	26	24
Chicken: dark and light meat, with skin	1 oz	28	70	0	7.7	4.2	1.2	1.4	1.0	25	—
Chicken fat	1 tbsp	14	126	0	0	14.0	4.6	6.4	2.5	9	0
Chicken liver: cooked, whole, 2 × 2 × ⅝"	1 liver	25	41	0.2	6.6	1.1	0.4	0.3	0.2	158	13
Chickpeas: see *Beans*											
Chocolate: bitter or baking	1 oz	28	143	8.2	3.0	15.0	8.4	5.6	0.3	0	1
Chocolate syrup (or topping): fudge type	2 tbsp	38	124	20.3	1.9	5.1	2.6	1.9	0.2	0	33
Clams: canned solids (chopped or minced)	1 cup	160	143	3.0	25.3	2.4	0.7	0.4	0.9	101	192
Cocoa: dry powder, medium fat, plain	1 tbsp	5	14	2.8	0.9	1.0	0.6	0.4	0	0	tr
Cocoa mix: 1 oz package	1 pkg	28	102	20.1	5.3	0.8	0.6	0.3	0	2	149
Coconut: shredded, fresh, meat only	1 cup	80	277	7.5	2.8	28.2	25.0	1.7	0.5	0	18
Cookie: commercial, chocolate chip, 2¼ × ⅜"	1 cookie	11	50	7.3	0.6	2.2	0.7	0.8	0.5	5	42
Cookie: commercial, fig bar, 1⅝ × 1⅝"	1 cookie	14	50	10.6	0.6	0.8	0.2	0.4	0.2	0	35

This information is current as of this printing. Check the manufacturer's label for updated analysis.

A dash (—) indicates that data are not available. Trace (tr) indicates that a very small amount of the constituent is present.

Abbreviations used in this table are: tbsp = tablespoon; tsp = teaspoon; oz = ounce; lb = pound; gm = gram; mg = milligrams; " = inches; Cal = calories; CHO = carbohydrate; Prot = protein; Sat fat = saturated fat; Mono fat = monounsaturated fat; Poly fat = polyunsaturated fat; Chol = cholesterol; Na = Sodium.

Food	Portion	gm	Cal	CHO	Prot	Fat	Sat fat	Mono fat	Poly fat	Chol	Na
Cookie: commercial, ginger snap, 2 × 1/4"	1 cookie	7	29	5.6	0.4	0.6	0.2	0.3	0.1	0	40
Cookie: commercial, macaroon, 2¾ × 1/4"	1 cookie	19	91	12.5	1.0	4.4	1.9	0.2	0.1	0	7
Cookie: commercial, marshmallow, chocolate-coated, 1¾ × ¾"	1 cookie	13	53	9.4	0.5	1.7	0.9	0.9	0	4	27
Cookie: commercial, oatmeal with raisins, 2⅝ × 1/4"	1 cookie	13	59	9.6	0.8	2.0	0.5	1.0	0.5	4	21
Cookie: commercial, peanut butter sandwich, 1¾ × 1/2"	1 cookie	12	58	8.2	1.2	2.4	0.6	1.2	0.6	5	21
Cookie: commercial, sandwich, round, 1¾ × 3/8"	1 cookie	10	50	6.9	0.5	2.3	0.6	1.1	0.5	5	48
Cookie: commercial, vanilla wafer, 1¾ × 1/4"	1 wafer	4	19	2.9	0.2	0.6	0.2	0.3	0.2	1	10
Cookie: prepared mix, brownies, 1¾ × 1¾ × 7/8"	1 piece	20	86	12.6	1.0	4.0	0.8	1.5	1.3	17	33
Cordial: apricot brandy, benedictine, anisette, creme de menthe, or curacao	4 tsp	20	66	6.3	0	0	0	0	0	0	0
Corn: canned, whole kernel	1 cup	165	139	32.7	4.3	1.3	0.4	0.1	0.7	0	389
Corn: canned, whole kernel, low sodium	1 cup	165	152	29.7	4.1	1.2	0.4	0.1	0.7	0	3
Corn: canned, cream style, low sodium	1 cup	256	210	47.4	6.7	2.8	0.8	0.3	1.7	0	5
Corn chips: 1½ oz package = 1¼ cups or 60 chips	1¼ cup	43	239	22.7	2.9	15.8	3.8	7.9	3.8	0	240
Corn meal: white and yellow, enriched, degermed	1 cup	138	502	108.2	10.9	1.7	0.5	0.2	1.0	0	1
Corned beef: see Beef											
Cornstarch: not packed	1 tbsp	8	29	7.0	0	0	0	0	0	0	tr
Cottage cheese: see Cheese											
Crab: fresh, cooked, not packed	1 cup	125	106	0.6	21.6	1.3	0.2	0.2	0.4	125	263
Crab: canned solids, packed	1 cup	160	149	1.8	27.8	2.6	0.4	0.5	0.9	162	1,600
Crackers: animal	10 whole	26	112	20.8	1.7	2.4	0.6	1.2	0.5	16	79
Cracker: graham, chocolate-coated, 2½ × 2 × 1/4"	1 whole	13	62	8.8	0.7	3.1	0.9	1.9	0.2	7	53
Crackers: graham, sugar honey, 2 squares, 2½" each	2 whole	14	58	10.8	1.0	1.6	0.4	0.8	0.4	1	72
Cracker: matzo	1 whole	30	118	26.1	3.2	0.3	0	0	0.1	0	10
Crackers: melba toast	3 whole	12	60	9.0	2.0	2.0	0.8	0.9	0.2	0.6	2
Crackers: melba toast, low sodium	3 whole	12	60	9.0	2.0	2.0	0.8	0.9	0.2	0.6	1

This information is current as of this printing. Check the manufacturer's label for updated analysis.

A dash (—) indicates that data are not available. Trace (tr) indicates that a very small amount of the constituent is present.

Abbreviations used in this table are: tbsp = tablespoon; tsp = teaspoon; oz = ounce; lb = pound; gm = gram; mg = milligrams; " = inches; Cal = calories; CHO = carbohydrate; Prot = protein; Sat fat = saturated fat; Mono fat = monounsaturated fat; Poly fat = polyunsaturated fat; Chol = cholesterol; Na = Sodium.

TABLE 2. *(continued)*

Food	Unit	Weight (g)	Cal	CHO (g)	Prot (g)	Fat (g)	Sat fat (g)	Mono fat (g)	Poly fat (g)	Chol (mg)	Na (mg)
Crackers: saltines, single crackers	4 whole	11	48	8.0	1.0	1.3	0.3	0.6	0.3	1	123
Crackers: sandwich, cheese and peanut butter (1 oz pack)	4 whole	28	139	15.9	4.3	6.8	1.8	3.1	1.6	6	281
Crackers: Triscuit®	1 whole	4	21	3.0	0.4	0.8	0.4	0.4	0.1	0	20
Cranberries: raw, chopped	1 cup	110	51	11.9	0.4	0.8	0	0	0.8	0	2
Cranberry juice: cocktail, sweetened	1 cup	253	164	41.7	0.3	0.3	0	0	0.3	0	3
Cranberry sauce: sweetened, canned	1 cup	277	404	103.9	0.3	0.6	0	0	0.6	0	3
Cream: fluid, half and half (11.7% fat)	1 tbsp	15	20	0.7	0.5	1.7	1.1	0.5	0.1	6	6
Cream: fluid, light (20.6% fat)	1 tbsp	15	29	0.6	0.4	2.9	1.8	0.8	0.1	10	6
Cream: fluid, light, whipping (31.3% fat), approximately 2 cups whipped	1 cup	239	699	7.1	5.2	73.9	46.2	21.7	2.1	265	82
Cream: fluid, heavy or whipping (37.6% fat), approximately 2 cups whipped	1 cup	238	821	6.6	4.9	88.1	54.8	25.4	3.3	326	89
Cream: sour	1 tbsp	14	31	0.6	0.5	3.0	1.9	0.9	0.1	6	8
Cream: sour, imitation (IMO®, Wonder®)	1 tbsp	15	26	0.7	0.5	2.4	2.0	0.3	0.1	1	7
Creamer: nondairy, powder, containing saturated fat (Creamora® and Coffee-Mate®)	1 tbsp	6	33	3.3	0.3	2.1	2.1	0	0	0	12
Creamer: nondairy, liquid, containing saturated fat (Coffee Rich®)	1 tbsp	15	20	1.7	0.2	1.5	1.4	0	0	0	12
Creamer: nondairy, liquid, containing polyunsaturated fat (Poly Perx® and Mocha Mix®)	1 tbsp	15	20	1.8	0.1	1.5	0.2	0.7	0.6	0	1
Cucumbers: raw, pared, whole, 2⅛ × 8¼"	1 whole	280	39	9.0	1.7	0.3	0	0	0.3	0	17
Dates: hydrated, without pits	10 whole	80	219	58.3	1.8	0.4	0	0	0.4	0	1
Dessert topping: frozen, semisolid (Cool Whip®)	1 tbsp	4	13	0.9	0.1	1.0	0.9	0.1	0	0	1
Dessert topping: nondairy, pressurized	1 tbsp	4	11	0.6	0	0.9	0.8	0.1	0	0	2
Doughnut: cake type, plain, 1½ × ¾"	1 whole	14	55	7.2	0.6	2.6	0.7	1.3	0.5	7	70
Doughnut: yeast leavened, plain, 3¾ × 1¼"	1 whole	42	176	16.0	2.7	11.3	2.8	5.6	2.5	12	99
Duck: flesh only, raw, domesticated	1 oz	28	47	0	6.1	2.3	0.5	1.1	0.3	—	21
Duck: flesh and skin, raw, domesticated	1 oz	28	92	0	4.5	8.1	1.9	4.1	0.9	—	21
Eclair: custard filling with chocolate, 5 × 2 × 1¾"	1 whole	100	239	23.2	6.2	13.6	4.4	6.2	2.1	145	82

This information is current as of this printing. Check the manufacturer's label for updated analysis.

A dash (—) indicates that data are not available. Trace (tr) indicates that a very small amount of the constituent is present.

Abbreviations used in this table are: tbsp = tablespoon; tsp = teaspoon; oz = ounce; lb = pound; gm = gram; mg = milligrams; " = inches; Cal = calories; CHO = carbohydrate; Prot = protein; Sat fat = saturated fat; Mono fat = monounsaturated fat; Poly fat = polyunsaturated fat; Chol = cholesterol; Na = Sodium.

Food	Portion	Weight (gm)	Cal	CHO (gm)	Prot (gm)	Fat (gm)	Sat fat (gm)	Mono fat (gm)	Poly fat (gm)	Chol (mg)	Na (mg)
Egg: chicken, fresh, medium	1 whole	50	79	0.6	6.1	5.6	1.7	2.2	0.7	274	69
Egg: chicken, white, fresh	1 white	33	16	0.4	3.4	tr	0	0	0	0	50
Egg: chicken, yolk, fresh	1 yolk	17	63	0	2.8	5.6	1.7	2.2	0.7	272	8
Eggnog: commercial	1 cup	254	342	34.4	9.7	19.0	11.3	5.7	0.9	149	138
Egg substitute: Eggbeaters®, 1 egg equivalent	¼ cup	60	40	3.0	7.0	0	0	0	0	0	130
Egg substitute: Second Nature®, 1 egg equivalent	3 tbsp	47	35	0.5	4.7	1.6	0.3	0.6	0.8	0	79
Egg substitute: Lucern®, 1 egg equivalent	¼ cup	60	50	2.0	6.0	2.0	—	—	—	tr	—
Eggplant: cooked, diced	1 cup	200	38	8.2	2.0	0.4	0	0	0.4	0	2
English muffin: see *Bread*											
Fig: raw, whole, 1½" diameter	1 small	40	32	8.1	0.5	0.1	0	0	0.1	0	1
Fish: see *Catfish, Haddock, Halibut, Herring, Snapper, Flounder, Sole*											
Fish sticks: breaded, cooked, frozen, 4 × 1 × ½"	1 oz	28	50	1.0	4.7	2.5	0.7	1.0	0.7	17	20
Flounder: raw	1 oz	28	22	0	4.7	0.2	0	0	0.1	14	22
Flour: white, all purpose, enriched, unsifted	1 cup	125	455	95.1	13.1	1.3	0.3	0.1	0.8	0	3
Flour: white, self-rising, enriched, unsifted	1 cup	125	440	92.8	11.6	1.3	0.4	0.1	0.8	0	1,349
Flour: whole wheat	1 cup	120	400	85.2	16.0	2.4	0.7	0.2	1.4	0	4
Frankfurter: 5 × ¾"	1 whole	45	139	0.8	5.6	12.4	4.7	5.9	0.8	27	495
Frosting mix: prepared	1 tbsp	15	61	13.2	0.3	1.5	0.4	0.8	0.1	0	9
Frosting: ready to spread (with animal or vegetable shortening)	1 tbsp	15	55	10.8	0.1	1.6	0.5	0.9	0.2	0	9
Fruit cocktail: canned, solids and liquid, water-packed	1 cup	245	91	23.8	1.0	0.2	0	0	0.2	0	12
Garbanzos: see *Beans*											
Gelatin: dry, unflavored, 1 envelope	1 pkg	7	23	0	6.0	0	0	0	0	0	0
Gelatin: sweetened dessert powder (JELL-O®), prepared with water, plain	½ cup	120	71	16.9	1.8	0	0	0	0	0	61
Gelatin: low calorie, prepared with water	½ cup	120	8	0	2.0	0	0	0	0	0	8
Gin: see *Liquor*											
Gizzard: chicken, all classes, cooked, chopped	¼ cup	36	54	0.3	9.8	1.2	0.4	0.5	0.3	71	21
Goose: flesh only, raw	1 oz	28	45	0	6.3	2.0	0.5	0.9	0.2	—	24
Grapes: raw, seedless (Thompson)	10 grapes	50	34	8.7	0.3	0.2	0	0	0.2	0	2

This information is current as of this printing. Check the manufacturer's label for updated analysis.

A dash (—) indicates that data are not available. Trace (tr) indicates that a very small amount of the constituent is present.

Abbreviations used in this table are: tbsp = tablespoon; tsp = teaspoon; oz = ounce; lb = pound; gm = gram; mg = milligrams; " = inches; Cal = calories; CHO = carbohydrate; Prot = protein; Sat fat = saturated fat; Mono fat = monounsaturated fat; Poly fat = polyunsaturated fat; Chol = cholesterol; Na = Sodium.

TABLE 2. *(continued)*

Food	Unit	Weight (g)	Cal	CHO (g)	Prot (g)	Fat (g)	Sat fat (g)	Mono fat (g)	Poly fat (g)	Chol (mg)	Na (mg)
Grape juice: frozen concentrate, sweetened, diluted	1 cup	250	133	33.3	0.5	0	0	0	0	0	3
Grapefruit: all varieties	1 whole	400	80	20.8	1.0	0.2	0	0	0.2	0	2
Grapefruit juice: unsweetened, frozen concentrate, diluted	1 cup	247	101	24.2	1.2	0.2	0	0	0.2	0	2
Greens, collard: frozen, cooked	1 cup	170	51	9.5	4.9	0.7	0	0	0.7	0	27
Haddock: raw	1 oz	28	29	0	6.6	0.1	0	0	0.1	17	17
Halibut: Atlantic or Pacific, broiled	1 oz	28	28	0	5.9	0.3	0.1	0	0.1	14	15
Ham: see *Pork*											
Hamburger: see *Beef*											
Herring: canned, solids and liquid, plain	1 oz	28	59	0	5.6	3.1	0.7	1.6	0.5	24	—
Honey: strained	1 tbsp	21	64	17.3	0.1	0	0	0	0	0	1
Honeydew: 7 × 2" wedge, 1/10 of melon	1 slice	226	49	11.5	1.2	0.4	0	0	0.4	0	18
Horseradish: prepared	1 tbsp	15	6	1.4	0.2	0	0	0	0	0	14
Ice cream: rich, approximately 16% fat, hardened	1 cup	148	349	32.0	4.1	23.7	14.7	6.8	0.9	88	108
Ice cream: regular, approximately 10% fat, hardened	1 cup	133	269	31.7	4.8	14.3	8.9	4.1	0.5	59	116
Ice cream bar: chocolate-covered (Eskimo Pie)	1 bar	85	270	22.0	2.9	19.1	14.7	2.8	0.5	35	—
Ice cream sandwich: 3 oz size	1 whole	85	238	35.8	4.3	8.5	4.0	2.2	0.4	34	—
Ice cream cone	1 cone	3	11	2.3	0.3	0.1	0	0.1	0	0	1
Ice milk: 5.1% fat, soft serve	1 cup	175	223	38.4	8.0	4.6	2.9	1.3	0.2	13	163
Ice milk: 5.1% fat, hardened	1 cup	131	184	29.0	5.2	5.6	3.5	1.6	0.2	18	105
Instant breakfast: dry powder, all flavors except eggnog	1¼ oz	36	130	23.4	7.2	0.9	0.5	0.3	0.1	4	tr
Jelly: sweetened	1 tbsp	18	49	12.7	0	0	0	0	0	0	3
Knockwurst link: 4 × 1⅛"	1 link	68	165	1.5	9.6	18.5	6.8	8.8	1.8	42	748
Ladyfingers	1 whole	11	40	7.1	0.9	0.9	0.3	0.4	0.1	39	8
Lamb: <7% fat, chop, leg, roast, sirloin chop (lean only)	1 oz	28	53	0	8.2	2.0	0.9	0.8	0.1	28	15
Lamb: 10% fat, shank, shoulder (lean only)	1 oz	28	58	0	7.6	2.8	1.4	1.2	0.2	28	15
Lamb: 20% fat, leg, roast, sirloin chop (lean only)	1 oz	28	79	0	7.2	5.4	2.8	2.4	0.4	28	14
Lamb: 30% fat, breast, chop, rib (lean and fat)	1 oz	28	96	0	6.2	7.7	3.6	3.1	0.4	28	14
Lard	1 tbsp	13	117	0	0	12.8	5.1	5.7	1.5	12	0

This information is current as of this printing. Check the manufacturer's label for updated analysis.

A dash (—) indicates that data are not available. Trace (tr) indicates that a very small amount of the constituent is present.

Abbreviations used in this table are: tbsp = tablespoon; tsp = teaspoon; oz = ounce; lb = pound; gm = gram; mg = milligrams; " = inches; Cal = calories; CHO = carbohydrate; Prot = protein; Sat fat = saturated fat; Mono fat = monounsaturated fat; Poly fat = polyunsaturated fat; Chol = cholesterol; Na = Sodium.

Food	Portion	gm	Cal	CHO	Prot	Fat	Sat fat	Mono fat	Poly fat	Chol	Na
Lemon: raw, 1 wedge (⅙ of 2⅛" lemon)	1 slice	18	3	1.0	0.1	0	0	0	0	0	0
Lemon juice: canned, unsweetened	1 tbsp	15	4	1.2	0.1	tr	0	0	tr	0	tr
Lemonade: concentrate, frozen, diluted	1 cup	248	88	22.9	0.2	0	0	0	0	0	0
Lentils: see *Beans*											
Lettuce: raw, crisp head varieties, chopped or shredded	1 cup	55	7	1.6	0.5	0.1	0	0	0.1	0	5
Liquor: gin, rum, vodka, whiskey	1 oz	28	70	0	0	0	0	0	0	0	0
Liver: see *Beef* or *Chicken*											
Lobster: northern, cooked, ½" cubes	1 cup	145	138	0.4	27.1	1.5	0.2	0.2	0.5	123	305
Luncheon meat: see *Salami, Bologna, Braunschweiger, Sausage, Turkey*											
Macadamia nuts: 15 whole nuts	1 oz	28	196	4.5	2.2	20.3	3.1	16.3	0.6	0	—
Macaroni: enriched, cooked, hot	1 cup	140	155	32.2	4.8	0.6	0	0.3	0.3	0	1
Mackerel: canned, solids and liquids	¼ cup	35	64	0	7.5	3.5	0.9	1.3	0.8	33	148
Mango: raw	1 whole	300	152	38.8	1.6	0.9	0	0	0.9	0	16
Margarine: P/S >3.1 (Promise® soft, Parkay soft safflower, Hains® soft, Saffola® soft)	1 tbsp	14	102	0.1	0.1	11.5	1.5	3.5	6.3	0	140
Margarine: P/S 2.6 to 3.0 (Mrs. Filbert's® soft corn oil, Promise® stick, Parkay liquid squeeze)	1 tbsp	14	102	0.1	0.1	11.5	1.7	4.6	4.9	0	140
Margarine: P/S 2.0 to 2.5 (Fleischmann's® soft, Chiffon® soft, Parkay corn oil soft)	1 tbsp	14	102	0.1	0.1	11.5	2.1	4.1	5.0	0	110
Margarine: P/S 1.6 to 1.9 (Fleischmann's® stick, Chiffon® stick, Meadow Gold® stick)	1 tbsp	14	102	0.1	0.1	11.5	2.1	5.0	3.6	0	110
Margarine: P/S 1.0 to 1.5 (Mazola® stick, Parkay corn oil stick, Imperial® stick)	1 tbsp	14	100	0.1	0.1	11.3	2.0	5.1	4.0	0	115
Margarine: low sodium, P/S 1.7 (Fleischmann's®, Mazola®)	1 tbsp	14	100	0.1	0.1	11.2	2.1	5.0	3.6	0	tr
Margarine: P/S <0.5, all vegetable fat (Kraft® all purpose stick, Swift® all purpose stick)	1 tbsp	14	102	0.1	0.1	11.5	2.2	7.5	1.5	0	140
Margarine: P/S <0.5, vegetable and animal or all animal (Gaylord® stick, Meadowlake® stick)	1 tbsp	14	102	0.1	0.1	11.5	4.7	5.6	1.0	0	140
Margarine: P/S 2.4, diet tub Fleischmann's® soft, Imperial® soft	1 tbsp	14	50	0.1	0	5.6	1.0	2.1	2.4	0	135
Mellorine	1 cup	131	244	30.8	5.9	11.1	9.5	0.6	0.2	18	105

This information is current as of this printing. Check the manufacturer's label for updated analysis.

A dash (—) indicates that data are not available. Trace (tr) indicates that a very small amount of the constituent is present.

Abbreviations used in this table are: tbsp = tablespoon; tsp = teaspoon; oz = ounce; lb = pound; gm = gram; mg = milligrams; " = inches; Cal = calories; CHO = carbohydrate; Prot = protein; Sat fat = saturated fat; Mono fat = monounsaturated fat; Poly fat = polyunsaturated fat; Chol = cholesterol; Na = Sodium.

TABLE 2. *(continued)*

Food	Unit	Weight (g)	Cal	CHO (g)	Prot (g)	Fat (g)	Sat fat (g)	Mono fat (g)	Poly fat (g)	Chol (mg)	Na (mg)
Milk: skim (less than 1% fat)	1 cup	245	86	11.9	8.4	0.4	0.3	0.1	0	4	126
Milk: low fat (1% to 2% fat)	1 cup	244	102	11.7	8.0	2.6	1.6	0.8	0.1	10	123
Milk: whole (3.3% fat)	1 cup	244	150	11.4	8.0	8.2	5.1	2.4	0.3	33	120
Milk: canned, evaporated, whole	1 cup	252	338	25.3	17.2	19.1	11.6	5.9	0.6	74	267
Milk: canned, evaporated, skim	1 cup	256	200	29.0	19.4	0.6	0.4	0.2	0	10	294
Milk: nonfat, dry powder, approximately 1 cup reconstituted	⅓ cup	23	81	11.8	8.0	0.2	0.1	0	0	4	124
Milk: canned, condensed, sweetened	1 cup	306	982	166.2	24.2	26.6	16.8	7.4	1.0	104	389
Milk: chocolate drink, fluid, commercial, made with whole milk	1 cup	250	213	27.5	8.5	8.5	5.3	2.5	0.3	30	118
Milk: low sodium (whole)	1 cup	244	149	10.9	7.6	8.4	5.3	2.4	0.3	33	6
Milkshake: chocolate	11 oz	311	369	65.9	9.5	8.4	5.2	2.4	0.3	33	346
Milkshake: vanilla	11 oz	313	350	55.6	12.1	9.5	5.9	2.7	0.4	37	299
Molasses: light	1 tbsp	21	52	13.3	0	0	0	0	0	0	3
Mushrooms: raw, sliced, chopped, or diced	1 cup	70	20	3.1	1.9	0.2	0	0	0.2	0	11
Mustard: prepared, yellow	1 tsp	5	4	0.3	0.2	0.2	0	0	0.2	0	63
Nectarine: raw, 2½" diameter	1 whole	150	88	23.6	0.8	0	0	0	0	0	8
Noodles: egg, enriched, cooked	1 cup	160	200	37.3	6.6	2.4	0.8	1.1	0.2	50	3
Noodles: chow mein, canned	1 cup	45	220	26.1	5.9	10.6	2.8	4.3	2.9	5	—
Oil: coconut	1 tbsp	14	120	0	0	13.6	11.7	0.8	0.2	0	0
Oil: cod liver	1 tbsp	14	120	0	0	13.6	2.4	7.0	3.5	—	0
Oil: corn	1 tbsp	14	120	0	0	13.6	1.7	3.4	7.9	0	0
Oil: cottonseed	1 tbsp	14	120	0	0	13.6	3.6	2.6	6.9	0	0
Oil: olive	1 tbsp	14	119	0	0	13.5	1.9	9.8	1.2	0	0
Oil: palm kernel	1 tbsp	14	120	0	0	13.6	11.1	1.6	0.2	0	0
Oil: peanut	1 tbsp	14	119	0	0	13.5	2.6	6.2	4.1	0	0
Oil: safflower	1 tbsp	14	120	0	0	13.6	1.3	1.7	10.0	0	0
Oil: soybean	1 tbsp	14	120	0	0	13.6	2.0	3.1	7.8	0	0
Oil: soybean-cottonseed blend	1 tbsp	14	120	0	0	13.6	2.2	3.1	7.7	0	0
Oil: sunflower	1 tbsp	14	120	0	0	13.6	1.4	2.8	8.7	0	0
Okra: frozen, cooked, cuts	1 cup	185	70	16.3	4.1	0.2	0	0	0.2	0	4
Olives: ripe, whole, extra large	10 whole	55	61	1.2	0.5	6.5	0.7	5.0	0.5	0	385
Olives: green, whole, large	10 whole	46	45	0.5	0.5	4.9	0.5	3.7	0.3	0	926
Onions: green, raw, 4⅛ × ⅝"	2 med	30	14	3.2	0.3	0.1	0	0	0.1	0	2
Onions: mature, raw, chopped	1 cup	170	65	14.8	2.6	0.2	0	0	0.2	0	17

This information is current as of this printing. Check the manufacturer's label for updated analysis.

A dash (—) indicates that data are not available. Trace (tr) indicates that a very small amount of the constituent is present.

Abbreviations used in this table are: tbsp = tablespoon; tsp = teaspoon; oz = ounce; lb = pound; gm = gram; mg = milligrams; " = inches; Cal = calories; CHO = carbohydrate; Prot = protein; Sat fat = saturated fat; Mono fat = monounsaturated fat; Poly fat = polyunsaturated fat; Chol = cholesterol; Na = Sodium.

Food	Measure	gm	Cal	CHO	Prot	Fat	Sat fat	Mono fat	Poly fat	Chol	Na
Onions: mature, cooked, whole or sliced	1 cup	210	61	13.7	2.5	0.2	0	0	0.2	0	15
Orange: Florida, medium, 2¹¹⁄₁₆″ diameter	1 whole	204	71	18.1	1.1	0.3	0	0	0.3	0	2
Orange juice: concentrate, frozen, unsweetened, diluted	1 cup	249	122	28.9	1.7	0.2	0	0	0.2	0	2
Oysters: canned, 18 to 27 medium or 27 to 44 small	12 oz	340	224	11.6	28.6	6.1	1.8	0.7	2.0	170	248
Oysters: raw, 13 to 19 medium or 19 to 31 small	1 cup	240	158	8.2	20.2	4.3	1.2	0.5	1.4	120	175
Pancake: made from mix, 6 × ½″	1 cake	73	164	23.7	5.3	5.3	—	—	—	—	412
Peach: raw, pared, 2¾″ diameter, approximately 2½ per lb	1 whole	175	51	12.9	0.8	0.1	0	0	0.1	0	1
Peaches: canned, syrup packed, halves, slices, or chunks	1 cup	256	200	51.5	1.0	0.3	0	0	0.3	0	5
Peanut butter	1 cup	258	1,520	48.5	65.0	130.5	27.1	60.7	39.0	0	1,561
Peanuts: roasted, salted, 10 Virginia, 20 Spanish, or 1 tbsp chopped	10 nuts	9	53	1.7	2.3	4.5	0.8	2.1	1.3	0	38
Pear: raw, Bartletts, 2½ × 3½″	1 whole	180	100	25.1	1.1	0.7	0	0	0.7	0	3
Pear: canned, syrup-packed, with 1⅔ tbsp liquid	1 half	76	58	14.9	0.2	0.2	0	0	0.2	0	1
Pear nectar: canned	1 cup	130	130	33.0	0.8	0.5	0	0	0.5	0	3
Peas: cow or blackeyed, canned, cooked	1 cup	255	179	31.6	12.8	0.8	0.2	0	0.3	0	602
Peas: green, immature, canned solids	1 cup	170	150	28.6	8.0	0.7	0	0.4	0.7	0	401
Peas: green, immature, canned solids, low sodium	1 cup	170	122	22.1	7.5	0.7	0	0.4	0.7	0	5
Pecans: chopped or pieces	1 tbsp	7	51	1.1	0.7	5.2	0.5	3.1	1.3	0	tr
Pepper: immature, green, raw, 3¾ × 3″	1 whole	200	36	7.9	2.0	0.3	0	0	0.3	0	21
Pepper: jalapeño, canned	1 whole	18	5	1.1	0.2	0	0	0	0	0	72
Pepper: jalapeño, fresh	1 whole	18	7	1.6	0.2	0	0	0	0	0	5
Pheasant: flesh only, raw	1 oz	28	46	0	6.7	1.9	0.5	0.8	0.2	0	—
Pickle: dill or sour, large, 4 × 1¾″	1 whole	135	15	3.0	0.9	0.3	0	0	0.3	0	1,928
Pickle: dill or sour, 3¾ × 1¼″, low sodium	1 whole	65	7	1.4	0.5	0.1	0	0	0.1	0	4
Pickles: fresh, sweetened (bread and butter), 1½ × ¼″	2 slices	15	11	2.7	0.1	0	0	0	0	0	101
Pickle: sweet, gherkins, large, 3 × 1″	1 whole	35	51	12.8	0.2	0.1	0	0	0.1	0	500
Pickle relish: finely chopped, sweet	1 tbsp	15	21	5.1	0.1	0.1	0	0	0.1	0	107

This information is current as of this printing. Check the manufacturer's label for updated analysis.

A dash (—) indicates that data are not available. Trace (tr) indicates that a very small amount of the constituent is present.

Abbreviations used in this table are: tbsp = tablespoon; tsp = teaspoon; oz = ounce; lb = pound; gm = gram; mg = milligrams; ″ = inches; Cal = calories; CHO = carbohydrate; Prot = protein; Sat fat = saturated fat; Mono fat = monounsaturated fat; Poly fat = polyunsaturated fat; Chol = cholesterol; Na = Sodium.

TABLE 2. (continued)

Food	Unit	Weight (g)	Cal	CHO (g)	Prot (g)	Fat (g)	Sat fat (g)	Mono fat (g)	Poly fat (g)	Chol (mg)	Na (mg)
Pie: frozen, baked, apple, 8" diameter	1 pie	550	1,386	219.0	10.6	54.8	13.6	27.3	12.2	0	1,168
Pie: frozen, baked, cherry, 8" diameter	1 pie	580	1,690	257.4	12.5	70.0	17.4	34.8	15.6	0	1,333
Pie: mix, baked, coconut custard (eggs and milk), 8" diameter	1 pie	797	1,618	231.9	34.3	63.0	27.1	31.1	8.0	837	1,873
Pineapple: raw, diced pieces	1 cup	155	81	21.2	0.6	0.3	0	0	0.3	0	2
Pineapple: canned, syrup-packed, chunk, tidbit, or crushed	1 cup	255	189	49.5	0.8	0.3	0	0	0.3	0	3
Pineapple: canned, water-packed, tidbits	1 cup	246	96	25.1	0.7	0.2	0	0	0.2	0	2
Pineapple: in its own juice (no sugar added) 4 slices with juice or 1 cup with juice	1 cup	227	140	35.0	1.0	1.0	0	0	1.0	0	2
Pineapple juice: canned, unsweetened	1 cup	250	138	33.8	1.0	0.3	0	0	0.3	0	3
Plum: hybrid, fresh, 2⅛" diameter	1 whole	70	32	8.1	0.3	0.1	0	0	0.1	0	1
Plums: canned, served with 2¾ tbsp syrup	3 whole	140	110	28.7	0.5	0.1	0	0	0.1	0	1
Popcorn: no salt or fat added to popped corn	1 cup	6	23	4.6	0.8	0.3	0	0.1	0.2	0	tr
Pork: fresh, 10% fat, ham or picnic ham (lean only)	1 oz	28	61	0	8.4	2.8	0.9	1.2	0.3	25	18
Pork: fresh 13–20% fat, Boston butt roast, chop, loin, shoulder (lean only)	1 oz	28	71	0	8.0	3.9	1.6	2.1	0.5	25	20
Pork: fresh, 23–30% fat, Boston butt, ground pork, ham, loin picnic, shoulder (lean and fat)	1 oz	28	103	0	6.6	8.3	2.9	3.8	0.9	25	16
Pork: spareribs, 37% fat (lean and fat)	1 oz	28	125	0	5.9	11.0	3.8	5.1	1.2	25	10
Pork: cured, 7–10% fat, ham or picnic ham (lean only)	1 oz	28	56	0	7.6	2.7	0.9	1.1	0.2	25	273
Pork: cured, 13–20% fat, Boston butt, shoulder (lean only)	1 oz	28	75	0	6.9	5.1	1.8	2.4	0.6	25	247
Pork: cured, 23–30% fat, ham, picnic, shoulder (lean and fat)	1 oz	28	93	0	6.4	7.2	2.5	3.4	0.8	25	230
Pork: deviled ham, canned	¼ cup	56	198	0	7.8	18.2	6.4	8.5	2.0	35	703
Potato chips	10 chips	20	114	10.0	1.1	8.0	2.0	1.7	4.0	0	200
Potatoes: fresh, boiled, diced, or sliced	1 cup	155	101	22.5	2.9	0.2	0	0	0.2	0	3
Potato: fresh, baked in skin, 2⅓ × 4¾"	1 whole	202	145	32.8	4.0	0.2	0	0	0.2	0	6
Potato: frozen, French fried, 4" strips (oven-heated)	10 strips	78	172	26.3	2.8	6.6	1.6	1.4	3.3	0	3
Potato, sweet: fresh, baked, 5 × 2"	1 whole	146	161	37.0	2.4	0.6	0	0	0.6	0	14
Potatoes, sweet: pieces, canned in syrup	1 cup	200	216	49.8	4.0	0.4	0	0	0.4	0	96

This information is current as of this printing. Check the manufacturer's label for updated analysis.
A dash (—) indicates that data are not available. Trace (tr) indicates that a very small amount of the constituent is present.
Abbreviations used in this table are: tbsp = tablespoon; tsp = teaspoon; oz = ounce; lb = pound; gm = gram; mg = milligrams; " = inches; Cal = calories; CHO = carbohydrate; Prot = protein; Sat fat = saturated fat; Mono fat = monounsaturated fat; Poly fat = polyunsaturated fat; Chol = cholesterol; Na = Sodium.

Food	Measure										
Pretzels: extruded type, rods, 7½" × ½"	1 whole	14	55	10.6	1.4	0.6	0.2	0.4	0.1	0	235
Pretzels: twisted type, rings (3), 1⅛ × 1¾ × ¼"	10 whole	30	117	22.8	2.9	1.4	0.3	0.8	0.2	0	504
Prunes: dried, uncooked, without pits	10 whole	102	260	68.7	2.1	0.6	0	0	0.6	0	8
Prunes: dried, cooked, no added sugar	1 cup	250	253	66.7	2.1	0.6	0	0	0.6	0	9
Prune juice: canned or bottled	1 cup	256	197	48.6	1.0	0.3	0	0	0.3	0	5
Pudding mix: chocolate, regular, prepared with whole milk	1 cup	260	322	59.3	8.8	7.8	4.3	2.6	0.2	36	335
Pudding mix: chocolate, instant, prepared with whole milk	1 cup	260	325	63.4	7.8	6.5	3.6	2.2	0.3	36	322
Pudding mix: low calorie, dry form, 1 package (all kinds)	4 oz	128	100	24.0	0	0	0	0	0	0	280
Pumpkin: canned	1 cup	245	81	19.4	2.5	0.7	0	0	0.7	0	5
Quail: flesh and skin, raw	1 oz	28	48	0	7.2	2.0	0.5	0.9	0.5	—	11
Raisins: natural, seedless, uncooked, whole, not packed	1 tbsp	9	26	7.0	0.2	tr	0	0	tr	0	2
Raspberries: raw, red	1 cup	123	70	16.7	1.5	0.6	0	0	0.6	0	1
Rhubarb: frozen, sweetened	1 cup	270	381	97.2	1.4	0.3	0	0	0.3	0	5
Rice: brown, cooked without salt	1 cup	195	232	49.7	4.9	1.2	0.3	0.3	0.6	0	5
Rice: white, enriched, cooked without salt	1 cup	205	221	49.6	4.1	0.4	0.1	0.1	0.1	0	5
Roll: hard, enriched	1 roll	25	78	14.9	2.5	0.8	0.2	0.4	0.2	0	157
Roll: soft, enriched, brown and serve, or Parker House	1 roll	28	83	14.8	2.3	1.6	0.4	0.7	0.4	0	142
Roll: enriched, hotdog (6 × 2") or hamburger (3½ × 1½")	1 whole	40	119	21.2	3.3	2.2	0.5	1.1	0.5	0	202
Rum: see *Liquor*											
Salad dressing: blue or roquefort	1 tbsp	15	76	1.1	0.7	8.0	1.6	1.8	3.8	10	164
Salad dressing: blue or roquefort, low calorie	1 tbsp	16	12	0.7	0.5	0.9	0.5	0.3	.0	1	177
Salad dressing: French	1 tbsp	16	66	2.8	0.1	6.2	1.1	1.3	3.2	0	219
Salad dressing: French, low calorie	1 tbsp	16	15	2.5	0.1	0.7	0.1	0.1	0.4	0	126
Salad dressing: Italian	1 tbsp	15	83	1.0	tr	9.0	1.5	1.9	4.6	0	314
Salad dressing: Italian, low calorie	1 tbsp	15	8	0.4	tr	0.7	0.1	0.2	0.4	0	118
Salad dressing: mayonnaise	1 tbsp	15	101	0.3	0.2	11.2	2.0	2.4	5.5	9	84
Salad dressing: mayonnaise, low sodium	1 tbsp	14	99	0.3	0.2	11.0	2.0	2.4	5.5	9	2
Salad dressing: mayonnaise type (Miracle Whip®)	1 tbsp	15	65	2.2	0.2	6.3	1.1	1.4	3.1	7	88

This information is current as of this printing. Check the manufacturer's label for updated analysis.

A dash (—) indicates that data are not available. Trace (tr) indicates that a very small amount of the constituent is present.

Abbreviations used in this table are: tbsp = tablespoon; tsp = teaspoon; oz = ounce; lb = pound; gm = gram; mg = milligrams; " = inches; Cal = calories; CHO = carbohydrate; Prot = protein; Sat fat = saturated fat; Mono fat = monounsaturated fat; Poly fat = polyunsaturated fat; Chol = cholesterol; Na = Sodium.

TABLE 2. *(continued)*

Food	Unit	Weight (g)	Cal	CHO (g)	Prot (g)	Fat (g)	Sat fat (g)	Mono fat (g)	Poly fat (g)	Chol (mg)	Na (mg)
Salad dressing: mayonnaise type, low calorie	1 tbsp	16	22	0.8	0.2	2.0	0.4	0.4	1.0	0	19
Salad dressing: Russian	1 tbsp	15	74	1.6	0.2	7.6	1.4	1.7	3.9	7	130
Salad dressing: Thousand Island	1 tbsp	16	80	2.5	0.1	8.0	1.4	1.7	3.9	7	112
Salad dressing: Thousand Island, low calorie	1 tbsp	15	27	2.3	0.1	2.1	0.4	0.5	1.1	0	105
Salami: cooked, 4½" diameter slice	1 oz	28	73	0.4	5.0	5.8	2.1	2.7	0.6	15	297
Salmon: fresh, broiled or baked, no added fat	1 oz	28	48	0	7.7	1.6	0.5	0.8	0.1	10	33
Salmon: canned, drained, pink	1 oz	28	49	0	5.7	1.9	0.2	0.3	1.0	10	135
Salmon: smoked (Lox)	1 oz	28	50	0	6.1	2.6	0.5	0.8	0.1	10	135
Salt: table	1 tsp	6	0	0	0	0				0	2,196
Salt pork	1 oz	28	219	0	1.1	24.0	8.5	11.3	2.7	20	340
Sandwich spread: with chopped pickle	1 tbsp	15	58	2.4	0.1	5.5	1.1	1.4	3.1	8	96
Sandwich spread: low calorie	1 tbsp	15	17	1.2	0.2	1.4	0.3	0.3	0.8	0	94
Sardine: canned in oil, 3 × 1 × ½"	1 whole	12	24	0.3	2.9	1.3	0.4	0.4	0.4	17	99
Sauerkraut: canned, solids and liquid	1 cup	235	42	9.4	2.4	0.5	0	0	0.5	0	1,755
Sausage, Polish: 5⅝ × 1"	1 link	76	231	0.9	11.9	19.6	6.9	9.1	1.7	47	836
Sausage, pork: 4 × ⅞" (uncooked)	1 link	13	49	0	2.4	4.2	1.5	2.0	0.5	8	125
Sausage, Vienna: canned, 2 × ⅞" diameter	1 whole	16	56	0	2.2	5.2	1.8	2.5	0.6	10	157
Scallops: fresh, cooked, steamed	1 oz	28	32	—	6.6	0.3	0	0	0.1	15	75
Sesame seeds: dry, hulled	1 tbsp	8	47	1.4	1.5	4.4	0.6	1.6	1.8	0	—
Sherbet: orange	1 cup	193	270	58.7	2.2	3.8	2.4	1.1	0.1	14	88
Shortening: animal	1 tbsp	13	111	0	0	12.5	6.3	5.5	0.8	10	0
Shortening: animal-vegetable	1 tbsp	13	111	0	0	12.5	5.6	5.5	1.1	6	0
Shortening: vegetable	1 tbsp	13	111	0	0	12.5	3.3	5.8	3.5	0	0
Shrimp: 4½ oz can drained	1 cup	128	148	0.8	31.0	1.5	0.2	0.2	0.6	192	—
Shrimp: canned, approximately 2" long	10 whole	17	20	0.1	4.1	0.2	0	0	0.1	26	—
Shrimp: fresh, cooked, 8 shrimp, each 3¼" long (small)	2 oz	58	67	0.4	14.0	0.7	0.1	0.1	0.3	87	81
Snapper: red or gray, raw	1 oz	28	26	0	5.6	0.3	0.1	0.1	0.1	—	19
Sole: raw	1 oz	28	22	0	4.7	0.2	0	0	0.1	—	22
Soup: canned, bean with pork, prepared with equal volume of water	1 cup	250	170	21.8	8.0	6.0	1.5	2.2	1.8	4	1,008
Soup: canned, beef broth, prepared with equal volume of water	1 cup	240	31	2.6	5.0	0	0	0	0	0	782
Soup: canned, cream of celery, prepared with equal volume of water	1 cup	240	86	8.9	1.7	5.5	1.4	1.2	2.4	7	955

This information is current as of this printing. Check the manufacturer's label for updated analysis.

A dash (—) indicates that data are not available. Trace (tr) indicates that a very small amount of the constituent is present.

Abbreviations used in this table are: tbsp = tablespoon; tsp = teaspoon; oz = ounce; lb = pound; gm = gram; mg = milligrams; " = inches; Cal = calories; CHO = carbohydrate; Prot = protein; Sat fat = saturated fat; Mono fat = monounsaturated fat; Poly fat = polyunsaturated fat; Chol = cholesterol; Na = Sodium.

Food	Measure	Grams	Cal	CHO	Prot	Fat	Sat fat	Mono fat	Poly fat	Chol	Na
Soup: canned, cream of chicken, prepared with equal volume of water	1 cup	240	94	7.9	2.9	5.8	2.0	3.2	1.4	8	970
Soup: canned, cream of mushroom, prepared with equal volume of water	1 cup	240	132	10.1	2.4	9.4	2.5	1.8	4.4	6	955
Soup: canned, chicken noodle, prepared with equal volume of water	1 cup	240	67	7.9	3.4	2.4	0.6	1.0	0.5	6	979
Soup: canned, clam chowder, Manhattan style, prepared with equal volume of water	1 cup	245	78	12.3	2.2	2.2	0.4	0.4	1.3	6	938
Soup: canned, minestrone, prepared with equal volume of water	1 cup	245	105	14.2	4.9	2.7	0.6	0.7	1.2	2	995
Soup: canned, onion, prepared with equal volume of water	1 cup	240	65	5.3	5.3	2.4	0.8	1.0	0.6	6	1,051
Soup: canned, split pea, prepared with equal volume of water	1 cup	245	145	20.6	8.6	3.2	1.0	1.5	0.3	6	941
Soup: canned, tomato, prepared with equal volume of water	1 cup	245	88	15.7	2.0	2.0	0.4	0.4	0.9	2	970
Soup: canned, vegetable beef, prepared with equal volume of water	1 cup	245	89	9.6	5.3	3.4	0.8	0.9	1.6	6	1,046
Soup: canned, vegetarian vegetable, prepared with equal volume of water	1 cup	245	80	13.2	2.2	2.2	0.5	0.6	0.9	2	838
Soup: dehydrated, onion, 1 package	1½ oz	43	150	23.2	6.0	4.6	1.0	2.0	1.0	0	2,871
Sour cream: see Cream											
Soy sauce	1 tbsp	18	12	1.7	1.0	0.2	0	0	0.2	0	1,319
Soybeans: mature seeds, cooked	1 cup	180	234	19.4	19.8	10.3	1.5	2.1	5.3	0	4
Soybean curd (tofu): 2½ × 2¾ × 1"	1 piece	120	86	2.9	9.4	5.0	0.8	1.0	2.6	0	8
Soybean seeds: sprouted, raw	1 cup	105	48	5.6	6.5	1.5	0.5	0.1	0.9	0	—
Soybean seeds: sprouted, cooked	1 cup	125	48	4.6	6.6	1.8	0.5	0.2	1.1	0	—
Spaghetti: enriched, cooked without salt	1 cup	140	155	32.2	4.8	0.6	0	0	0.6	0	1
Spaghetti with meat balls and tomato sauce: canned, rings	1 cup	250	258	28.5	12.3	10.3	2.2	3.3	3.9	39	1,220
Spinach: frozen, cooked	1 cup	205	47	7.6	6.2	0.6	0	0	0.6	0	107
Spinach: canned, low sodium	1 cup	205	53	8.2	6.6	1.0	0.3	0.1	0.6	0	66
Squash, summer: fresh, cooked, sliced	1 cup	180	25	5.6	1.6	0.2	0	0	0.2	0	2
Squash, winter: frozen, cooked	1 cup	240	91	22.1	2.9	0.7	0	0	0.7	0	2
Steak: see Beef											

This information is current as of this printing. Check the manufacturer's label for updated analysis.

A dash (—) indicates that data are not available. Trace (tr) indicates that a very small amount of the constituent is present.

Abbreviations used in this table are: tbsp = tablespoon; tsp = teaspoon; oz = ounce; lb = pound; gm = gram; mg = milligrams; " = inches; Cal = calories; CHO = carbohydrate; Prot = protein; Sat fat = saturated fat; Mono fat = monounsaturated fat; Poly fat = polyunsaturated fat; Chol = cholesterol; Na = Sodium.

TABLE 2. (continued)

Food	Unit	Weight (g)	Cal	CHO (g)	Prot (g)	Fat (g)	Sat fat (g)	Mono fat (g)	Poly fat (g)	Chol (mg)	Na (mg)
Stew: beef and vegetable, canned	1 cup	245	194	17.4	14.2	7.6	3.2	3.1	0.2	36	1,007
Strawberries: fresh, whole	1 cup	149	55	12.5	1.0	0.7	0	0	0.7	0	1
Sugar: brown, packed	1 cup	220	821	212.1	0	0	0	0	0	0	66
Sugar: granulated	1 tbsp	12	46	11.9	0	0	0	0	0	0	tr
Sugar: powdered (confectioner's), unsifted	1 tbsp	8	31	8.0	0	0	0	0	0	0	tr
Sunflower seed kernels: dry, hulled	1 tbsp	9	51	1.8	2.2	4.3	0.5	0.9	2.7	0	3
Sweet roll: Danish pastry, without nuts or fruit, 4½ × 1"	1 whole	65	274	29.6	4.8	15.3	4.5	7.1	2.8	17	238
Sweetbreads (thymus), beef	1 oz	28	90	0	7.3	6.6	—	—	—	132	99
Syrup: cane and maple	1 tbsp	20	50	12.8	0	0	0	0	0	0	tr
Taco shell: fried tortilla	1 whole	30	146	19.7	2.6	5.6	1.5	2.3	1.5	0	tr
Tangerine: large, 2½" diameter	1 whole	136	46	11.7	0.8	0.2	0	0	0.2	0	2
Tapioca: dry	1 tbsp	10	33	8.2	0.1	tr	0	0	tr	0	tr
Tartar sauce	1 tbsp	14	76	0.6	0.2	8.3	1.0	2.1	4.1	7	102
Tofu: see Soybean Curd											
Tomatoes: canned, solids and liquid	1 cup	241	51	10.4	2.4	0.5	0	0	0.5	0	313
Tomatoes: fresh, raw, 3 × 2⅛" high (tomato = 6 slices)	1 whole	200	40	8.6	2.0	0.4	0	0	0.4	0	5
Tomatoes: fresh, cooked	1 cup	241	63	13.3	3.1	0.5	0	0	0.5	0	10
Tomatoes: canned, solids and liquid, low sodium	1 cup	241	48	10.1	2.4	0.5	0	0	0.5	0	7
Tomato catsup: canned or bottled	1 cup	273	289	69.3	5.5	1.1	0	0	1.1	0	2,845
Tomato chili sauce: bottled	1 cup	273	284	67.7	6.8	0.8	0	0	0.8	0	3,653
Tomato juice: canned or bottled	1 cup	243	46	10.4	2.2	0.2	0	0	0.2	0	486
Tomato juice: canned or bottled, low sodium	1 cup	242	46	10.4	1.9	0.2	0	0	0.2	0	7
Tomato paste: canned	1 cup	262	215	48.7	8.9	1.0	0.3	0.1	0.6	0	100
Tomato paste: low sodium	1 cup	262	215	48.7	8.9	1.0	0.3	0.1	0.6	0	40
Tomato sauce	1 cup	240	80	18.0	3.0	0	0	0	0	0	882
Tomato sauce: low sodium	1 cup	240	80	18.0	3.0	0	0	0	0	0	13
Tortilla: corn, 6" diameter	1 whole	30	70	13.4	1.6	0.6	0	0	0	0	tr
Tortilla: flour	1 whole	30	108	22.4	2.9	1.2	0.6	0.8	0.3	0	120
Tuna: water-packed, canned, chunk style, solids and liquid, low sodium	6½ oz	184	234	0	51.5	1.5	0.4	0.3	0.4	115	75
Tuna: oil-packed, canned (drained), 1 cup	4½ oz	127	295	0	46.1	10.9	3.6	2.8	2.9	104	1,280
Turkey: light meat, without skin	1 oz	28	45	0	9.3	0.7	0.2	0.2	0.2	22	23
Turkey: dark meat, without skin	1 oz	28	48	0	8.5	1.5	0.4	0.4	0.4	29	28

This information is current as of this printing. Check the manufacturer's label for updated analysis.

A dash (—) indicates that data are not available. Trace (tr) indicates that a very small amount of the constituent is present.

Abbreviations used in this table are: tbsp = tablespoon; tsp = teaspoon; oz = ounce; lb = pound; gm = gram; mg = milligrams; " = inches; Cal = calories; CHO = carbohydrate; Prot = protein; Fat = fat; Sat fat = saturated fat; Mono fat = monounsaturated fat; Poly fat = polyunsaturated fat; Chol = cholesterol; Na = Sodium.

Food	Measure	gm	Cal	CHO (gm)	Prot (gm)	Fat (gm)	Sat fat (gm)	Mono fat (gm)	Poly fat (gm)	Chol (mg)	Na (mg)
Turkey: light and dark with skin	1 oz	28	63	0	9.0	2.9	0.8	1.0	0.8	30	—
Turkey bologna or franks	1 oz	28	71	2.1	3.5	5.4	2.4	2.1	0.9	37	336
Turkey ham	1 oz	28	40	0.5	5.5	1.5	0.4	0.4	0.4	28	280
Turkey pastrami	1 oz	28	34	0.8	5.2	1.6	0.4	0.4	0.4	29	525
Turkey salami: with skin	1 oz	28	50	0.5	4.6	3.6	0.8	1.0	0.8	26	454
Turnip greens: frozen, chopped, cooked	1 cup	165	38	6.4	4.1	0.5	0	0	0.5	0	28
Turnips: fresh, cooked, cubes	1 cup	155	36	7.6	1.2	0.3	0	0	0.3	0	53
Veal: <6% fat, breast riblet, cutlet, leg, loin, rump, shank, shoulder steak (lean only)	1 oz	28	40	0	5.7	1.7	0.9	0.8	0.1	28	16
Veal: 10% fat, cutlet, leg, rump, shank, shoulder, steak (lean and fat)	1 oz	28	61	0	8.2	3.0	1.4	1.3	0.2	28	13
Veal: 15% fat, loin (lean and fat)	1 oz	28	67	0	7.5	3.8	1.8	1.6	0.2	29	13
Veal: 20% fat, rib (lean and fat)	1 oz	28	86	0	7.4	6.0	3.2	2.9	0.3	29	14
Veal: 25% fat, breast riblet (lean and fat)	1 oz	28	89	0	4.7	7.7	3.6	3.1	0.4	29	14
Vodka: see Liquor											
Vinegar: cider	1 cup	240	34	14.2	0	0	0	0	0	0	2
Waffle: made from mix, 7 × ⅝"	1 waffle	75	206	27.2	6.6	8.0	—	—	—	—	515
Walnuts: English, chopped pieces	1 tbsp	8	49	1.2	1.1	4.8	0.5	0.7	3.1	0	tr
Water chestnuts	4 nuts	25	20	4.8	0.4	0.1	0	0	0.1	0	5
Watermelon: diced pieces	1 cup	160	42	10.2	0.8	0.3	0	0	0.3	0	2
Watermelon: 10 × 1" wedge, or 4" arc × 8" radius	1 slice	926	111	27.3	2.1	0.9	0	0	0.9	0	4
Whiskey: see Liquor											
Weiner: 5 × ¾"	1 whole	45	139	0.8	5.6	12.4	4.7	5.9	0.8	27	495
Wine: dessert (port, madeira, sweet sherry)	1 oz	30	41	2.3	0	0	0	0	0	0	1
Wine: table (burgundy, rosé, white, dry sherry)	1 oz	29	25	1.2	0	0	0	0	0	0	1
Worcestershire sauce	1 tbsp	15	6	1.4	0.1	0	0	0	0	0	267
Yeast: bakers, dry package, scant tbsp	¼ oz	7	20	2.7	2.6	0.1	0	0.1	0.1	0	4
Yogurt: skim, home recipe	1 cup	227	127	17.4	13.0	0.4	0.3	0.1	0	4	174
Yogurt: plain, low fat	1 cup	227	144	16.0	11.9	3.5	2.3	1.0	0.1	14	159
Yogurt: whole milk	1 cup	227	139	10.6	7.9	7.4	4.8	2.0	0.2	29	105
Yogurt: with fruit (1–2% fat)	1 cup	227	225	42.3	9.0	2.6	1.7	0.7	0.1	10	121
Yogurt: frozen (2% fat)	1 cup	227	244	48.0	6.0	3.0	1.9	0.7	0.1	10	121

This information is current as of this printing. Check the manufacturer's label for updated analysis.

A dash (—) indicates that data are not available. Trace (tr) indicates that a very small amount of the constituent is present.

Abbreviations used in this table are: tbsp = tablespoon; tsp = teaspoon; oz = ounce; lb = pound; gm = gram; mg = milligrams; " = inches; Cal = calories; CHO = carbohydrate; Prot = protein; Sat fat = saturated fat; Mono fat = monounsaturated fat; Poly fat = polyunsaturated fat; Chol = cholesterol; Na = Sodium.

TABLE 2. *(continued)*

Information used in this table is from the following sources.

Adams, C. F.: *Nutritive Value of American Foods In Common Units.* USDA Handbook No. 456, 1975.

Anderson, B. A.: Comprehensive evaluation of fatty acids in foods. VII. Pork products. *Journal of the American Dietetic Association,* 69:44–49, 1976.

Anderson, B. A.: Comprehensive evaluation of fatty acids in foods. XIII. Sausages and luncheon meats. *Journal of the American Dietetic Association,* 72:48–52, 1978.

Anderson, B. A., Fristrom, G. A., and Weihrauch, J. L.: Comprehensive evaluation of fatty acids in foods. X. Lamb and veal. *Journal of the American Dietetic Association,* 70:53–58, 1977.

Anderson, B. A., Kinsella, J. E., and Watt, B. K.: Comprehensive evaluation of fatty acids in foods. II. Beef products. *Journal of the American Dietetic Association,* 67:35–41, 1975.

Brignoli, C. A., Kinsella, J. E., and Weihrauch, J.–L.: Comprehensive evaluation of fatty acids in foods. V. Unhydrogenated fats and oils. *Journal of the American Dietetic Association,* 68:224–229, 1976.

Consumer and Food Economics Institution: *Composition of Foods—Dairy and Egg Products—Raw, Processed, Prepared.* USDA Agricultural Handbook No. 8–1, 1976.

Exler, J., Avena, R. M., and Weihrauch, J. L.: Comprehensive evaluation of fatty acids in foods. XI. Leguminous seeds. *Journal of the American Dietetic Association,* 71:412–415, 1977.

Exler, J., and Weihrauch, J. L.: Comprehensive evaluation of fatty acids in foods. VIII. Finfish. *Journal of the American Dietetic Association,* 69:243–248, 1976.

Exler, J., and Weihrauch, J. L.: Comprehensive evaluation of fatty acids in foods. XII. Shellfish. *Journal of the American Dietetic Association,* 71:518–521, 1977.

Feeley, R. M., Criner, P. E., and Watt, B. K.: Cholesterol content of foods. *Journal of the American Dietetic Association,* 61:134–149, 1972.

Food manufacturers' and distributors' product information.

Fristrom, G. A., Stewart, B. C., Weihrauch, J. L., and Posati, L. P.: Comprehensive evaluation of fatty acids in foods. IV. Nuts, peanuts, and soups. *Journal of the American Dietetic Association,* 67:351–355, 1975.

Fristrom, G. A., and Weihrauch, J. L.: Comprehensive evaluation of fatty acids in foods. IX. Fowl. *Journal of the American Dietetic Association,* 69:517–522, 1976.

National Dairy Council: Composition and nutritive value of dairy foods. *Dairy Council Digest,* 47:25–30, No. 5, September–October, 1976.

Posati, L. P., Kinsella, J. E., and Watt, B. K.: Comprehensive evaluation of fatty acids in foods. I. Dairy products. *Journal of the American Dietetic Association,* 66:482–488, 1975.

Posati, L. P., Kinsella, J. E., and Watt, B. K.: Comprehensive evaluation of fatty acids in foods. III. Eggs and egg products. *Journal of the American Dietetic Association,* 67:111–115, 1975.

Weihrauch, J. L., Kinsella, J. E., and Watt, B. K.: Comprehensive evaluation of fatty acids in foods. VI. Cereal products. *Journal of the American Dietetic Association,* 68:335–340, 1976.

TABLE 3. *Ratio of polyunsaturated to saturated fatty acids*

Food	P/S ratio[a]
Oils[b]	
Coconut oil	0.02
Corn oil	4.58
Cottonseed oil	1.94
Olive oil	0.63
Palm kernel oil	0.02
Peanut oil[c]	1.78
Safflower oil (high linoleic acid)	7.85
Soybean oil	3.84
Sunflower seed oil (southern)	4.60
Nuts[d]	
Almond	2.33
Brazil nut	1.47
Cashew	0.81
Coconut	0.02
Filbert	1.46
Macadamia	0.21
Peanut	1.58
Pecan	2.94
Pistachio	0.95
Walnut, black	8.02
Walnut, English	5.99
Animal fats[b]	
Beef tallow	0.09
Chicken fat	0.54
Lard	0.30
Mutton fat	0.19

[a]P = sum of all fatty acids with two or more double bonds; S = sum of the saturated fatty acids (6:0 to 20:0).

[b]Adapted from Brignoli, C. A., Kinsella, J. E., and Weihrauch, J. L.: Comprehensive evaluation of fatty acids in foods. V. Unhydrogenated fats and oils. *Journal of the American Dietetic Association*, 68:224–229, 1976.

[c]Adapted from Exler, J., Avena, R. M., and Weihrauch, J. L.: Comprehensive evaluation of fatty acids in food. VI. Leguminous seeds. *Journal of the American Dietetic Association*, 71:412–415, 1977.

[d]Adapted from Fristrom, G. A., Steward, B. C., Weihrauch, J. L., and Posati, L. P.: Comprehensive evaluation of fatty acids in foods. IV. Nuts, peanuts, and soups. *Journal of the American Dietetic Association*, 67:351–355, 1975.

TABLE 4. *Good sources of vitamin A*

Food	Measure	Weight (grams)	Vitamin A (International Units)
Apricots			
Fresh, whole or halves	1 cup	155	4,190
Canned	1 cup	246	4,500
Broccoli, cooked			
Stalks	1 cup	155	3,880
Chopped	1 cup	185	4,810
Cantaloupe			
Cubed	1 cup	160	5,440
Carrots			
Raw, grated	1 cup	110	12,000
Cooked, sliced	1 cup	155	16,280
Chard, Swiss—leaves and stalks, cooked	1 cup	145	7,830
Endive (curly endive or escarole), raw	1 cup	50	1,650
Greens			
Beet, cooked	1 cup	145	7,400
Collard, cooked	1 cup	190	14,820
Dandelion, cooked	1 cup	105	12,290
Mustard, cooked	1 cup	140	8,120
Turnip, cooked	1 cup	145	9,140
Kale, cooked	1 cup	110	9,130
Mango, sliced	1 cup	165	7,920
Papaya, cubed	1 cup	140	2,450
Rutabaga			
Raw	1 cup	140	810
Cooked	1 cup	170	940
Spinach			
Raw	1 cup	55	4,460
Cooked	1 cup	180	14,580
Squash, winter, cooked	1 cup	205	8,610
Sweet potatoes, cooked, canned, pieces	1 cup	200	15,600
Watercress, whole	1 cup	35	1,720

Adapted from Adams, C. F.: *Nutritive Value of American Foods—In Common Units*. USDA Agriculture Handbook No. 456, 1975.

TABLE 5. *Good sources of vitamin C*

Food	Measure	Weight (grams)	Vitamin C (milligrams)
Broccoli, chopped, frozen, cooked	1 cup	185	105
Cantaloupe, cubed pieces	1 cup	160	53
Cauliflower			
Raw, flowerbuds	1 cup	100	78
Cooked	1 cup	125	69
Grapefruit			
Sections	1 cup	200	76
Juice	1 cup	246	93
Peppers			
Green			
Raw, strips	1 cup	100	128
Cooked, strips	1 cup	135	130
Mature red, raw, chopped	1 cup	100	204
Greens			
Collard, cooked	1 cup	190	144
Mustard, cooked	1 cup	140	67
Turnip, cooked	1 cup	145	100
Kale, cooked	1 cup	110	102
Mango, sliced whole	1 cup	165	58
Lemon juice	1 cup	244	112
Orange			
Sections	1 cup	180	90
Juice	1 cup	248	124
Papaya, cubed	1 cup	140	78
Rutabaga			
Raw whole	1 cup	140	60
Cooked	1 cup	170	44
Spinach, cooked	1 cup	180	50
Strawberries, sliced	1 cup	255	135
Sweet potato, canned, cooked	1 cup	200	28
Tangerine			
Sections, whole	1 cup	195	60
Juice, canned	1 cup	247	54
Tomato			
Cooked	1 cup	241	58
Raw, whole	1 medium	100	21
Juice	1 cup	243	39

Adapted from Adams, C. F.: *Nutritive Value of American Foods—In Common Units*. USDA Agriculture Handbook No. 456, 1975.

TABLE 6. *Metric conversions*

To change	To	Multiply by
Weights		
Ounces	Grams	28.35
Pounds	Kilograms	0.45
Grams	Ounces	0.035
Kilograms	Pounds	2.2
Volumes		
Teaspoons	Milliliters	5
Tablespoons	Milliliters	15
Fluid ounces	Milliliters	30
Cups	Liters	0.24
Pints	Liters	0.47
Quarts	Liters	0.95
Gallons	Liters	3.8
Milliliters	Fluid ounces	0.03
Liters	Pints	2.1
Liters	Quarts	1.06
Liters	Gallons	0.26
Lengths		
Inches	Centimeters	2.5
Feet	Centimeters	30
Yards	Meters	0.9
Miles	Kilometers	1.6
Millimeters	Inches	0.04
Centimeters	Inches	0.4
Meters	Feet	3.3
Meters	Yards	1.1
Kilometers	Miles	0.6
Temperatures		
Fahrenheit	Celsius	5/9 (after subtracting 32)
Celsius	Fahrenheit	9/5 (then add 32)

TABLE 7. *Point system for calculating sodium*

Food	Unit	Calories	Sodium points	Food	Unit	Calories	Sodium points
1 point = 1 milliequivalent sodium = 23 milligrams sodium				Beans: lima, canned, low sodium	1 cup	162	0
Aimonds: dried, shelled, slivered (not packed)	1 tbsp	43	0	Beans: pinto, calico, red Mexican	1 cup	218	0
Anchovy: 1–4″ flat	1 whole	5	1	Beans: mung, sprouts, cooked and drained	1 cup	35	0
Angel food cake: see *Cake*				Beans: mung, sprouts, uncooked	1 cup	37	0
Apple: raw with skin	1 whole	80	0	Beans: green, snap, fresh, frozen, cooked	1 cup	31	0
Apple: raw, pared, ¼″ slices or diced pieces	1 cup	59	0	Beans: green, snap, canned	1 cup	32	14
Apple butter	1 tbsp	33	0	Beans: green, snap, canned, low sodium	1 cup	30	0
Apple juice: canned or bottled	1 cup	117	0	Beans: white, Great Northern, navy, cooked	1 cup	212	1
Applesauce: canned, sweetened	1 cup	232	0	Beans: yellow or wax, frozen, cooked	1 cup	28	0
Apricots: raw	3 whole	55	0	Beans: yellow or wax, canned	1 cup	32	14
Apricot nectar: canned or bottled	1 cup	143	0	Beans: yellow or wax, canned, low sodium	1 cup	28	0
Artichoke: frozen, cooked, bud or globe	1 whole	52	2	Beef: dried, chipped, uncooked	1 oz	58	53
Asparagus: canned spears, ½″ diameter	4 spears	17	8	Beef: <6% fat; flank, round, Pike's Peak (lean only)	1 oz	53	1
Asparagus: canned, cut spears, low sodium	1 cup	47	0	Beef: 10% fat; chuck, filet mignon, New York strip, porterhouse, t-bone, tenderloin, ground round, choice grade (lean only)	1 oz	61	1
Avocado: California, raw, 3⅛″ diameter	1 whole	369	0				
Avocado: California, raw, puréed, mashed, or sieved	1 tbsp	25	0	Beef: 15% fat; club, rib eye roast, choice grade (lean only)	1 oz	74	1
Bacon: Canadian, cooked, 3⅜ × ³⁄₁₆″	1 oz	78	32	Beef: 20% fat; ground chuck	1 oz	82	1
Bacon: cooked (approximately 20 slices/pound raw)	2 slices	86	7	Beef: 25% fat; ground beef (hamburger), chuck, steak, pot roast (lean and fat)	1 oz	93	1
Bacon bits: with coconut oil	1 tsp	15	5				
Bacon bits: with soy oil	1 tsp	14	5	Beef: >30% fat; brisket, rib eye steak, standing rib roast, spareribs (lean and fat)	1 oz	110	1
Bagel: water	1 whole	212	5				
Baking powder: double acting	1 tsp	3	13				
Baking powder: low sodium	1 tsp	7	0	Beef: corned	1 oz	110	11
Baking soda	¼ tsp	0	15	Beef tongue: medium-fat, cooked, 3 × 2 × ⅛″	1 slice	49	1
Banana: raw, medium	1 whole	101	0	Beef kidney: cooked, ½ × ½ × ¼″	1 oz	353	15
Barbecue sauce: commercial (corn oil)	1 tbsp	14	6				
Beans: garbanzos or chickpeas	1 cup	248	1	Beef liver	1 oz	40	2
Beans: pork and beans in tomato sauce, canned	1 cup	311	51	Beef tallow: suet	1 tbsp	120	0
Beans: kidney	1 cup	218	0	Beer: regular	12 oz	151	1
Beans: lentils	1 cup	212	0				
Beans: lima, frozen, cooked	1 cup	168	7				
Beans: lima, canned	1 cup	163	17				

This information is current as of this printing. Check the manufacturer's label for updated analysis.

Abbreviations used in this table are: tbsp = tablespoon; oz = ounce; tsp = teaspoon; (—) = data not available.

TABLE 7. *Point system for calculating sodium (continued)*

Food	Unit	Calories	Sodium points	Food	Unit	Calories	Sodium points
Beets: red, canned, diced, sliced, or whole	1 cup	63	17	Cake: gingerbread (mix), 2¾ × 2¾ × 1⅜"	1 slice	174	8
Beets: red, canned, diced, sliced, or whole, low sodium	1 cup	63	3	Cake: marble with white icing (mix), ¹⁄₁₂ of layer cake	1 slice	288	10
Biscuit: made with shortening	1 whole	103	8	Cake: yellow with chocolate icing (mix), ¹⁄₁₂ of layer cake	1 slice	310	9
Blackberries: raw (also boysenberries, dewberries)	1 cup	84	0	Candy: candy corn, approximately 72 pieces	¼ cup	182	5
Bologna: 1 slice	1 oz	86	12	Candy*a*: chocolate, bittersweet	1 oz	135	0
Bouillon cube: all kinds (1 tsp instant bouillon)	1 cube	5	42	Candy*a*: chocolate, sweet	1 oz	150	0
Braunschweiger (liver sausage)	1 oz	90	12	Candy: chocolate-covered mint, 1⅜ × ⅜"	1 small	45	1
Bread: cracked wheat	1 slice	66	6	Candy: chocolate-covered raisins	1 cup	808	5
Bread: English muffin	1 whole	133	11	Candy: chocolate-covered vanilla cream	1 piece	56	1
Bread: French, enriched; 2½ × 2 × ½"	1 slice	44	4	Candy: fudge, plain, 1 cubic inch	1 piece	84	2
Bread: pita, pocket	1 large	145	4	Candy: gum drops, 1 large or 8 small	1 large	34	0
Bread: pumpernickel (dark rye)	1 slice	79	8	Candy: jellybeans	10 pieces	104	0
Bread: raisin	1 slice	66	4	Candy: M & M® type	¼ cup	230	2
Bread: rye (light)	1 slice	61	6	Candy: peanut brittle, 2½ × 2½ × ⅓" piece	1 oz	119	0
Bread: white, enriched	1 slice	68	6	Candy: chocolate-flavored roll (Tootsie Roll®) 1 × ½"	1 piece	28	1
Bread: whole wheat, firm crumb	1 slice	61	6	Candy: chocolate-flavored roll (Tootsie Roll®) 1 × ½"			
Bread: white, low sodium	1 slice	76	0	Candy bar*a*: chocolate-coated almonds, or peanut bar (Mr. Goodbar®)	1 oz	161	1
Broccoli: medium stalk, fresh, cooked and drained	1 stalk	47	1	Candy bar*a*: chocolate-coated almonds, or peanut bar (Mr. Goodbar®)			
Brussels sprouts: frozen, cooked, and drained	1 cup	51	1	Candy bar*a*: chocolate-coated with coconut center (Mound®)	1 oz	124	2
Butter: 1 pat	1 tsp	36	2	Candy bar*a*: fudge, peanut, caramel (O'Henry®, Snickers®, Rally®, Baby Ruth®)	1 oz	130	2
Buttermilk: made from skim milk	1 cup	88	14	Candy bar*a*: fudge, peanut, caramel (O'Henry®, Snickers®, Rally®, Baby Ruth®)			
Buttermilk: made from low-fat milk	1 cup	99	11	Candy bar*a*: Hershey Krackel® or Nestlés Crunch®	1 oz	144	2
Cabbage: common or Chinese; shredded, cooked, and drained	1 cup	29	1	Candy bar*a*: Hershey Krackel® or Nestlés Crunch®			
Cabbage: common or Chinese, raw, shredded	1 cup	22	1	Candy bar*a*: milk chocolate bar or 7 chocolate kisses	1 oz	147	1
Cake: angel food, ¹⁄₁₂ of 10" tube cake	1 slice	161	7	Cantaloupe: 5" diameter	1 whole	159	3
Cake: coffeecake (mix), 2⅝ × 2¾ × 1¼"	1 slice	232	13	Cantaloupe: cubed or diced, approximately 20/cup	1 cup	48	1
Cake: cream cheese, without crust or topping	1 slice	368	8	Carbonated beverage: Coca-Cola®, Mr. Pibb®	12 oz	144	1
Cake: devil's food (frozen), ⅙ of 7½" cake	1 slice	323	16	Carbonated beverage: ginger ale	12 oz	108	—
Cake: devil's food cupcake with icing (mix), 2½" diameter	1 whole	119	4				

TABLE 7. *Point system for calculating sodium (continued)*

Food	Unit	Calories	Sodium points	Food	Unit	Calories	Sodium points
Carbonated beverage: Sprite®	12 oz	143	3	Cereal: granola, cooked (¼ cup dry = ½ cup cooked)	½ cup	100	1
Carbonated beverage: Sprite® without sugar	12 oz	5	3	Cereal: Grape-Nuts®	1 cup	430	35
Carbonated beverage: Mr. Pibb® without sugar	12 oz	2	2	Cereal: oatmeal, cooked without salt	1 cup	132	0
Carbonated beverage: Fresca®	12 oz	3	4	Cereal: puffed rice	1 cup	60	0
Carbonated beverage: Tab®	12 oz	1	2	Cereal: puffed wheat	1 cup	54	0
Carrot: raw, approximately 1⅛ × 7½"	1 whole	30	1	Cereal: raisin bran	1 cup	144	9
				Cereal: Rice Krispies®	1 cup	117	12
Carrots: fresh, cooked, sliced	1 cup	48	2	Cereal: Spoon Size Shredded Wheat®, approximately 50 biscuits per cup	1 cup	180	0
Carrots: canned solids, sliced	1 cup	47	16				
Carrots: canned solids, sliced, low sodium	1 cup	39	3	Cereal: shredded wheat biscuit, 3¾ × 2¼ × 1"	1 whole	90	0
Cashew: roasted in oil, unsalted (14 large, 18 medium, or 26 small)	1 oz	159	0	Cereal: sugar-coated corn flakes	1 cup	154	12
Catfish: freshwater, raw	1 oz	29	1	Cereal: Wheat Chex®	⅔ cup	110	9
Cauliflower: frozen, cooked, approximately 7 flowerettes	1 cup	32	1	Cereal: wheat germ	1 tbsp	23	0
				Cereal: Wheaties® or Total®	1 cup	104	13
Caviar: sturgeon, granular	1 tbsp	42	15	Cheese: American	1 oz	106	18
Celery: green, raw, 8 × 1½" stalk	1 stalk	7	2	Cheese: blue	1 oz	100	17
				Cheese: brick	1 oz	105	7
Cereal: bran, unprocessed, 1.17 cup	1 oz	91	0	Cheese: brie	1 oz	95	8
				Cheese: camembert	1 oz	85	10
Cereal: bran buds	1 cup	144	21	Cheese: cheddar	1 oz	114	8
Cereal: 40% bran flakes	1 cup	106	9	Cheese: colby	1 oz	112	7
Cereal: Cheerios® or puffed oats	1 cup	99	14	Cheese: cottage, creamed (4% fat)	¼ cup	54	9
Cereal: corn flakes	1 cup	97	11	Cheese: cottage, low fat (2% fat)	¼ cup	51	10
Cereal: corn grits, enriched, cooked without salt	1 cup	125	0	Cheese: cottage, dry curd	¼ cup	31	0
Cereal: cream of rice, cooked without salt	1 cup	123	0	Cheese: cream cheese, 2 tbsp	1 oz	99	4
Cereal: cream of wheat, cooked without salt	1 cup	180	0	Cheese: edam	1 oz	101	12
Cereal: farina, enriched, regular, cooked without salt	1 cup	103	0	Cheese: feta	1 oz	75	14
				Cheese: gouda	1 oz	101	10
				Cheese: gruyere	1 oz	117	4
Cereal: farina, enriched, quick-cooking, cooked with salt	1 cup	105	20	Cheese: monterey	1 oz	106	7
				Cheese: mozzarella, part-skim, low moisture	1 oz	79	7
Cereal: farina, enriched, instant-cooking, cooked without salt	1 cup	135	1	Cheese: mozzarella, whole milk	1 oz	80	5
Cereal: granola, without coconut or other saturated fat	¼ cup	139	1				

*a*The weight of candy bars often changes; the analysis is given for 1 ounce and can be calculated for the total unit (1 piece of candy).

This information is current as of this printing. Check the manufacturer's label for updated analysis.

Abbreviations used in this table are: tbsp = tablespoon; oz = ounce; tsp = teaspoon; (—) = data not available.

TABLE 7. *Point system for calculating sodium (continued)*

Food	Unit	Calories	Sodium points	Food	Unit	Calories	Sodium points
Cheese: muenster	1 oz	104	8	Cocoa: dry powder, medium fat, plain	1 tbsp	14	0
Cheese: neufchatel	1 oz	74	5				
Cheese: parmesan, grated	1 tbsp	23	4	Cocoa mix: 1 oz package	1 pkg	102	6
Cheese: provolone	1 oz	100	11	Coconut: shredded, fresh, meat only	1 cup	277	1
Cheese: ricotta, whole milk (13% fat)	¼ cup	108	2				
Cheese: ricotta, part skim milk (8% fat)	¼ cup	86	3	Cookie: commercial, chocolate chip, 2¼ × ⅜"	1 cookie	50	2
Cheese: romano	1 oz	110	15	Cookie: commercial, fig bar, 1⅝ × 1⅝"	1 cookie	50	2
Cheese: roquefort	1 oz	105	22				
Cheese: swiss	1 oz	95	17	Cookie: commercial, ginger snap, 2 × ¼"	1 cookie	29	2
Cheese: Velveeta® (cheese spread)	1 oz	82	17	Cookie: commercial, macaroon, 2¾ × ¼"	1 cookie	91	0
Cheese: 1% butterfat (Countdown®)	1 oz	40	18	Cookie: commercial, marshmallow, chocolate-coated, 1¾ × ¾"	1 cookie	53	1
Cheese: 4–8% butterfat, processed (Breeze®, Chef's Delight®, Country Club®, Mellow Age®, Tasty®, Lite-Line®, low-fat DI-ET®)	1 oz	50	19	Cookie: commercial, oatmeal with raisins, 2⅝ × ¼"	1 cookie	59	1
				Cookie: commercial, peanut butter sandwich, 1¾ × ½"	1 cookie	58	1
Cheese: 5% butterfat, natural (St. Otho)	1 oz	49	—	Cookie: commercial, sandwich, round 1¾ × ⅜"	1 cookie	50	2
Cheese: 19–32% polyunsaturated fat (Golden Image®, Cheez-ola®, Dorman®, Nutrend®, Scandic®, Unique®)	1 oz	98	14	Cookie: commercial, vanilla wafer, 1¾ × ¼"	1 wafer	19	0
				Cookie: prepared mix, brownies, 1¾ × 1¾ × ⅞"	1 piece	86	1
Cheese: 23% polyunsaturated fat, low sodium (Cheez-ola®)	1 oz	90	7	Cordial: apricot brandy, benedictine, anisette, creme de menthe, curacao	4 tsp	66	0
Cherries: raw, sweet, unpitted	10 whole	47	0				
Cherries: canned, sweet, syrup-packed, pitted	1 cup	208	0	Corn: canned, whole kernel	1 cup	139	17
Chicken: gizzard, all classes, cooked, chopped	1 cup	215	4	Corn: canned, whole kernel, low sodium	1 cup	152	0
				Corn: canned, cream style, low sodium	1 cup	210	0
Chicken: light meat, no skin	1 oz	51	1	Corn chips: 1½ oz package = 1¼ cups or 60 chips	1¼ cup	239	10
Chicken: dark meat, no skin	1 oz	52	1				
Chicken: dark and light meat, with skin	1 oz	70	—	Corn meal: white and yellow, enriched, degermed	1 cup	502	0
Chicken fat	1 tbsp	126	0	Corned beef: see *Beef*			
Chicken liver: cooked, whole, 2 × 2 × ⅝"	1 liver	41	1	Cornstarch: not packed	1 tbsp	29	0
Chickpeas: see *Beans*				Cottage cheese: see *Cheese*			
Chocolate: bitter or baking	1 oz	143	0	Crab: fresh, cooked, not packed	1 cup	106	11
Chocolate syrup (or topping): fudge type	2 tbsp	124	1	Crab: canned solids, packed	1 cup	149	70
Clams: canned solids (chopped or minced)	1 cup	143	8				

TABLE 7. *Point system for calculating sodium (continued)*

Food	Unit	Calories	Sodium points	Food	Unit	Calories	Sodium points
Crackers: animal	10 whole	112	3	Dessert topping: nondairy, pressurized	1 tbsp	11	0
Cracker: graham, chocolate-coated, 2½ × 2 × ¼"	1 whole	62	2	Doughnut: cake type, plain, 1½ × ¾"	1 whole	55	3
Crackers: graham, sugar, honey, 2 squares, 2½" each	2 whole	58	3	Doughnut: yeast-leavened, plain, 3¾ × 1¼"	1 whole	176	4
Cracker: matzo	1 whole	118	0	Duck: flesh only, raw, domesticated	1 oz	47	1
Crackers: melba toast	3 whole	60	0	Duck: flesh and skin, raw, domesticated	1 oz	92	1
Crackers: melba toast, low sodium	3 whole	60	0	Eclair: custard filling with chocolate, 5 × 2 × 1¾"	1 whole	239	4
Crackers: saltines, single crackers	4 whole	48	5	Egg: chicken, whole, fresh, medium	1 whole	79	3
Crackers: sandwich, cheese and peanut butter (1 oz pack)	4 whole	139	12	Egg: chicken, fresh	1 white	16	2
Crackers: Triscuit®	1 whole	21	1	Egg: chicken, fresh	1 yolk	63	0
Cranberries: raw, chopped	1 cup	51	0	Eggnog: commercial	1 cup	342	6
Cranberry juice: cocktail, sweetened	1 cup	164	0	Egg substitute: Eggbeaters®, 1 egg equivalent	¼ cup	40	6
Cranberry sauce: sweetened, canned	1 cup	404	0	Egg substitute: Second Nature®, 1 egg equivalent	3 tbsp	35	3
Cream: fluid, half and half (11.7% fat)	1 tbsp	20	0	Egg substitute: Lucern®, 1 egg equivalent	¼ cup	50	0
Cream: fluid, light (20.6% fat)	1 tbsp	29	0	Eggplant: cooked, diced	1 cup	38	0
Cream: fluid, light, whipping (31.3% fat), approximately 2 cups whipped	1 cup	699	4	English muffin: see *Bread* Fig: raw, whole, 1½" diameter	1 small	32	0
Cream: fluid, heavy, or whipping (37.6% fat), approximately 2 cups whipped	1 cup	821	4	Fish: see *Catfish, Haddock, Halibut, Herring, Snapper, Flounder, Sole* Fish sticks: breaded, cooked, frozen, 4 × 1 × ½"	1 oz	50	1
Cream: sour	1 tbsp	31	0	Flounder: raw	1 oz	22	1
Cream: sour, imitation (IMO®, Wonder®)	1 tbsp	26	0	Flour: white, all purpose, enriched, unsifted	1 cup	455	0
Creamer: nondairy, powder, containing saturated fat (Creamora® and Coffee-Mate®)	1 tbsp	33	1	Flour: white, self-rising, enriched, unsifted	1 cup	440	59
Creamer: nondairy, liquid, containing saturated fat (Coffee Rich®)	1 tbsp	20	1	Flour: whole wheat	1 cup	400	0
				Frankfurter: 5 × ¾"	1 whole	139	22
				Frosting mix: prepared	1 tbsp	61	0
Creamer: nondairy, liquid, containing polyunsaturated fat (Poly Perx® and Mocha Mix®)	1 tbsp	20	0	Frosting: ready to spread (with animal or vegetable shortening)	1 tbsp	55	0
Cucumber: raw, pared, whole, 2⅛ × 8¼"	1 whole	39	1	Fruit cocktail: canned, solids and liquid, water-packed	1 cup	91	1
Dates: hydrated, without pits	10 whole	219	0				
Dessert topping: frozen, semisolid (Cool Whip®)	1 tbsp	13	0				

This information is current as of this printing. Check the manufacturer's label for updated analysis.

Abbreviations used in this table are: tbsp = tablespoon; oz = ounce; tsp = teaspoon; (—) = data not available.

TABLE 7. *Point system for calculating sodium (continued)*

Food	Unit	Calories	Sodium points	Food	Unit	Calories	Sodium points
Garbanzos: see *Beans*				Jelly: sweetened	1 tbsp	49	0
Gelatin: dry, unflavored, 1 envelope	1 pkg	23	0	Knockwurst link: 4 × 1⅛"	1 link	165	33
				Ladyfingers	1 whole	40	0
Gelatin: sweetened dessert powder (JELL-O®), prepared with water, plain	½ cup	71	3	Lamb: <7% fat, chop, leg, roast, sirloin chop (lean only)	1 oz	53	1
Gelatin: low calorie, prepared with water	½ cup	8	0	Lamb: 10% fat, shank, shoulder (lean only)	1 oz	58	1
Gin: see *Liquor*				Lamb: 20% fat, leg, roast, sirloin chop (lean and fat)	1 oz	79	1
Gizzard: chicken, all classes, cooked, chopped	¼ cup	54	1	Lamb: 30% fat, breast, chop, rib (lean and fat)	1 oz	96	1
Goose: flesh only, raw	1 oz	45	1	Lard	1 tbsp	117	0
Grapes: raw, seedless (Thompson)	10 grapes	34	0	Lemon: raw, 1 wedge (⅙ of 2⅛" lemon)	1 slice	3	0
Grape juice: frozen concentrate, sweetened, diluted	1 cup	133	0	Lemon juice: canned, unsweetened	1 tbsp	4	0
Grapefruit: all varieties	1 whole	80	0	Lemonade: concentrate, frozen, diluted	1 cup	88	0
Grapefruit juice: unsweetened, frozen concentrate, diluted	1 cup	101	0	Lentils: see *Beans*			
				Lettuce: raw, crisp head varieties, chopped or shredded	1 cup	7	0
Greens, collard: frozen, cooked	1 cup	51	1	Liquor: gin, rum, vodka, whiskey	1 oz	70	0
Haddock: raw	1 oz	29	1	Liver: see *Beef* or *Chicken*			
Halibut: Atlantic or Pacific, broiled	1 oz	28	1	Lobster: northern, cooked, ½" cubes	1 cup	138	13
Ham: see *Pork*				Luncheon meat: see *Salami, Bologna, Braunschweiger, Sausage, Turkey*			
Hamburger: see *Beef*							
Herring: canned, solids and liquid, plain	1 oz	59	0				
Honey: strained	1 tbsp	64	0				
Honeydew: 7 × 2" wedge, 1/10 of melon	1 slice	49	1	Macadamia nuts: 15 whole nuts	1 oz	196	—
Horseradish: prepared	1 tbsp	6	1	Macaroni: enriched, cooked, hot	1 cup	155	0
Ice cream: rich, approximately 16% fat, hardened	1 cup	349	5	Mackerel: canned, solids and liquids	¼ cup	64	6
Ice cream: regular, approximately 10% fat, hardened	1 cup	269	5	Mango: raw	1 whole	152	1
Ice cream bar: chocolate-covered (Eskimo Pie®)	1 bar	270	—	Margarine: P/S >3.0 (Promise® soft, Parkay® soft safflower, Hains® soft, Saffola® soft)	1 tbsp	102	6
Ice cream sandwich: 3 oz size	1 whole	238	—	Margarine: P/S 2.6 to 3.0 (Mrs. Filbert's® soft corn oil, Promise® stick, Parkay® liquid squeeze)	1 tbsp	102	6
Ice cream cone	1 cone	11	0				
Ice milk: 5.1% fat, soft serve	1 cup	223	7				
Ice milk: 5.1% fat, hardened	1 cup	184	5	Margarine: P/S 2.0 to 2.5 (Fleischmann's® soft, Chiffon® soft, Parkay® corn oil soft)	1 tbsp	102	5
Instant breakfast: dry powder, all flavors except eggnog	1¼ oz	130	0				

TABLE 7. *Point system for calculating sodium (continued)*

Food	Unit	Calories	Sodium points	Food	Unit	Calories	Sodium points
Margarine: P/S 1.6 to 1.9 (Fleischmann's® stick, Chiffon® stick, Meadow Gold® stick)	1 tbsp	102	5	Oil: cod liver	1 tbsp	120	0
				Oil: corn	1 tbsp	120	0
				Oil: cottonseed	1 tbsp	120	0
				Oil: olivo	1 tbsp	119	0
Margarine: P/S 1.0 to 1.5 (Mazola® stick, Parkay® corn oil stick, Imperial® stick)	1 tbsp	100	5	Oil: palm kernel	1 tbsp	120	0
				Oil: peanut	1 tbsp	119	0
				Oil: safflower	1 tbsp	120	0
				Oil: soybean	1 tbsp	120	0
Margarine: low sodium, P/S 1.7 (Fleischmann's®, Mazola®)	1 tbsp	100	0	Oil: soybean-cottonseed blend	1 tbsp	120	0
				Oil: sunflower	1 tbsp	120	0
Margarine: P/S <0.5, all vegetable fat (Kraft® all purpose stick, Swift® all purpose stick)	1 tbsp	102	6	Okra: frozen, cooked, cuts	1 cup	70	0
				Olives: ripe, whole, extra large	10 whole	61	17
				Olives: green, whole, large	10 whole	45	40
Margarine: P/S <0.5, vegetable and animal or all animal (Gaylord® stick, Meadowlake® stick)	1 tbsp	102	6	Onions: green, raw, 4⅛ × ⅝"	2 med	14	0
				Onions: mature, raw, chopped	1 cup	65	1
				Onions: mature, cooked, whole or sliced	1 cup	61	1
Margarine: P/S 2.4, diet tub (Fleischmann's® soft, Imperial® soft)	1 tbsp	50	6	Orange: Florida, medium, 2¹¹⁄₁₆" diameter	1 whole	71	0
Mellorine	1 cup	244	5	Orange juice: concentrate, frozen, unsweetened, diluted	1 cup	122	0
Milk: skim (less than 1% fat)	1 cup	86	5				
Milk: low fat (1–2% fat)	1 cup	102	5	Oysters: canned, 18 to 27 medium or 27 to 44 small	12 oz	224	11
Milk: whole (3.3% fat)	1 cup	150	5				
Milk: canned, evaporated, whole	1 cup	338	12	Oysters: raw, 13 to 19 medium or 19 to 31 small	1 cup	158	8
Milk: canned, evaporated, skim	1 cup	200	13				
Milk: nonfat, dry powder, approximately 1 cup reconstituted	⅓ cup	81	5	Pancake: made from mix, 6 × ½"	1 cake	164	18
Milk: canned, condensed, sweetened	1 cup	982	17	Peach: raw, pared, 2¾" diameter, approximately 2½ per pound	1 whole	51	0
Milk: chocolate drink, fluid, commercial made with whole milk	1 cup	213	5	Peaches: canned, syrup-packed, halves, slices, or chunks	1 cup	200	0
Milk: low sodium (whole)	1 cup	149	0	Peanut butter	1 cup	1,520	68
Milkshake: chocolate	11 oz	369	15	Peanuts: roasted, salted, 10 Virginia, 20 Spanish, or 1 tbsp chopped		53	2
Milkshake: vanilla	11 oz	350	13				
Molasses: light	1 tbsp	52	0	Pear: raw, Bartlett, 2½ × 3½" diameter	1 whole	100	0
Mushrooms: raw, sliced, chopped, or diced	1 cup	20	0				
Mustard: prepared, yellow	1 tsp	4	3	Pear: canned, syrup-packed, with 1⅔ tbsp liquid	1 half	58	0
Nectarine: raw, 2½" diameter	1 whole	88	0				
Noodles: egg, enriched, cooked	1 cup	200	0				
Noodles: chow mein, canned	1 cup	220	—				
Oil: coconut	1 tbsp	120	0				

This information is current as of this printing. Check the manufacturer's label for updated analysis.

Abbreviations used in this table are: tbsp = tablespoon; oz = ounce; tsp = teaspoon; (—) = data not available.

TABLE 7.   *Point system for calculating sodium (continued)*

Food	Unit	Calories	Sodium points	Food	Unit	Calories	Sodium points
Pear nectar: canned	1 cup	130	0	Pork: fresh, 13–20% fat, Boston butt roast, chop, loin, shoulder (lean only)	1 oz	71	1
Peas: cow or blackeyed, canned, cooked	1 cup	179	26				
Peas: green, immature, canned solids	1 cup	150	17	Pork: fresh, 23–30% fat, Boston butt, ground pork, ham, loin picnic, shoulder (lean and fat)	1 oz	103	1
Peas: green, immature, canned solids, low sodium	1 cup	122	0				
Pecans: chopped or pieces	1 tbsp	51	0	Pork: spareribs, 37% fat (lean and fat)	1 oz	125	0
Pepper: immature, green, raw, 3¾ × 3″ diameter	1 whole	36	1	Pork: cured, 7–10% fat, ham or picnic ham (lean only)	1 oz	56	12
Pepper: jalapēno, canned	1 whole	5	3				
Pepper: jalapēno, fresh	1 whole	7	0	Pork: cured, 13–20% fat, Boston butt, shoulder (lean only)	1 oz	75	11
Pheasant: flesh only, raw	1 oz	46	—				
Pickle: dill or sour, whole, large, 4 × 1¾″	1 whole	15	84	Pork: cured, 23–30% fat, ham, picnic, shoulder (lean and fat)	1 oz	93	10
Pickle: dill or sour, whole, 3¾ × 1¼″, low sodium	1 whole	7	0				
Pickle: fresh, sweetened (bread and butter), 1½ × ¼″	2 slices	11	4	Pork: deviled ham, canned	¼ cup	198	31
				Potato chips	10 chips	114	9
Pickle: sweet, gherkins, large, 3 × 1″	1 whole	51	22	Potatoes: fresh, boiled, diced or sliced	1 cup	101	0
Pickle relish: finely chopped, sweet	1 tbsp	21	5	Potato: fresh, baked in skin, 2⅓ × 4¾″	1 whole	145	0
Pie: frozen, baked, apple, 8″ diameter	1 pie	1,386	51	Potatoes: frozen, French fried, 4″ strips (oven-heated)	10 strips	172	0
Pie: frozen, baked, cherry, 8″ diameter	1 pie	1,690	58				
Pie: mix, baked, coconut custard (eggs and milk), 8″ diameter	1 pie	1,618	81	Potato, sweet: fresh, baked, 5 × 2″	1 whole	161	1
				Potatoes, sweet: pieces, canned in syrup	1 cup	216	4
Pineapple: raw, diced pieces	1 cup	81	0	Pretzels: extruded type, rods, 7½ × ½″	1 whole	55	10
Pineapple: canned, syrup packed, chunk, tidbit, or crushed	1 cup	189	0	Pretzels: twisted type, rings (3), 1⅞ × 1¾ × ¼″	10 whole	117	22
Pineapple: canned, water-packed, tidbits	1 cup	96	0	Prunes: dried, uncooked, without pits	10 whole	260	0
Pineapple: in its own juice (no sugar added), 4 slices with juice or 1 cup with juice	1 cup	140	0	Prunes: dried, cooked, no added sugar	1 cup	253	0
				Prune juice: canned or bottled	1 cup	197	0
Pineapple juice: canned, unsweetened	1 cup	138	0	Pudding mix: chocolate, regular, prepared with whole milk	1 cup	322	15
Plum: hybrid, fresh, 2⅛″ diameter	1 whole	32	0	Pudding mix: chocolate, instant, prepared with whole milk	1 cup	325	14
Plums: canned, served with 2¾ tbsp syrup	3 whole	110	0				
Popcorn: no salt or fat added to popped corn	1 cup	23	0	Pudding mix: low calorie, dry form, 1 package (all kinds)	4 oz	100	12
Pork: fresh, 10% fat, ham or picnic ham (lean only)	1 oz	61	1	Pumpkin: canned	1 cup	81	0
				Quail: flesh and skin, raw	1 oz	48	1
				Raisins: natural, seedless, uncooked, whole, not packed	1 tbsp	26	0

TABLE 7. *Point system for calculating sodium (continued)*

Food	Unit	Calories	Sodium points	Food	Unit	Calories	Sodium points
Raspberries: raw, red	1 cup	70	0	Sardine: canned in oil, 3 × 1 × ½″	1 whole	24	4
Rhubarb: frozen, sweetened	1 cup	381	0	Sauerkraut: canned, solids and liquid	1 cup	42	76
Rice: brown, cooked without salt	1 cup	232	0	Sausage, Polish: 5⅝ × 1″	1 link	231	36
Rice: white, enriched, cooked without salt	1 cup	221	0	Sausage, pork: 4 × ⅞″ (uncooked)	1 patty	49	5
Roll: hard, enriched	1 roll	78	7	Sausage, Vienna: canned, 2 × ⅞″ diameter	1 whole	56	7
Roll: soft, enriched, brown and serve, or Parker House	1 roll	83	6	Scallops: fresh, cooked, steamed	1 oz	32	3
Roll: enriched, hotdog (6 × 2″) or hamburger (3½ × 1½″)	1 whole	119	9	Sesame seeds: dry, hulled	1 tbsp	47	—
				Sherbet: orange	1 cup	270	4
Rum: see *Liquor*				Shortening: animal	1 tbsp	111	0
Salad dressing: blue or roquefort	1 tbsp	76	7	Shortening: animal-vegetable	1 tbsp	111	0
Salad dressing: blue or roquefort, low calorie	1 tbsp	12	8	Shortening: vegetable	1 tbsp	111	0
				Shrimp: 4½ oz can, drained	1 cup	148	—
Salad dressing: French	1 tbsp	66	10	Shrimp: canned, approximately 2″ long (small)	10 whole	20	—
Salad dressing: French, low calorie	1 tbsp	15	5				
Salad dressing: Italian	1 tbsp	83	14	Shrimp: fresh, cooked, 8 shrimp, each 3¼″ long	2 oz	67	4
Salad dressing: Italian, low calorie	1 tbsp	8	5	Snapper: red or gray, raw	1 oz	26	1
Salad dressing: mayonnaise	1 tbsp	101	4	Sole: raw	1 oz	22	1
Salad dressing: mayonnaise, low sodium	1 tbsp	99	0	Soup: canned, bean with pork, prepared with equal volume of water	1 cup	170	44
Salad dressing: mayonnaise type (Miracle Whip®)	1 tbsp	65	4	Soup: canned, beef broth, prepared with equal volume of water	1 cup	31	34
Salad dressing: mayonnaise type, low calorie	1 tbsp	22	1	Soup: canned, cream of celery, prepared with equal volume of water	1 cup	86	42
Salad dressing: Russian	1 tbsp	74	6	Soup: canned, cream of chicken, prepared with equal volume of water	1 cup	94	42
Salad dressing: Thousand Island	1 tbsp	80	5	Soup: canned, cream of mushroom, prepared with equal volume of water	1 cup	132	42
Salad dressing: Thousand Island, low calorie	1 tbsp	27	5				
Salami: cooked, 4½″ diameter slice	1 oz	73	13	Soup: canned, chicken noodle, prepared with equal volume of water	1 cup	67	43
Salmon: fresh, broiled or baked, no added fat	1 oz	48	1				
Salmon: canned, drained, pink	1 oz	49	6	Soup: canned, clam chowder, Manhattan style, prepared with equal volume of water	1 cup	78	41
Salmon: smoked (Lox)	1 oz	50	6				
Salt: table	1 tsp	0	95				
Salt pork	1 oz	219	15				
Sandwich spread: with chopped pickle	1 tbsp	58	4				
Sandwich spread: low calorie	1 tbsp	17	4				

This information is current as of this printing. Check the manufacturer's label for updated analysis.
Abbreviations used in this table are: tbsp = tablespoon; oz = ounce; tsp = teaspoon; (—) = data not available.

TABLE 7. *Point system for calculating sodium (continued)*

Food	Unit	Calories	Sodium points	Food	Unit	Calories	Sodium points
Soup: canned, minestrone, prepared with equal volume of water	1 cup	105	43	Sweet roll: Danish pastry, without nuts or fruit, 4½ × 1″	1 whole	274	10
Soup: canned, onion, prepared with equal volume of water	1 cup	65	46	Sweetbreads (thymus), beef	1 oz	90	4
Soup: canned, split pea, prepared with equal volume of water	1 cup	145	41	Syrup: cane and maple	1 tbsp	50	0
				Taco shell: fried tortilla	1 whole	146	0
Soup: canned, tomato, prepared with equal volume of water	1 cup	88	42	Tangerine: large, 2½″ diameter	1 whole	46	0
				Tapioca: dry	1 tbsp	33	0
				Tartar sauce	1 tbsp	76	4
Soup: canned, vegetable beef, prepared with equal volume of water	1 cup	89	45	Tofu: see *Soybean Curd*			
				Tomatoes: canned, solids and liquid	1 cup	51	14
Soup: canned, vegetarian vegetable, prepared with equal volume of water	1 cup	80	36	Tomatoes: fresh, raw, 3 × 2⅛″	1 whole	40	0
				Tomatoes: fresh, cooked	1 cup	63	0
Soup: dehydrated, onion, 1 package	1½ oz	150	125	Tomatoes: canned, solids and liquid, low sodium	1 cup	48	0
Sour cream: see *Cream*				Tomato catsup: canned or bottled	1 cup	289	124
Soy sauce	1 tbsp	12	57	Tomato chili sauce: bottled	1 cup	284	159
Soybeans: mature seeds, cooked	1 cup	234	0	Tomato juice: canned or bottled	1 cup	46	21
Soybean curd (tofu): 2½ × 2¾ × 1″	1 piece	86	0	Tomato juice: canned or bottled, low sodium	1 cup	46	0
Soybean seeds: sprouted, raw	1 cup	48	0	Tomato paste: canned	1 cup	215	4
				Tomato paste: low sodium	1 cup	215	2
Soybean seeds: sprouted, cooked	1 cup	48	0	Tomato sauce	1 cup	80	38
				Tomato sauce: low sodium	1 cup	80	1
Spaghetti: enriched, cooked without salt	1 cup	155	0	Tortilla: corn, 6″ diameter	1 whole	70	0
				Tortilla: flour	1 whole	108	5
Spaghetti with meat balls and tomato sauce: canned, rings	1 cup	258	53	Tuna: water-packed, canned, chunk style, solids and liquid, low sodium	6½ oz	234	3
Spinach: frozen, cooked	1 cup	47	5				
Spinach: canned, low sodium	1 cup	53	3				
Squash, summer: fresh, cooked, sliced	1 cup	25	0	Tuna: oil-packed, canned (drained), 1 cup	4½ oz	295	56
Squash, winter: frozen, cooked	1 cup	91	0	Turkey: light meat, without skin	1 oz	45	1
Steak: see *Beef*				Turkey: dark meat, without skin	1 oz	48	1
Stew: beef and vegetable, canned	1 cup	194	44	Turkey: light and dark with skin	1 oz	63	—
Strawberries: fresh, whole	1 cup	55	0	Turkey bologna or franks	1 oz	71	15
Sugar: brown, packed	1 cup	821	3	Turkey ham	1 oz	40	12
Sugar: granulated	1 tbsp	46	0	Turkey pastrami	1 oz	34	23
Sugar: powdered (confectioner's), unsifted	1 tbsp	31	0	Turkey salami: with skin	1 oz	50	20
				Turnip greens: frozen, chopped, cooked	1 cup	38	1
Sunflower seed kernels: dry, hulled	1 tbsp	51	2	Turnips: fresh, cooked, cubed	1 cup	36	2

TABLE 7. *Point system for calculating sodium (continued)*

Food	Unit	Calories	Sodium points	Food	Unit	Calories	Sodium points
Veal: <6% fat, breast riblet, cutlet, leg, loin, rump, shank, shoulder steak (lean only)	1 oz	40	1	Water chestnuts	4 nuts	20	0
				Watermelon: diced pieces	1 cup	42	0
				Watermelon: 10 × 1" wedge or 4" arc × 8" radius	1 slice	111	0
Veal: 10% fat, cutlet, leg, rump, shank, shoulder, steak (lean and fat)	1 oz	61	1	Whiskey: see *Liquor*			
				Weiner: 5 × ¾"	1 whole	139	22
Veal: 15% fat, loin (lean and fat)	1 oz	67	1	Wine: dessert (port, madeira, sweet sherry)	1 oz	41	0
Veal: 20% fat, rib (lean and fat)	1 oz	86	1	Wine: table (burgundy, rosé, white, dry sherry)	1 oz	25	0
Veal: 25% fat, breast riblet (lean and fat)	1 oz	89	1	Worcestershire sauce	1 tbsp	6	12
Vodka: see *Liquor*				Yeast: bakers, dry package, scant tbsp	¼ oz	20	0
Vinegar: cider	1 cup	34	0	Yogurt: skim, home recipe	1 cup	127	8
Waffle: made from mix, 7 × ⅝"	1 waffle	206	22	Yogurt: plain, low fat	1 cup	144	7
				Yogurt: whole milk	1 cup	139	5
Walnuts: English, chopped pieces	1 tbsp	49	0	Yogurt: with fruit (1–2% fat)	1 cup	225	5
				Yogurt: frozen (2% fat)	1 cup	244	5

Information used in this table is from the following sources.

Adams, C. F.: *Nutritive Value of American Foods In Common Units.* USDA Handbook No. 456, 1975.

Anderson, B. A.: Comprehensive evaluation of fatty acids in foods. VII. Pork products. *Journal of the American Dietetic Association,* 69:44–49, 1976.

Anderson, B. A.: Comprehensive evaluation of fatty acids in foods. XIII. Sausages and luncheon meats. *Journal of the American Dietetic Association,* 72:48–52, 1978.

Anderson, B. A., Fristrom, G. A., and Weihrauch, J. L.: Comprehensive evaluation of fatty acids in foods. X. Lamb and veal. *Journal of the American Dietetic Association,* 70:53–58, 1977.

Anderson, B. A., Kinsella, J. E., and Watt, B. K.: Comprehensive evaluation of fatty acids in foods. II. Beef products. *Journal of the American Dietetic Association,* 67:35–41, 1975.

Brignoli, C. A., Kinsella, J. E., and Weihrauch, J. L.: Comprehensive evaluation of fatty acids in foods. V. Unhydrogenated fats and oils. *Journal of the American Dietetic Association,* 68:224–229, 1976.

Consumer and Food Economics Institution: *Composition of Foods—Dairy and Egg Products—Raw, Processed, Prepared.* USDA Agricultural Handbook No. 8–1, 1976.

Exler, J., Avena, R. M., and Weihrauch, J. L.: Comprehensive evaluation of fatty acids in foods. XI. Leguminous seeds. *Journal of the American Dietetic Association,* 71:412–415, 1977.

Exler, J., and Weihrauch, J. L.: Comprehensive evaluation of fatty acids in foods. VIII. Finfish. *Journal of the American Dietetic Association,* 69:243–248, 1976.

Exler, J., and Weihrauch, J. L.: Comprehensive evaluation of fatty acids in foods. XII. Shellfish. *Journal of the American Dietetic Association,* 71:518–521, 1977.

Feeley, R. M., Criner, P. E., and Watt, B. K.: Cholesterol content of foods. *Journal of the American Dietetic Association,* 61:134–149, 1972.

Food manufacturers' and distributors' product information.

Fristrom, G. A., Stewart, B. C., Weihrauch, J. L., and Posati, L. P.: Comprehensive evaluation of fatty acids in foods. IV. Nuts, peanuts, and soups. *Journal of the American Dietetic Association,* 67:351–355, 1975.

Fristrom, G. A., and Weihrauch, J. L.: Comprehensive evaluation of fatty acids in foods. IX. Fowl. *Journal of the American Dietetic Association,* 69:517–522, 1976.

National Dairy Council: Composition and nutritive value of dairy foods. *Dairy Council Digest,* 47:25–30, No. 5, September-October, 1976.

Posati, L. P., Kinsella, J. E., and Watt, B. K.: Comprehensive evaluation of fatty acids in foods. I. Dairy products. *Journal of the American Dietetic Association,* 66:482–488, 1975.

Posati, L. P., Kinsella, J. E., and Watt, B. K.: Comprehensive evaluation of fatty acids in foods. III. Eggs and egg products. *Journal of the American Dietetic Association,* 67:111–115, 1975.

Weihrauch, J. L., Kinsella, J. E., and Watt, B. K.: Comprehensive evaluation of fatty acids in foods. VI. Cereal products. *Journal of the American Dietetic Association,* 68:335–340, 1976.

This information is current as of this printing. Check the manufacturer's label for updated analysis.

Abbreviations used in this table are: tbsp = tablespoon; oz = ounce; tsp = teaspoon; (—) = data not available.

Glossary

Adventitia: The outermost layer of the artery's wall, rich in connective tissue and nerve fibers.

Aerobic Exercises: A type of physical activity that results in the so-called "training effect," which means that an individual's maximum oxygen consumption is increased. "Training" results in a heart being able to achieve a given level of work at a lower pulse and blood pressure than before "training."

Amino Acids: The building blocks of proteins; raw materials from which the body makes proteins.

Aneurysm: Balloon-like sac formed by the abnormal expansion of the walls of an artery resulting from atherosclerosis or other causes of damage to the artery.

Angina Pectoris: Chest pains usually resulting from decreased blood flow to the heart caused by atherosclerotic disease of the coronary arteries.

Arteriosclerosis: Disease of the arteries often referred to as "hardening of the arteries." It includes, and is often used synonymously with, atherosclerosis. Whereas atherosclerosis refers primarily to disease of the innermost layer of the artery called the intima (Figure 1, Chapter 1), arteriosclerosis may include disease of the middle arterial layer (media) as well.

Artery: A vessel that carries blood from the heart to the tissues of the body, ending in small branches called arterioles, which in turn branch to form capillaries.

Atherosclerosis: A form of arteriosclerosis in which there is a characteristic deposit of fatty material initially within the innermost layer of the artery (the intima). It is associated with the growth of smooth-muscle cells, the formation of plaque, and other changes in the arterial wall. This form of arteriosclerosis causes most strokes and heart attacks.

Atrophy: The wasting away or decrease in size of an organ, tissue, or cell.

Behavior Modification: A set of principles, methods, and techniques derived primarily from research in experimental and social psychology. The objective of these methods is to change undesirable habits or behavior to those better suited to the well-being of the individual.

Behavioral Treatment: An approach which relies on meticulous observation of behavior, careful testing of ideas, and constant re-examination and reappraisal of results.

Beta-Blocking Agents: Drugs used to combat the consequences (chest pain or angina pectoris) of increased constriction of arteries in the heart or to lower blood pressure.

Capillaries: Small vessels, only one cell in thickness, from which blood supplies oxygen and nutrients to tissues. They are formed by the branching of arterioles. Capillaries combine into larger vessels called venules.

373

Cardiovascular: Pertaining to the heart and blood vessels.

Cerebrovascular: Pertaining to the blood vessels of the brain.

Cholesterol: A type of animal fat. Cholesterol is consumed in the diet and is also manufactured by the body.

Chylomicrons: Large lipoproteins which are carriers of newly absorbed fat from the diet. In the normal individual chylomicrons are cleared from the blood after fasting for 12 hours.

Circulatory System: The system which pumps blood through the blood vessels to the vital organs of the body, with the heart playing the central role.

Collagen Tissue: A type of fibrous connective protein tissue that supports the skin, tendons, artery walls, etc.

Complementary Proteins: A combination of incomplete proteins (see *Incomplete Proteins*) from different sources (e.g., beans and rice) which together yield complete protein.

Complete Proteins: Proteins which provide the essential amino acids (those the body cannot make). Eggs, milk, cheese, and meat are sources of complete proteins.

Coronary Thrombosis: See *Myocardial Infarction.*

Diabetes Mellitus: A deficiency or inappropriate secretion of insulin by the beta cells of the pancreas and an elevation of blood sugar.

Diastole: The phase of the heart's cycle during which it relaxes and fills its chambers with blood.

Elastin: A type of elastic tissue seen in the wall of arteries and other tissues of the body.

Electrocardiogram: A recording of a tracing of the heart's electrical activities.

Emphysema: The loss of elasticity of the bronchi in the lungs. This loss results in a chronic overexpansion in the lungs, leading to shortness of breath.

Endothelium: The innermost layer of cells lining a blood vessel.

Enriched: Federally regulated additions of certain nutrients to processed foods. Thiamin, riboflavin, niacin, and iron are commonly added.

Essential Amino Acids: The nine amino acids which cannot be manufactured by the body and must be supplied by the diet. They are lysine, tryptophan, phenylalanine, threonine, valine, methionine, leucine, isoleucine, and histidine.

Essential Fatty Acids: Fatty acids that the body cannot make and which must be supplied by the diet. The three most important ones are: linoleic, linolenic, and arachidonic.

Fatty Acids: Chains of carbon atoms with hydrogen attached. They are used as a source of energy by cells.

Fiber, Dietary: The indigestible carbohydrate components of plant food.

Framingham Study: This study began in Framingham, Massachusetts in 1949 with more than 5,000 men and women aged 30 to 60 years who had never had a heart attack. It is an ongoing study that is investigating the risk factors in cardiovascular disease by testing and measuring and then waiting to see which factors increase or decrease the risk. Every 2 years, each participant has a routine medical checkup. High density lipoproteins (HDL) have emerged as the most powerful predictor of coronary artery disease with low HDL being associated with a high incidence of coronary artery disease in men and women. Such factors as high blood pressure, cigarette smoking, obesity, and diabetes are monitored. Today 3,200 of the original participants are still in the study, with 2,000 of their children and 1,000 of their children's spouses.

Heart Attack: See *Myocardial Infarction.*

Hemoglobin: A protein within the red blood cells that is capable of transporting oxygen to the cells and carbon dioxide (a waste product) away from the cells.

High Density Lipoproteins (HDL): A type of lipoprotein made in the liver and intestine. They transport cholesterol from all parts of the body to the liver. High levels are correlated with a decreased risk of coronary heart disease. See *Lipoproteins.*

Hydrogenation: A procedure used to harden fat, enhance its stability, and prolong its shelf life.

Hypercholesterolemia: An elevation of the cholesterol concentration in the blood plasma.

Hyperlipidemia: An abnormally high concentration of fats (lipids) in the blood; usually refers to an elevation of blood cholesterol and/or triglycerides.

Hypertension: The condition in which the blood pressure within the arteries is elevated.

Hypertriglyceridemia: An elevation of the concentration of the triglycerides in the blood plasma.

Incomplete Proteins: Proteins which do not contain all of the nine essential amino acids. Care must be taken to "complement" foods adequately to ensure that all of the essential amino acids (those the body cannot make) are consumed daily.

Insulin: A protein hormone formed by the beta cells of the pancreas secreted into the blood where it regulates the metabolism of carbohydrate, especially sugar.

Intima: The innermost layer of the artery wall, separated from the blood by a layer of (endothelial) cells.

Linoleic Acid: The most common of several polyunsaturated fatty acids that occur in foods, accounting for about 60% of the total fatty acids. It is one of the essential fatty acids.

Lipids: Fatty substances—including cholesterol, triglycerides, and phospholipid—that are present in the blood and in tissues.

Lipoproteins, Plasma: Complexes of fat and protein that transport all of the fats, including cholesterol, triglycerides, and phospholipid, in the blood plasma.

Lobeline: An alkaloid from the leaves of tobacco plants—a nicotine substitute that is taken orally by smokers as a means of trying to stop smoking.

Low Density Lipoproteins (LDL): A type of lipoprotein formed in the body by a breakdown of the very low density lipoproteins (VLDL), and the main cholesterol carriers in the blood. High concentrations of LDL in the blood plasma are strongly correlated with premature atherosclerosis and coronary heart disease. See *Lipoproteins.*

Lumen: The inner diameter of a vessel through which the blood flows.

Media: The middle layer of the artery wall. It contains smooth-muscle cells, elastic tissue, and collagen, which allow the artery to contract and expand.

Medium-Chain Triglyceride (MCT) Oil: A type of fat that can be absorbed directly into the blood and does not require transport by chylomicrons, which normally carry triglycerides. MCT oil is absorbed by blood from certain parts of the alimentary and intestinal tract and is carried directly to the liver. It is used in diseases where chylomicrons and VLDL cannot be cleared from the blood and absorbed by the liver.

Monounsaturated Fat: Fatty acids with one double bond in their chemical structures.

Myocardial Infarction: Used synonymously with "heart attack" or "coronary thrombosis." It refers specifically, however, to the death of part of the heart muscle (myocardium). The diagnosis is established by physical symptoms, changes in the electrocardiogram, and measurement of blood enzymes released from the damaged heart muscle.

Myocardium: The muscular tissue of the heart.

Nicotine: A part of cigarette smoke which is a poison that can damage the blood vessels, heart, kidneys, and gastrointestinal tract.

Nitroglycerin: A member of the nitrate group of drugs, which has been used for many years to treat angina pectoris. It usually provides rapid relief of chest pain (within 1 to 3 minutes) in a patient suffering an attack of angina pectoris. Nitroglycerin is placed under the tongue where it is absorbed directly into the blood vessels and goes immediately to the arteries in the heart, causing them to dilate (expand), thus relieving the pressure and pain.

Obesity: An excess of body fat which can be determined by precise measurement.

Oleic Acid: A monounsaturated fatty acid.

Pancreatitis: An inflammation of the pancreas which can be caused by hyperlipidemia. (The pancreas secretes digestive enzymes and insulin.)

Phospholipid: A fatty constituent of the blood and cell membranes that contains glycerol, two fatty acids, and a phosphorus-containing component. It is essential to the structure of the cell membrane. In the blood it probably functions to keep cholesterol and triglycerides in solution. Lecithin and sphingomyelin are the two most common phospholipids in the body.

Plaque: A well-demarcated area, raised patch, or swelling on a body surface. The plaque associated with atherosclerosis is a deposit of fatty material and cholesterol on the inner surface (intima) of the artery that may progress to narrow or block the interior diameter of the artery. It is the most common cause of heart attacks.

Plasma: The fluid part of the blood.

Platelet: A cellular element of the blood that may participate in the clotting mechanism and which produces chemical substances that may contribute to the development of atherosclerosis.

Polyunsaturated Fats: Fatty acids that have two or more double bonds in their chemical structure. They are liquid at room temperature.

P/S Ratio: The ratio of polyunsaturated to saturated fats in the diet. The P/S ratio can be determined in any food containing these fats by measuring the amount of polyunsaturated fat and dividing this value by the amount of saturated fat.

Saturated Fat: Fat that hardens at room temperature. It is usually found in foods of animal origin and rarely in some foods of vegetable origin. The chemical structure of saturated fatty acids makes them extremely stable and thus more difficult to break down.

Stroke: An interruption of circulation in one of the arteries supplying the brain. It may be caused by a hemorrhage, blood clot, or by part of a clot or atherogenic plaque breaking off and being carried to the brain from a distant site.

Systole: The phase of the heart's cycle during which the heart muscle contracts to pump blood to the body.

Tar: A substance present in cigarette smoke which may damage the lungs and lead to cancer.

Thrombus: A clot in a blood vessel or in one of the cavities of the heart formed by clotting of the blood; when such a clot obstructs an artery in the heart, a heart attack may result. The obstruction of an artery which supplies blood to the brain by a thrombus may cause a stroke.

Triglycerides: A type of fat containing a backbone of glycerol to which fatty acids are attached. They may be of either animal or vegetable origin or may be manufactured by the body.

Type A Personality: The hard-driving, time-conscious person who is thought by some physicians and psychologists to have an increased risk of developing premature coronary artery disease.

Type B Personality: The relaxed, less-compulsive person who some physicians believe has a lower risk of developing coronary artery disease than does the hard-driving Type A personality.

Type I Diabetes: Insulin-dependent diabetes which usually begins in childhood.

Type II Diabetes: Non-insulin-dependent diabetes; usually begins after age 40 or 50.

Type I Hyperlipoproteinemia: A deficiency of a protein in fat cells that breaks down the triglycerides in the chylomicrons and very low density lipoproteins (VLDL). Triglycerides and chylomicrons are always elevated; cholesterol may be elevated.

Type IIa Hyperlipoproteinemia: An increase in the concentration of low density lipoproteins (LDL) with normal concentrations of the very low density lipoproteins (VLDL). Cholesterol is always elevated. It is often caused by an inherited disease called familial hypercholesterolemia and is marked by severe premature atherosclerosis.

Type IIb Hyperlipoproteinemia: Elevated levels of low density lipoproteins (LDL) and very low density lipoproteins (VLDL). Cholesterol and triglycerides are always elevated.

Type III Hyperlipoproteinemia: A rare disease characterized by an elevation of very low density lipoproteins (VLDL) and low density lipoproteins (LDL).

Type IV Hyperlipoproteinemia: An elevation of very low density lipoproteins (VLDL) in the blood plasma which represents triglycerides made in the body.

Type V Hyperlipoproteinemia: An elevation primarily of triglycerides from the diet, although triglycerides made in the body are also elevated. Chylomicrons, very low density lipoproteins (VLDL), and cholesterol are all elevated. Acute abdominal pain is frequently a symptom.

Unsaturated Fat: Fatty acids which contain one or more double bonds. See *Polyunsaturated Fat* and *Monounsaturated Fat.*

Very Low Density Lipoproteins (VLDL):   A type of lipoprotein that transports triglycerides made by the body. See *Lipoproteins.*

Subject Index

Recipe Index

Page numbers in italics refer to low-sodium recipes.